ELSEVIER

NETTER:
It's How You Know Anatomy.

D1291302

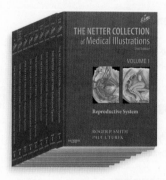

THE NETTER COLLECTION
of Medical Illustrations

VOLUME 1

Reproductive System

ROGER P. SMITH
PAUL J. TUREK

The Netter Green Book Series

In this legendary series, we are delighted to offer Netter's timeless work, now arranged and informed by modern text and radiologic imaging contributed by field-leading doctors and teachers from world-renowned medical institutions, and supplemented with new illustrations created by artists working in the Netter tradition.

Inside the classic green covers, students and practitioners will find hundreds of original works of art—the human body in pictures—paired with the latest in expert medical knowledge and innovation, and anchored in the sublime style of Frank Netter.

Visit **www.NetterReference.com/greenbooks** to learn more!

Netter's Correlative Imaging Series

The *Netter's Correlative Imaging* series pairs classic Netter and Netter-style illustrations with imaging studies and succinct descriptions to provide you with a richer understanding of human anatomy. These comprehensive, normal anatomy atlases cover all major sections of the body, featuring illustrated plates side-by-side with the most common imaging modalities for each region.

Learn more at MyNetter.com!

ELSEVIER

Explore more essential resources in the
NETTER BASIC SCIENCE COLLECTION!

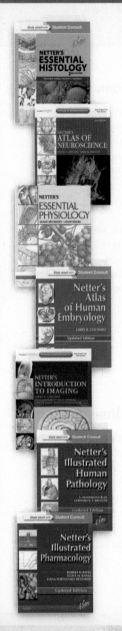

Netter's Essential Histology
With **Student Consult** Access

By William K. Ovalle, PhD and Patrick C. Nahirney, PhD
Bring histologic concepts to life through beautiful Netter illustrations!

Netter's Atlas of Neuroscience
With **Student Consult** Access

By David L. Felten, MD, PhD and Anil Shetty, PhD
Master the neuroscience fundamentals needed
for the classroom and beyond.

Netter's Essential Physiology
With **Student Consult** Access

By Susan Mulroney and Adam Myers, MD
Enhance your understanding of physiology the Netter way!

Netter's Atlas of Human Embryology
With **Student Consult** Access

By Larry R. Cochard, PhD
A rich pictorial review of normal and abnormal human
prenatal development.

Netter's Introduction to Imaging
With **Student Consult** Access

By Larry R. Cochard, PhD et al.
Finally...an accessible introduction to diagnostic imaging!

Netter's Illustrated Human Pathology
With **Student Consult** Access

By Maximilian L. Buja, MD and Gerhard R. F. Krueger
Gain critical insight into the structure-function relationships
and the pathological basis of human disease!

Netter's Illustrated Pharmacology
With **Student Consult** Access

*By Robert B. Raffa, PhD, Scott M. Rawls
and Elena Portyansky Beyzarov*
Take a distinct visual approach to understanding both
the basic science and clinical applications of pharmacology.

Learn more at MyNetter.com!

Netter's Concise Orthopaedic Anatomy

Jon C. Thompson, MD

Staff Orthopaedic Surgeon

Irwin Army Community Hospital

Fort Riley, Kansas

Illustrations by Frank H. Netter, MD

Contributing Illustrators

Carlos A. G. Machado, MD

John A. Craig, MD

SECOND EDITION—UPDATED EDITION

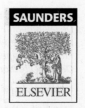

SAUNDERS

ELSEVIER

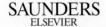

SAUNDERS
ELSEVIER

1600 John F. Kennedy Blvd. Ste 1800
Philadelphia, PA 19103-2899

NETTER'S CONCISE ORTHOPAEDIC ANATOMY,
SECOND EDITION—UPDATED EDITION   ISBN: 978-0-323-42970-2

Copyright © 2016, 2010, 2002 by Saunders, an imprint of Elsevier Inc.

All rights reserved. No part of this book may be produced or transmitted in any form or by any means, electronic or mechanical, including photocopying, recording or any information storage and retrieval system, without permission in writing from the publishers.

Permissions for Netter Art figures may be sought directly from Elsevier's Health Science Licensing Department in Philadelphia PA, USA: phone 1-800-523-1649, ext. 3276 or (215) 239-3276; or email H.Licensing@elsevier.com.

Notice

Knowledge and best practice in this field are constantly changing. As new research and experience broaden our knowledge, changes in practice, treatment and drug therapy may become necessary or appropriate. Readers are advised to check the most current information provided (i) on procedures featured or (ii) by the manufacturer of each product to be administered, to verify the recommended dose or formula, the method and duration of administration, and contraindications. It is the responsibility of the practitioner, relying on their own experience and knowledge of the patient, to make diagnoses, to determine dosages and the best treatment for each individual patient, and to take all appropriate safety precautions. To the fullest extent of the law, neither the Publisher nor the Author assumes any liability for any injury and/or damage to persons or property arising out of or related to any use of the material contained in this book.

—The Publisher

International Standard Book Number: 978-0-323-42970-2

Acquisitions Editor: Elyse O'Grady
Developmental Editor: Marybeth Thiel
Publishing Services Manager: Patricia Tannian
Project Manager: John Casey
Design Direction: Louis Forgione

Printed in India

Last digit is the print number 9 8 7

Working together to grow
libraries in developing countries

www.elsevier.com | www.bookaid.org | www.sabre.org

ELSEVIER   BOOK AID International   Sabre Foundation

Preface

I suppose there is always a question regarding the reception a first edition of any text will receive before its publication. The response and enthusiasm for the first edition of this text have been rewarding and exceeded my optimistic expectations. Inasmuch as imitation is a form of flattery, I am also pleased with the development of multiple other titles in the *Netter's Concise* series that were based on the format of this text. Despite this encouragement, it quickly became clear that the first edition of this text, written predominantly while I was a medical student, was in need of an update. Although the anatomy is a constant, our understanding of it, our terminology, and its clinical application continue to advance.

I received considerable feedback, both positive and negative, on the first edition. Much of it was constructive, and I am grateful for all of it. The revision has been both challenging and rewarding. Formatting this enormous volume of material was a painstaking process, and I would like to thank John Casey, the production team, and all of those at Elsevier for their patience, hard work, and professionalism. With their help I was able to develop my vision of this project. It has been a pleasure to work with them.

In this revision, I have tried to strike a balance between being thorough and yet concise while staying true to the original concept of the text, which was to allow the incomparable Netter artwork to do a majority of the teaching. Knowing it's impossible to please everyone, I look forward to hearing how well the balance was or was not achieved.

In this second edition, every table, both anatomic and clinical, was updated or revised. We were also able to enhance the text with radiographs, additional sections, and new artwork including additional surgical approaches. In the preface to the first edition I noted that the text embodied the book that I unsuccessfully tried to find on the shelves of medical bookstores as a medical student. That failed search originally prompted me to write the text. With the above-mentioned updates and additions, I feel that statement should be amended. *This* edition is, in fact, the text for which I had originally searched and fulfills the vision of the initial undertaking that began over 10 years ago. I hope the readers find it so.

Jon C. Thompson, MD

About the Author

Jon C. Thompson, MD, received his undergraduate degree from Dartmouth College and his medical degree from the Uniformed Services University of the Health Sciences in Bethesda, Maryland. Having recently completed his orthopaedic residency at Brooke Army Medical Center in San Antonio, Texas, he is now board certified in orthopaedic surgery and sports medicine. He is currently continuing his military service at Irwin Army Community Hospital, Fort Riley, Kansas. Dr. Thompson is glad to no longer have to answer questions regarding why he published an orthopaedic text before doing any formal orthopaedic training, as well as being able to spend more time with his family. His wife and four young children, though very supportive, are not looking forward to Dr. Thompson's future publishing projects.

To the men and women of the armed forces
who bravely serve our country

To the readers
whose enthusiasm for the text has
motivated me to do better

To my children,
Taylor, Turner, Jax, and Judson,
constant and perfect reminders
of the truly important and joyful aspects of life

To my wife,
Tiffany, the foundation
of every good thing in my life

About the Artists

Frank H. Netter, MD

Frank H. Netter was born in 1906, in New York City. He studied art at the Art Student's League and the National Academy of Design before entering medical school at New York University, where he received his medical degree in 1931. During his student years, Dr. Netter's notebook sketches attracted the attention of the medical faculty and other physicians, allowing him to augment his income by illustrating articles and textbooks. He continued illustrating as a sideline after establishing a surgical practice in 1933, but he ultimately opted to give up his practice in favor of a full-time commitment to art. After service in the United States Army during World War II, Dr. Netter began his long collaboration with the CIBA Pharmaceutical Company (now Novartis Pharmaceuticals). This 45-year partnership resulted in the production of the extraordinary collection of medical art so familiar to physicians and other medical professionals worldwide.

In 2005, Elsevier, Inc., purchased the Netter Collection and all publications from Icon Learning Systems. There are now over 50 publications featuring the art of Dr. Netter available through Elsevier, Inc. (in the US: www.us.elsevierhealth.com/Netter and outside the US: www.elsevierhealth.com)

Dr. Netter's works are among the finest examples of the use of illustration in the teaching of medical concepts. The 13-volume *Netter Collection of Medical Illustrations,* which includes the greater part of the more than 20,000 paintings created by Dr. Netter, became and remains one of the most famous medical works ever published. *The Netter Atlas of Human Anatomy,* first published in 1989, presents the anatomical paintings from the Netter Collection. Now translated into 16 languages, it is the anatomy atlas of choice among medical and health professions students the world over.

The Netter illustrations are appreciated not only for their aesthetic qualities, but also, more important, for their intellectual content. As Dr. Netter wrote in 1949, ". . . clarification of a subject is the aim and goal of illustration. No matter how beautifully painted, how delicately and subtly rendered a subject may be, it is of little value as a *medical illustration* if it does not serve to make clear some medical point." Dr. Netter's planning, conception, point of view, and approach are what inform his paintings and what makes them so intellectually valuable.

Frank H. Netter, MD, physician and artist, died in 1991.

Learn more about the physician-artist whose work has inspired the Netter Reference collection:

http://www.netterimages.com/artist/netter.htm

Carlos Machado, MD

Carlos Machado was chosen by Novartis to be Dr. Netter's successor. He continues to be the main artist who contributes to the Netter collection of medical illustrations.

Self-taught in medical illustration, cardiologist Carlos Machado has contributed meticulous updates to some of Dr. Netter's original plates and has created many paintings of his own in the style of Netter as an extension of the Netter collection. Dr. Machado's photorealistic expertise and his keen insight into the physician/patient relationship informs his vivid and unforgettable visual style. His dedication to researching each topic and subject he paints places him among the premier medical illustrators at work today.

Learn more about his background and see more of his art at:

http://www.netterimages.com/artist/machado.htm

Contents

Introduction

Netter's Concise Orthopaedic Anatomy is an easy-to-use reference and compact atlas of orthopaedic anatomy for students and clinicians. Using images from both the *Atlas of Human Anatomy* and the 13-volume *Netter Collection of Medical Illustrations,* this book brings over 450 Netter images together.

Tables are used to highlight the Netter images and offer key information on bones, joints, muscles, nerves, and surgical approaches. Clinical material is presented in a clear and straightforward manner with emphasis on trauma, minor procedures, history and physical exam, and disorders.

Users will appreciate the unique color-coding system that makes information look-up even easier. Key material is presented in black, red, and green to provide quick access to clinically relevant information.

BLACK: standard text

GREEN: key/testable information

RED: key information that if missed could result in morbidity or mortality

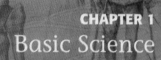

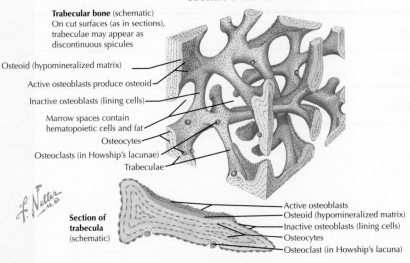

Epiphysis
Growth plate (physis)
Metaphysis
Shaft (diaphysis)
Metaphysis
Intraarticular

Section through diaphysis. Composed mostly of solid, hard, cortical bone

Section through metaphysis. Composed mostly of spongy, cancellous bone

Structure of Cancellous Bone

Trabecular bone (schematic) On cut surfaces (as in sections), trabeculae may appear as discontinuous spicules

Osteoid (hypomineralized matrix)
Active osteoblasts produce osteoid
Inactive osteoblasts (lining cells)
Marrow spaces contain hematopoietic cells and fat
Osteocytes
Osteoclasts (in Howship's lacunae)
Trabeculae

Active osteoblasts
Osteoid (hypomineralized matrix)
Inactive osteoblasts (lining cells)
Osteocytes
Osteoclast (in Howship's lacuna)

Section of trabecula (schematic)

STRUCTURE	COMMENT
BONE	
Function	• Serves as attachment sites for muscles • Protection for organs (e.g., cranium, ribs, pelvis) • Reservoir for minerals in the body: 99% of body's calcium stored as hydroxyapatite crystals • Hematopoiesis site
BONE FORMS	

Long bones	• Form by enchondral ossification (except clavicle): primary (in shaft) and secondary growth centers
	• Have physes ("growth plates") at each end where it grows in length (metacarpals, metatarsals, and phalanges of hand and feet typically have only one physis)
	• 3 parts of long bone:
	  ○ **Diaphysis:** shaft, made of thick cortical bone, filled with bone marrow
	  ○ **Metaphysis:** widening of bone near the end, typically made of cancellous bone
	  ○ **Epiphysis:** end (usually articular) of bone, forms from secondary ossification centers

Flat bones	• Form by intramembranous ossification (e.g., pelvis, scapula)
MICROSCOPIC BONE TYPES	
Woven	• Immature or pathologic bone; poorly organized, not stress oriented • Examples: Immature—bones in infants, fracture callus; Pathologic—tumors
Lamellar	• Mature bone; highly organized with stress orientation • Mature (>4y.o.) cortical and cancellous bone are both made up of lamellar bone

Structure of Cortical (Compact) Bone

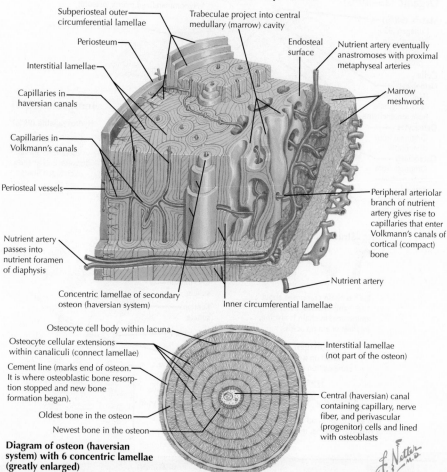

Subperiosteal outer circumferential lamellae

Periosteum

Interstitial lamellae

Capillaries in haversian canals

Capillaries in Volkmann's canals

Periosteal vessels

Nutrient artery passes into nutrient foramen of diaphysis

Concentric lamellae of secondary osteon (haversian system)

Trabeculae project into central medullary (marrow) cavity

Endosteal surface

Nutrient artery eventually anastromoses with proximal metaphyseal arteries

Marrow meshwork

Peripheral arteriolar branch of nutrient artery gives rise to capillaries that enter Volkmann's canals of cortical (compact) bone

Nutrient artery

Inner circumferential lamellae

Osteocyte cell body within lacuna

Osteocyte cellular extensions within canaliculi (connect lamellae)

Cement line (marks end of osteon. It is where osteoblastic bone resorption stopped and new bone formation began).

Oldest bone in the osteon

Newest bone in the osteon

Interstitial lamellae (not part of the osteon)

Central (haversian) canal containing capillary, nerve fiber, and perivascular (progenitor) cells and lined with osteoblasts

Diagram of osteon (haversian system) with 6 concentric lamellae (greatly enlarged)

STRUCTURE	COMMENT
STRUCTURAL BONE TYPES	
Cortical (compact)	• Strong, dense bone, makes up 80% of the skeleton • Composed of multiple osteons (haversian systems) with intervening interstitial lamellae • **Osteons** are made up of concentric bone lamellae with a central canal (haversian canal) containing osteoblasts (new bone formation) and an arteriole supplying the osteon. Lamellae are connected by canaliculi. Cement lines mark outer limit of osteon (bone resorption ended). • Volkmann's canals: radially oriented, have arteriole, and connect adjacent osteons • Thick cortical bone is found in the diaphysis of long bones
Cancellous (spongy/trabecular)	• Crossed lattice structure, makes up 20% of the skeleton • High bone turnover rate. Bone is resorbed by osteoclasts in Howship's lacunae and formed on the opposite side of the trabeculae by osteoblasts. • Osteoporosis is common in cancellous bone, making it susceptible to fractures (e.g., vertebral bodies, femoral neck, distal radius, tibial plateau). • Commonly found in the metaphysis and epiphysis of long bones

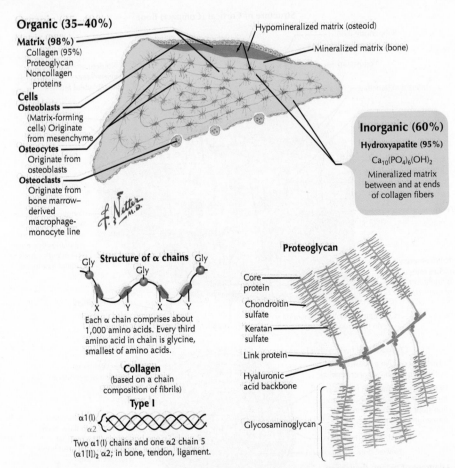

Organic (35–40%)

Matrix (98%)
Collagen (95%)
Proteoglycan
Noncollagen
  proteins

Cells
Osteoblasts
(Matrix-forming
cells) Originate
from mesenchyme
Osteocytes
Originate from
osteoblasts
Osteoclasts
Originate from
bone marrow–
derived
macrophage-
monocyte line

Hypomineralized matrix (osteoid)

Mineralized matrix (bone)

Inorganic (60%)

Hydroxyapatite (95%)
$Ca_{10}(PO_4)_6(OH)_2$
Mineralized matrix
between and at ends
of collagen fibers

Structure of α chains
Gly   Gly
Gly

X   Y   X   Y

Each α chain comprises about
1,000 amino acids. Every third
amino acid in chain is glycine,
smallest of amino acids.

Collagen
(based on a chain
composition of fibrils)

Type I

α1(I)
α2

Two α1(I) chains and one α2 chain 5
$(α1[I])_2$ α2; in bone, tendon, ligament.

Proteoglycan

Core
protein
Chondroitin
sulfate
Keratan
sulfate
Link protein
Hyaluronic
acid backbone

Glycosaminoglycan

COMPONENT	COMMENT
BONE COMPOSITION	
Bone is composed of multiple components: 1. Organic phase ("matrix:" proteins, macromolecules, cells); 2. Inorganic phase (minerals, e.g., Ca++); 3. Water	
Inorganic phase • Calcium hydroxyapatite • Osteocalcium phosphate	• Approximately 60% of bone weight • $Ca_{10}(PO_4)_6(OH)_2$. Primary mineral in bone. Adds compressive strength. • "Brushite" is a secondary/minor mineral in bone.
Organic phase • Collagen • Proteoglycans • Noncollagen proteins • Cells	• Also known as "osteoid" before its mineralization; approximately 35% of bone weight • Type 1 collagen gives tensile strength and is 90% of organic phase. Mineralization occurs at ends (hole zones) and along sides (pores) of the collagen fibers. • Macromolecules made up of a hyaluronic backbone w/ multiple glycosaminoglycans • Glycosaminoglycans (GAG): made of core protein w/ chondroitin & keratin branches • Gives bone compressive strength • Osteocalcin #1, is indicator of increased bone turnover (e.g., Paget's disease) • Others: osteonectin, osteopontin • Osteoblasts, osteocytes, osteoclasts
Water	• Approximately 5% of bone weight (varies with age and location)
Periosteum surrounds the bone, is thicker in children, and responsible for the growing diameter (width) of long bones.	

Four Mechanisms of Bone Regulation

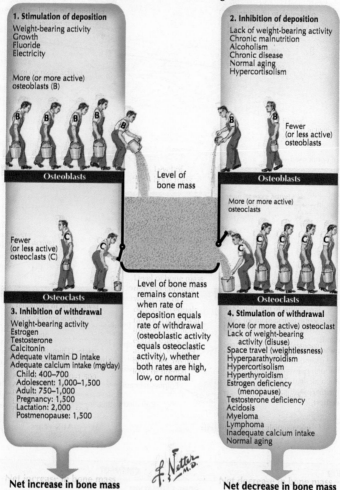

1. Stimulation of deposition

Weight-bearing activity
Growth
Fluoride
Electricity

More (or more active) osteoblasts (B)

Osteoblasts

Fewer (or less active) osteoclasts (C)

Osteoclasts

2. Inhibition of deposition

Lack of weight-bearing activity
Chronic malnutrition
Alcoholism
Chronic disease
Normal aging
Hypercortisolism

Fewer (or less active) osteoblasts

Osteoblasts

More (or more active) osteoclasts

Osteoclasts

Level of bone mass

3. Inhibition of withdrawal

Weight-bearing activity
Estrogen
Testosterone
Calcitonin
Adequate vitamin D intake
Adequate calcium intake (mg/day)
  Child: 400–700
  Adolescent: 1,000–1,500
  Adult: 750–1,000
  Pregnancy: 1,500
  Lactation: 2,000
  Postmenopause: 1,500

Level of bone mass remains constant when rate of deposition equals rate of withdrawal (osteoblastic activity equals osteoclastic activity), whether both rates are high, low, or normal

4. Stimulation of withdrawal

More (or more active) osteoclast
Lack of weight-bearing activity (disuse)
Space travel (weightlessness)
Hyperparathyroidism
Hypercortisolism
Hyperthyroidism
Estrogen deficiency (menopause)
Testosterone deficiency
Acidosis
Myeloma
Lymphoma
Inadequate calcium intake
Normal aging

Net increase in bone mass

Net decrease in bone mass

CELL	COMMENT
BONE CELL TYPES	
Osteoblasts	• Function: produce bone matrix ("osteoid"). Make type 1 collagen and other matrix proteins • Line new bone surfaces and follow osteoclasts in cutting cones • Receptors: **PTH** (parathyroid hormone), vitamin D, glucosteroids, estrogen, PGs, ILs
Osteocytes	• Osteoblast surrounded by bone matrix. Represent 90% of all bone cells • Function: maintain & preserve bone. Long cell processes communicate via canaliculi. • Receptors: **PTH** (release calcium), **calcitonin** (do not release calcium)
Osteoclasts	• Large, multinucleated cells derived from the same line of cells as monocytes & macrophages • Function: when active, use a "ruffled border" to resorb bone; found in Howship's lacunae • Receptors: **calcitonin,** estrogen, IL-1, RANK L. Inhibited by bisphosphonates

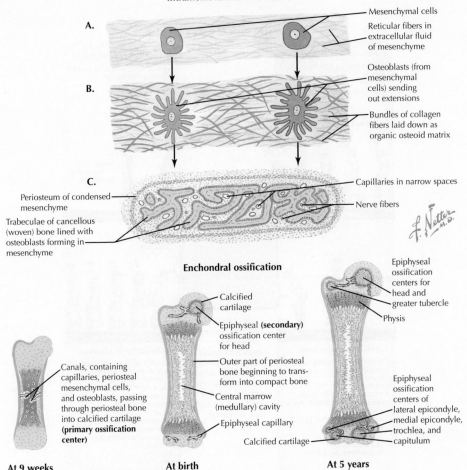

Intramembranous ossification

A.
Mesenchymal cells

Reticular fibers in extracellular fluid of mesenchyme

B.
Osteoblasts (from mesenchymal cells) sending out extensions

Bundles of collagen fibers laid down as organic osteoid matrix

C.
Periosteum of condensed mesenchyme

Trabeculae of cancellous (woven) bone lined with osteoblasts forming in mesenchyme

Capillaries in narrow spaces

Nerve fibers

Enchondral ossification

At 9 weeks

Canals, containing capillaries, periosteal mesenchymal cells, and osteoblasts, passing through periosteal bone into calcified cartilage (**primary ossification center**)

At birth

Calcified cartilage

Epiphyseal (**secondary**) ossification center for head

Outer part of periosteal bone beginning to transform into compact bone

Central marrow (medullary) cavity

Epiphyseal capillary

Calcified cartilage

At 5 years

Epiphyseal ossification centers for head and greater tubercle

Physis

Epiphyseal ossification centers of lateral epicondyle, medial epicondyle, trochlea, and capitulum

OSSIFICATION	COMMENT
BONE FORMATION	
Bone formation (ossification) occurs in 3 different ways: enchondral, intramembranous, appositional	
Enchondral	• Bone replaces a cartilage anlage (template). Osteoclasts remove the cartilage, and osteoblasts make the new bone matrix, which is then mineralized. • Typical in long bones (except clavicle). • Primary ossification centers (in shaft) typically develop in prenatal period. • Secondary ossification centers occur at various times after birth, usually in the epiphysis. • Longitudinal growth at the physis also occurs by enchondral ossification. • Also found in fracture callus
Intramembranous	• Bone develops directly from mesenchymal cells without a cartilage anlage. • Mesenchymal cells differentiate into osteoblasts, which produce bone. • Examples: flat bones (e.g., the cranium) and clavicle
Appositional	• Osteoblasts make new matrix/bone on top of existing bone. • Example: periosteal-mediated bone diameter (width) growth in long bones

Epiphysis and Physis

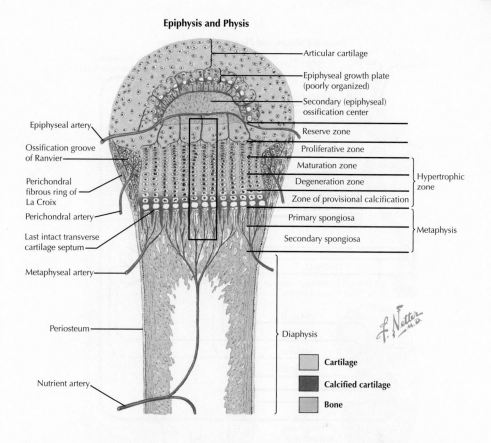

Articular cartilage

Epiphyseal growth plate (poorly organized)

Secondary (epiphyseal) ossification center

Epiphyseal artery

Reserve zone

Ossification groove of Ranvier

Proliferative zone

Maturation zone

Degeneration zone

Hypertrophic zone

Perichondral fibrous ring of La Croix

Zone of provisional calcification

Perichondral artery

Primary spongiosa

Secondary spongiosa

Metaphysis

Last intact transverse cartilage septum

Metaphyseal artery

Periosteum

Diaphysis

Nutrient artery

Cartilage

Calcified cartilage

Bone

STRUCTURE	COMMENT
ANATOMY OF THE PHYSIS	
The physis provides longitudinal growth in long bones. It is divided into multiple zones, each with a different function. • There is another physis in each epiphysis (similar organization) responsible for epiphyseal growth (not longitudinal). • There is typically also a physis at the site of an immature apophysis (e.g., tibial tubercle). It fuses at bone maturity.	
Reserve zone	• Loosely organized cells produce abundant matrix and store metabolites.
Proliferative zone	• Longitudinal growth occurs here as chondrocytes divide and stack into columns. • Achondroplasia is result of dysfunction of this zone.
Hypertrophic zone Maturation zone Degenerative zone Zone of provisional Ca^{++}	• Has 3 subzones. Function is to prepare the matrix for calcification and calcify it. • Cells (chondrocytes) mature and enlarge 5-10x in size. • Chondrocytes die, proteoglycans are degraded, allowing for mineralization of matrix. • Released calcium mineralizes the cartilage matrix (radiographically dense zone).
Metaphysis Primary spongiosa Secondary spongiosa	• Osteoblasts make immature (woven) bone on the calcified cartilage. • Osteoclasts remove cartilage & immature bone; osteoblasts make new (lamellar) bone.
Other Groove of Ranvier Perichondral ring	• Peripheral chondrocytes allow for widening/growth of the physis. • AKA "perichondral ring of La Croix." Provides peripheral support for cartilaginous physis.

Normal Calcium and Phosphate Metabolism

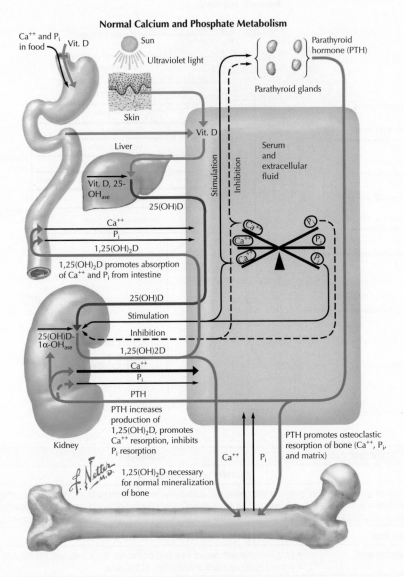

MINERAL	COMMENT
BONE METABOLISM	
Bone plays a critical role in maintaining proper serum calcium and phosphate levels.	
Calcium	• Calcium (Ca^{++}) plays a critical role in cardiac, skeletal muscle, and nerve function. • Normal dietary requirement 500-1300mg. More is required during pregnancy, lactation, fractures. • 99% of body's stored calcium is in the bone. • Calcium levels directly regulated by PTH and Vitamin D 1,25.
Phosphate	• Important component of bone mineral (hydroxyapatite) and body metabolic functions • 85% of body's stored phosphate is in the bone.

Regulation of Calcium and Phosphate Metabolism

	Parathyroid hormone (PTH) (peptide)	1,25-D$_3$ (steroid)	Calcitonin (peptide)
Hormone	From chief cells of parathyroid glands	From proximal tubule of kidney	From parafollicular cells of thyroid gland
Factors stimulating production	Decreased serum Ca^{++}	Elevated PTH Decreased serum Ca^{++} Decreased serum P$_i$	Elevated serum Ca^{++}
Factors inhibiting production	Elevated serum Ca^{++} Elevated 1,25(OH)$_2$D	Decreased PTH Elevated serum Ca^{++} Elevated serum P$_i$	Decreased serum Ca^{++}
End organs for hormone action — Intestine	No direct effect Acts indirectly on bowel by stimulating production of 1,25(OH)$_2$D in kidney	Strongly stimulates intestinal absorption of Ca^{++} and P$_i$	
End organs for hormone action — Kidney	Stimulates 25(OH)D-1α-OH$_{ase}$ in mitochondria of proximal tubular cells to convert 25(OH)D to 1,25(OH)$_2$D Increases fractional reabsorption of filtered Ca^{++} Promotes urinary excretion of P$_i$		Increases renal calcium excretion
End organs for hormone action — Bone	Increases bone resorption indirectly by up-regulating osteoblast production of autocrine cytokines such as interleukin-6, which results in increased production of paracrine cytokines that stimulate osteoclast production and activity. PTH also has an anabolic effect on osteoblasts that results in overproduction of osteoid in chronic hyperparathyroidism	Stimulates bone resorption in a similar fashion to PTH and also other membrane receptors	Inhibits bone resorption by direct inhibition of osteoclast differentiation and activity
Net effect on calcium and phosphate concentrations in extracellular fluid and serum	Increased serum calcium Decreased serum phosphate	Increased serum calcium	Decreased serum calcium (transient)

HORMONE	COMMENT
BONE REGULATION	
Parathyroid hormone (PTH)	• Low serum calcium triggers PTH release. PTH binds 1. osteoblasts (which stimulate osteoclasts to resorb bone), 2. osteocytes (to release Ca^{++}), 3. kidney (increase Ca^{++} reabsorption)
Vitamin D 1,25 (OH)	• Vitamin D from skin (UV light) or diet is hydroxylated twice ([1-liver], [25-kidney]) • Vit. D 1,25 triggered by low serum Ca^{++} stimulates uptake in intestine and bone resorption
Calcitonin	• Released when serum Ca^{++} is elevated. Directly inhibits osteoclasts (bone resorption) and increases urinary excretion from kidneys, thus lowering serum levels
Other hormones	• Estrogen, corticosteroids, thyroid hormone, insulin, growth hormone

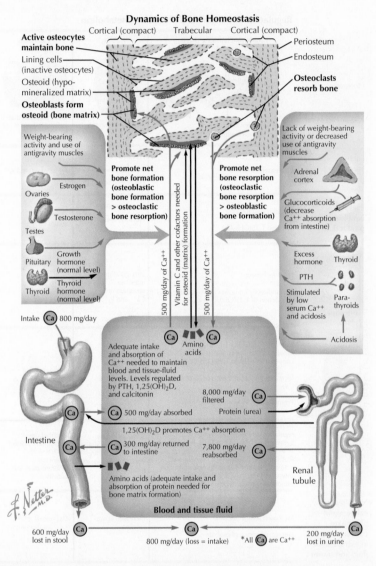

Dynamics of Bone Homeostasis

CONDITION	COMMENT
METABOLIC DISORDERS	
Hypercalcemia 1° Hyperparathyroidism	• Symptoms: constipation, nausea, abdominal pain, confusion, stupor, coma • Typically from parathyroid adenoma and/or overproduction of PTH hormone • "Brown tumors" form. Labs: increased serum calcium, decreased serum phosphate
2° Hyperparathyroidism	• Malignancy (lung CA produces PTH-like protein), MEN syndromes
Hypocalcemia Hypoparathyroidism	• Symptoms: hyperreflexia, tetany, +Chvostek's/Trousseau sign(s), papilledema • Due to decreased PTH production, results in decreased serum calcium levels • Can occur after thyroidectomy with inadvertent excision of parathyroid glands
Renal osteodystrophy Rickets/osteomalacia	• Due to one of many diseases resulting in chronic renal failure • Failure to properly mineralize the bone matrix (qualitative problem) • Due to Vitamin D deficiency (nutritional) or receptor defect (usually hereditary)

Comparison of Osteoporosis and Osteomalacia

		Osteoporosis	Osteomalacia
Definition	Unmineralized matrix / Mineralized matrix / Normal	Unmineralized matrix / Mineralized matrix / Bone mass decreased, mineralization normal	Unmineralized matrix / Mineralized matrix / Bone mass variable, mineralization decreased
Age at onset		Generally elderly, postmenopause	Any age
Etiology		Endocrine abnormality, age, idiopathic, inactivity, disuse, alcoholism, calcium deficiency	Vitamin D deficiency, abnormality of vitamin D pathway, hypophosphatemic syndromes, renal tubular acidosis, hypophosphatasia
Symptomatology		Pain referable to fracture site	Generalized bone pain
Signs		Tenderness at fracture site	Tenderness at fracture site and generalized tenderness
Radiographic features		Axial predominance	Often symmetric, pseudofractures, or completed fractures / Appendicular predominance
Laboratory findings	Serum Ca^{++}	Normal	Low or normal (high in hypophosphatasia)
	Serum P_i	Normal $Ca^{++} \times P_i > 30$	Low or normal $Ca^{++} \times P_i > 30$ if albumin normal (high in renal osteodystrophy)
	Alkaline phosphatase	Normal	Elevated, except in hypophosphatasia
	Urinary Ca^{++}	High or normal	Normal or low (high in hypophosphatasia)
	Bone biopsy	Tetracycline labels normal	Tetracycline labels abnormal

CONDITION	COMMENT
METABOLIC DISORDERS	
Osteoporosis	• Decrease in bone mass (quantitative problem). Most common in elderly patients • 2 types: Type 1: most common, affects cancellous bone (femoral neck, vertebral body, etc); Type 2: age related, >70y.o. Both cancellous and cortical bone mass are deficient. • DEXA scan is standard for evaluation. Hormone replacement or bisphosphonates may be used.
Scurvy	• Vitamin C deficiency leads to defective collagen, resulting in a constellation of symptoms.
Osteopetrosis	• "Marble bone disease". Osteoclast dysfunction results in too much bone density.
Paget's disease	• Simultaneous osteoblast & osteoclast activity results in dense, but brittle bones.

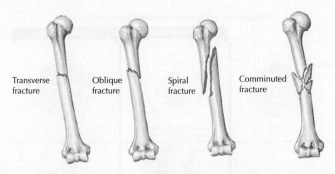

Transverse fracture

Oblique fracture

Spiral fracture

Comminuted fracture

—— **Gustilo and Anderson classification of open fracture** ——

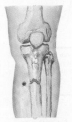

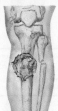

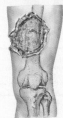

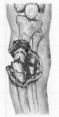

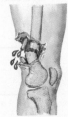

Type I. Wound <1 cm long. No evidence of deep contamination

Type II. Wound >1 cm long. No extensive soft tissue damage

Type IIIA. Large wound. Good soft tissue coverage

Type IIIB. Large wound. Exposed bone fragments, extensive stripping of periosteum. Needs coverage

Type IIIC. Large wound with major arterial injury

f. Netter
M.D.

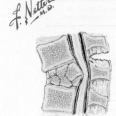

Compression fracture

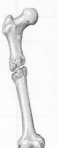

Pathologic fracture (tumor or bone disease)

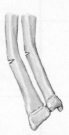

Greenstick fracture

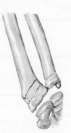

Torus (buckle) fracture

—— In children ——

DESCRIPTION	COMMENT
FRACTURES	
Type/description	• Transverse, oblique, spiral, comminuted, segmental, impacted, avulsion
Displacement	• Nondisplaced, minimally displaced, displaced
Angulation	• Direction of distal fragment (e.g., dorsal displacement) or direction of apex (e.g., apex volar)
Open vs closed	• Open if bone penetrated skin resulting in open wound (surgical emergency for infection risk) • Gustilo & Anderson classification of open fractures (I, II, III a,b,c) is commonly used
Other	• Compression: failure of bone due to compressive load. • Salter-Harris: pediatric fracture involving an open physis (growth plate) • Greenstick: pediatric fracture with disruption of a single cortex • Buckle/torus: pediatric fracture involving an impacted cortex • Pathologic: fracture resulting from a diseased bone/bone tumor

Injury to Growth Plate (Salter-Harris Classification, Rang Modification)

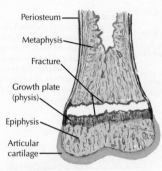
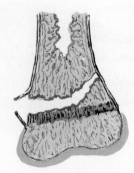

Periosteum

Metaphysis

Fracture

Growth plate (physis)

Epiphysis

Articular cartilage

Type I. Complete separation of epiphysis from shaft through calcified cartilage (growth zone) of growth plate. No bone actually fractured; periosteum may remain intact. Most common in newborns and young children

Type II. Most common. Line of separation extends partially across deep layer of growth plate and extends through metaphysis, leaving triangular portion of metaphysis attached to epiphyseal fragment

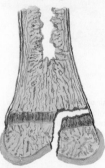
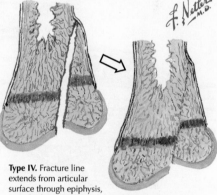

Type III. Uncommon. Intra-articular fracture through epiphysis, across deep zone of growth plate to periphery. Open reduction and fixation often necessary

Type IV. Fracture line extends from articular surface through epiphysis, growth plate, and metaphysis. If fractured segment not perfectly realigned with open reduction, osseous bridge across growth plate may occur, resulting in partial growth arrest and joint angulation

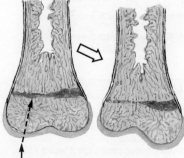
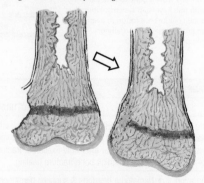

Type V. Severe crushing force transmitted across epiphysis to portion of growth plate by abduction or adduction stress or axial load. Minimal or no displacement makes radiographic diagnosis difficult; growth plate may nevertheless be damaged, resulting in partial growth arrest or shortening and angular deformity

Type VI. Portion of growth plate sheared or cut off. Raw surface heals by forming bone bridge across growth plate, limiting growth on injured side and resulting in angular deformity

Healing of fracture

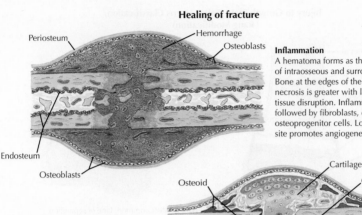

Inflammation
A hematoma forms as the result of disruption of intraosseous and surrounding vessels. Bone at the edges of the fracture dies. Bone necrosis is greater with larger amounts of soft tissue disruption. Inflammatory cells are followed by fibroblasts, chondroblasts, and osteoprogenitor cells. Low pO_2 at the fracture site promotes angiogenesis.

Repair of soft callus formation
Soft callus forms, initially composed of collagen; this is followed by progressive cartilage and osteoid formation.

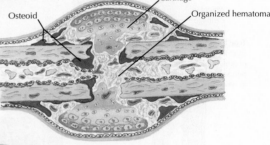

Repair of hard callus formation
Osteoid and cartilage of external, periosteal, and medullary soft callus become mineralized as they are converted to woven bone (hard callus)

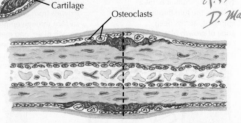

Remodeling
Osteoclastic and osteoblastic activity converts woven bone to lamellar bone with true haversian systems. Normal bone contours are restored; even angulation may be partially or completely corrected.

STAGE	COMMENT
FRACTURE HEALING	
Fracture healing occurs as a continuum with three stages: inflammation, repair (callus formation), remodeling. • To heal, most fractures require good blood supply (most important) and stability. • Callus formation does not occur after rigid fixation of fractures (ORIF); instead primary/direct healing occurs. • Smoking and NSAIDs both inhibit bone/fracture healing.	
Inflammation	• Hematoma develops & supplies hematopoietic/osteoprogenitor cells. Granulation tissue forms.
Repair	• Soft callus: cells produce a cartilage (soft) callus that bridges the bone ends (bridging callus) • Hard callus: replacement of soft callus into immature (woven) bone (enchondral ossification)
Remodeling	• Immature (woven) bone is replaced by mature (lamellar) bone

Factors That Promote or Delay Bone Healing

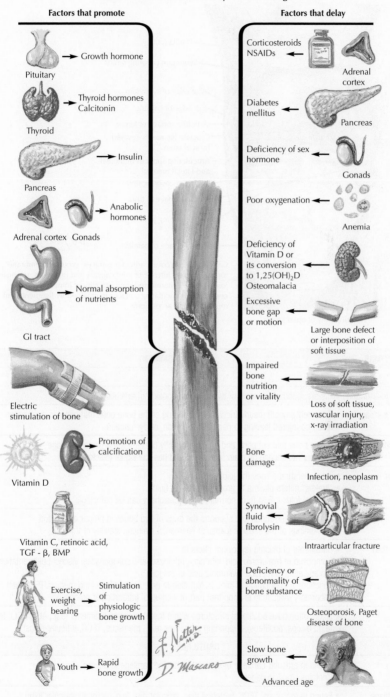

Factors that promote

Growth hormone
Pituitary

Thyroid hormones
Calcitonin
Thyroid

Insulin
Pancreas

Anabolic hormones
Adrenal cortex   Gonads

Normal absorption of nutrients
GI tract

Electric stimulation of bone

Promotion of calcification
Vitamin D

Vitamin C, retinoic acid, TGF - β, BMP

Exercise, weight bearing → Stimulation of physiologic bone growth

Youth → Rapid bone growth

Factors that delay

Corticosteroids
NSAIDs
Adrenal cortex

Diabetes mellitus
Pancreas

Deficiency of sex hormone
Gonads

Poor oxygenation
Anemia

Deficiency of Vitamin D or its conversion to 1,25(OH)₂D
Osteomalacia

Excessive bone gap or motion
Large bone defect or interposition of soft tissue

Impaired bone nutrition or vitality
Loss of soft tissue, vascular injury, x-ray irradiation

Bone damage
Infection, neoplasm

Synovial fluid fibrolysin
Intraarticular fracture

Deficiency or abnormality of bone substance
Osteoporosis, Paget disease of bone

Slow bone growth
Advanced age

Synovial joints

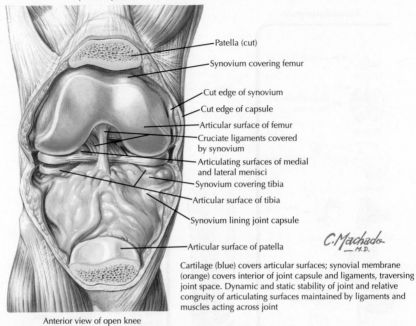

Patella (cut)

Synovium covering femur

Cut edge of synovium

Cut edge of capsule

Articular surface of femur

Cruciate ligaments covered by synovium

Articulating surfaces of medial and lateral menisci

Synovium covering tibia

Articular surface of tibia

Synovium lining joint capsule

Articular surface of patella

C. Machado
—M.D.

Cartilage (blue) covers articular surfaces; synovial membrane (orange) covers interior of joint capsule and ligaments, traversing joint space. Dynamic and static stability of joint and relative congruity of articulating surfaces maintained by ligaments and muscles acting across joint

Anterior view of open knee

STRUCTURE	COMMENT
JOINTS	
Synovial (diarthrodial) joints are found at the ends of two adjacent bones that articulate.	
Articular cartilage	• Extremely smooth (nearly frictionless) covering of the bone ends that glide on each other • It can be injured leading to pain, degeneration, or dysfunction
Subchondral bone	• Dense bone that supports and is found directly beneath the articular cartilage • Appears radiodense on plain film x-rays and has low signal (black) on MR
Synovium	• Inner membrane lines the joint capsule • "Makes" (filters plasma to produce) synovial fluid • Synovial folds (plica) form normally but occasionally can be pathologic
Capsule	• Outer layer, surrounds and supports the ends of two bones in proper orientation • Thickenings of the capsule (capsular ligaments) maintain stability of the joint
Synovial fluid	• Ultrafiltrate of plasma (synovium filters it) • Composed of hyaluronic acid, lubricin, proteinase, and collagenases. Viscosupplementation therapy aims to replace hyaluronic acid in the joint • Function: 1. Lubrication of joint. 2. Nutrition to articular cartilage (and menisci/TFCC, etc) • Laboratory evaluation is important part of workup of intraarticular processes
Other	• Joints often have additional structures within them, including ligaments (e.g., ACL, PCL), tendons (e.g., biceps, popliteus), supporting structures (e.g., meniscus, TFCC, articular discs)
CARTILAGE	
Hyaline	• Found in articular cartilage of synovial joints and cartilage in physes • Contains type II collagen
Fibrocartilage	• Found in meniscus, TFCC, vertebral disc, articular disc (e.g., acromioclavicular joint) • Contains type I collagen

Structure of synovial joints

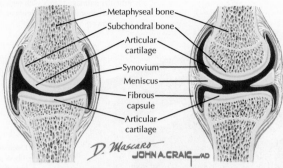

Typical synovial joints exhibit congruent articular cartilage surfaces supported by subchondral and metaphyseal bone and stabilized by joint capsule and ligaments. Inner surfaces, except for articular cartilage, covered by synovial membrane (synovium)

Degrees of sprain

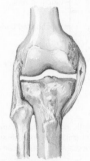 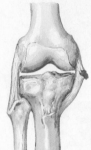 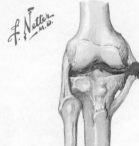

Grade I. Stretching of ligament with minimal disruption of fibers

Grade II. Tearing of up to 50% of ligament fibers; small hematoma. Hemarthrosis may be present

Grade III. Complete tear of ligament and separation of ends, hematoma, and hemarthrosis

STRUCTURE	COMMENT
LIGAMENTS	
Function	• Attach two bones to each other (usually at a joint [ACL] or b/w 2 prominences [suprascapular]) • Ligaments provide stability to a joint allowing for physiologic range of motion
Types	• Ligaments can be discrete structures (e.g., ACL or PCL) • Many ligaments are thickenings of the fibrous joint capsule (e.g., ATFL in ankle)
Insertion	• 1. Ligamentous tissue (primarily type 1 collagen) attaches to fibrocartilage • 2. Fibrocartilage attaches to calcified fibrocartilage (most injuries occur here) • 3. Calcified fibrocartilage (Sharpey's fibers) attaches to bone/periosteum

Injury	• Ligament injuries are termed "sprains" and are graded 1-3
	  ○ Grade 1: stretching of ligament.
	  ○ Grade 2: partial tear of ligament
	  ○ Grade 3: complete tear of ligament
	• Adults tend to have midsubstance injuries; children have more avulsion injuries

Treatment	• Depending on ligament: 1. immobilization, 2. therapy, 3. surgical repair, 4. surgical reconstruction
Ligament strength	• Pediatrics: ligament is stronger than physis, so physis usually injured. Sprains are less common. • Adults: ligament is weakest portion of joint, so sprains are common. • Geriatrics: ligament is stronger than weaker bone, so fracture more common than sprain.

Articular cartilage matrix with regional organization based on chondrocyte proximity and matrix composition (high power)

Gliding surface

Superficial zone (fibers parallel to surface)

Middle zone (random fibers)

Deep zone (fibers perpendicular to surface)

Tidemark (calcification line)
Calcified zone

Subchondral bone

Cancellous bone

Collagen fibrils form structural framework for articular cartilage and provide support for chondrocytes and proteoglycan aggregates

Articular cartilage and subchondral bone with lamellar organization (low power)

STRUCTURE	COMMENT
ARTICULAR CARTILAGE	
Hyaline cartilage covering of intraarticular ends of bones.	
Function	• Smooth (nearly frictionless) surface covering the ends of articulating bones • Allows for pain-free range of motion • Avascular (nutrition from synovial fluid), aneural, alymphatic
Composition	• Water: up to 80% of weight. Changes with load/compression; decr. with age, increases with OA • Collagen: 90+% is type II (also types V, VI, IX, X, XI); gives tensile strength • Proteoglycans: gives compressive strength; decreases with age and allows softening • Chondrocytes: maintains cartilage, produces collagen and proteoglycans
Zones (layers)	• Superficial: thin layer, fibers have tangential orientation (parallel to surface), resists shear • Middle: moderate-sized layer, fibers are randomly/obliquely oriented • Deep: thick layer, fibers are vertical (perpendicular to surface), resists compression • Tidemark: ultrathin line separating deep zone from calcified zone • Calcified zone: transitional zone that attaches cartilage to subchondral bone
Injury & healing	• Articular cartilage is avascular; limited healing capacity, making treatment of injuries problematic • Injuries extending deep to the tidemark may heal with fibrocartilage (not hyaline) • Microfracture surgery is based on stimulating the differentiation of mesenchymal cells within the bone into chondrocytes to produce fibrocartilage healing of articular cartilage injuries

Early degenerative changes

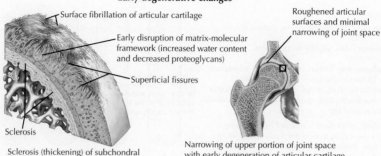

Surface fibrillation of articular cartilage

Early disruption of matrix-molecular framework (increased water content and decreased proteoglycans)

Superficial fissures

Sclerosis

Sclerosis (thickening) of subchondral bone early sign of degeneration

Roughened articular surfaces and minimal narrowing of joint space

Narrowing of upper portion of joint space with early degeneration of articular cartilage

Advanced degenerative changes

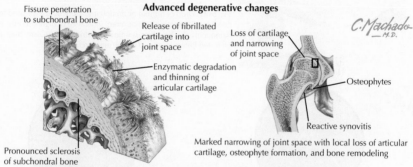

Fissure penetration to subchondral bone

Release of fibrillated cartilage into joint space

Enzymatic degradation and thinning of articular cartilage

Pronounced sclerosis of subchondral bone

Loss of cartilage and narrowing of joint space

Osteophytes

Reactive synovitis

C. Machado —M.D.

Marked narrowing of joint space with local loss of articular cartilage, osteophyte formation, and bone remodeling

End-stage degenerative changes

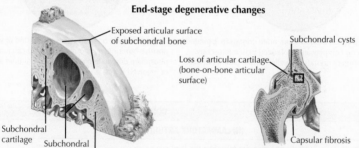

Exposed articular surface of subchondral bone

Loss of articular cartilage (bone-on-bone articular surface)

Subchondral cartilage

Subchondral cysts

Subchondral sclerosis

Subchondral cysts

Capsular fibrosis

Articular cartilage lost and joint space narrowed. Bone shows remodeling osteophyte and subchondral cysts.

STRUCTURE	COMMENT
OSTEOARTHRITIS	
Pathophysiology	• Diffuse wear, erosion, or degeneration of articular cartilage • Microscopically: increase in water content, disorganized collagen, proteoglycan breakdown
Etiology	• Primary: idiopathic, no other identifiable cause; common in elderly patient population • Secondary: due to other underlying condition (e.g., posttraumatic, joint dysplasia, etc)
Incidence	• Most common type of arthritis • Common in weight-bearing joints (knee #1, hip), also in spine, DIPJ, PIPJ, & thumb CMCJ
Symptoms	• Worsening pain and disability (cartilage loss allows bones to directly articulate on each other)
Radiographs	• 1. Joint space narrowing, 2. osteophytes, 3. subchondral sclerosis, 4. subchondral cysts
Treatment	• Rest, activity modification, NSAIDs, therapy (ROM), steroid injection, arthrodesis or arthroplasty

Synovial fluid analysis

Analysis

A. Normal. Clear to pale yellow, transparent.
WBC < 200
B. Osteoarthritis. Slightly deeper yellow, transparent.
WBC <2000
C. Inflammatory. Darker yellow, cloudy, translucent
(type blurred or obscured). WBC < 80,000
D. Septic. Purulent, dense, opaque. WBC > 80,000
E. Hemarthrosis. Red, opaque. Must be differentiated
from traumatic tap

The clarity of the fluid is assessed by expressing a
small amount of fluid out of the plastic syringe into a
glass tube. Printed words viewed through normal and
noninflammatory joint fluid can be read easily.

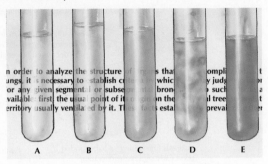

A   B   C   D   E

Viscosity. Drop of normal or noninflammatory fluid expressed from
needle will string out 1 in or more, indicative of high viscosity. Inflammatory fluid evidences little or no stringing. Viscosity may also
be tested between *gloved* thumb and forefinger.

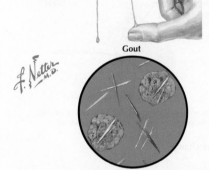

Gout

Free and phagocytized monosodium urate crystals in aspirated
joint fluid seen on compensated polarized light microscopy.
Negatively birefrigent crystals are yellow when parallel to axis.

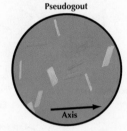

Pseudogout

Axis

Diagnosis made on basis of demonstration of weakly
positive birefringent, rhomboid-shaped calcium pyro-
phosphate dihydrate crystals in synovial fluid aspirate
of involved joints

TYPE	COMMENT
INFLAMMATORY ARTHRITIS	
Rheumatoid arthritis	• Autoimmune disorder targeting the joint synovium • Chronic synovitis and pannus formation lead to articular surface degeneration and eventually joint destruction • Women 3:1; Labs: +RF, HLA-DR4; monocytes mediate the disease effect • Multiple extraarticular manifestations: ocular, skin nodules, vasculitis • Characterized by warm, painful joints with progressive deformity (e.g., ulnar deviation of fingers) • Radiographic findings: 1. joint space narrowing, 2. osteopenia, 3. bone/joint erosion • Treatment: primarily medical until advanced stages necessitate surgical reconstruction
Gout	• Monosodium urate crystal deposition in joint/synovium • Labs: elevated serum uric acid; synovial analysis: negatively birefringent crystals • Typical presentation: monoarticular arthritis (1st MTPJ #1 site); symptoms can be self-limiting • Treatment consists of indomethacin (NSAID) & colchicine
Pseudogout	• Deposition of calcium pyrophosphate dihydrate crystals (CPPD) in the joint • Chondrocalcinosis (calcification of cartilage) can also occur (e.g., calcification of meniscus) • Monoarticular arthritis in older patient is typical presentation; women>men • Synovial analysis shows weakly positive birefringent crystals
Reiter's syndrome	• Triad: urethritis, conjunctivitis, arthritis. Labs: +HLA-B27

Anatomy of Peripheral Nerve

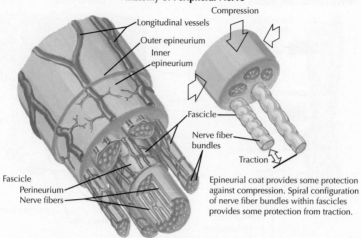

Epineurial coat provides some protection against compression. Spiral configuration of nerve fiber bundles within fascicles provides some protection from traction.

Nerve Fiber Types

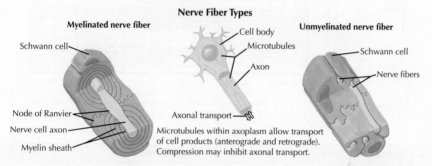

Microtubules within axoplasm allow transport of cell products (anterograde and retrograde). Compression may inhibit axonal transport.

JOHN A.CRAIG—AD

STRUCTURE	COMMENT
NERVE ANATOMY	
Neuron	• A nerve cell made up of cell body (in dorsal root ganglion [DRG] for afferent fibers, in ventral horn for efferent fibers), dendrites (receive signal), axon (transmit signal), presynaptic terminal
Glial cells	• Schwann cell produces myelin to cover the axon; myelin increases conduction speed
Node of Ranvier	• Gap between Schwann cells; facilitates conduction of action potentials/impulse signals
Nerve fiber	• A single axon. 3 types: large/myelinated fibers are fast, small/unmyelinated are slow • Efferent fibers (axons) transmit motor signals from CNS via ventral horn to peripheral muscles • Afferent fibers (axons) transmit sensory signals from peripheral receptor via DRG to CNS
Fascicle	• A group of nerve fibers surrounded by perineurium • Fascicles unite and divide (form plexi) continuously along the course of the nerve
Peripheral nerve	• One or more fascicles surrounded by epineurium • Most peripheral nerves have both motor and sensory fascicles
Epineurium	• Surrounds all fascicles of peripheral nerve; protects and nourishes fascicles
Perineurium	• Surrounds individual fascicles; provides tensile strength to peripheral nerve
Endoneurium	• Surrounds nerve fibers (axons); protects and nourishes nerve fibers
Blood supply	• Intrinsic: vascular plexus within the endoneurium, perineurium, and epineurium • Extrinsic: vessels that enter the epineurium along its course

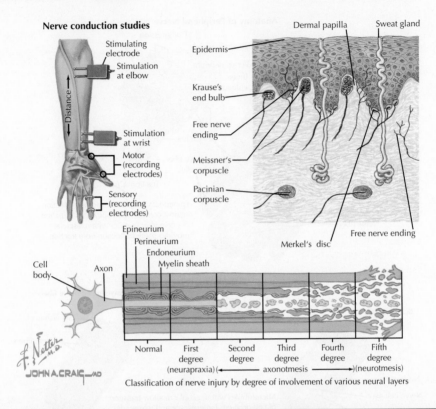

Nerve conduction studies

Classification of nerve injury by degree of involvement of various neural layers

STRUCTURE	COMMENT
NERVE FUNCTION	
Nerve conduction	• Resting potential: a polar difference is maintained between intracellular & extracellular environments • Action potential: change in Na$^+$ permeability depolarizes cells, produces signal conduction
Nerve conduction study (NCS)	• Measures nerve conduction velocity by using a combination of stimulating & recording electrodes • Velocity can be decreased by compression or demyelination (injury or disease)
Receptors	• Multiple types: pain, pressure, thermal, mechanical, etc • Pacinian corpuscle: pressure; Meissner: dynamic 2pt (rapid); Merkel: static 2pt (static)
Disorders	• **Guillain-Barré:** ascending motor weakness/paralysis. Caused by demyelination of peripheral nerves. Typically follows a viral syndrome. Most cases are self-limiting. May need IV IG. • **Charcot-Marie-Tooth:** Autosomal dominant disorder. Demyelinating disorder affecting motor>sensory nerves. Peroneals, hand & foot intrinsics commonly affected: cavus feet, claw toes.
NERVE INJURY	
Classification	• Seddon: 3 categories of injury: neurapraxia, axonotmesis, and neurotmesis • Sunderland: 5 degrees (axonotmesis subdivided into 3 based on intact endo, peri, or epineurium)
Neurapraxia	• Local myelin damage (often from compression), axon is intact; no distal degeneration
Axonotmesis	• Disruption of axon & myelin, epineurium is intact; Wallerian degeneration occurs
Neurotmesis	• Complete disruption of the nerve; poor prognosis; nerve repair typically needed

Physiology of Neuromuscular Junction

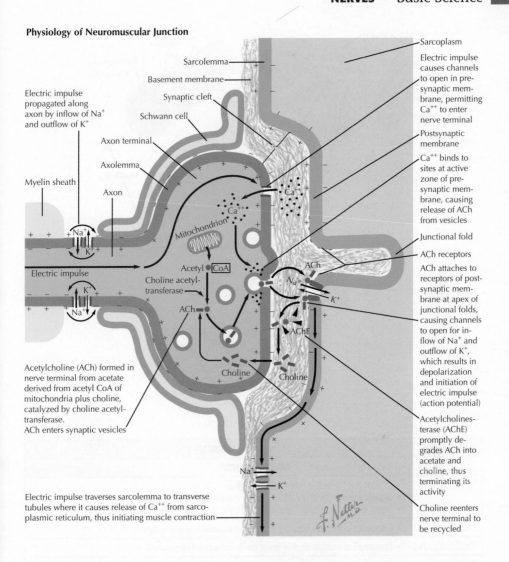

Sarcoplasm

Sarcolemma

Basement membrane

Synaptic cleft

Schwann cell

Electric impulse causes channels to open in pre-synaptic membrane, permitting Ca++ to enter nerve terminal

Electric impulse propagated along axon by inflow of Na+ and outflow of K+

Axon terminal

Axolemma

Myelin sheath

Axon

Postsynaptic membrane

Ca++ binds to sites at active zone of pre-synaptic membrane, causing release of ACh from vesicles

Na+

K+

Mitochondrion

Ca++

Ca++

Junctional fold

ACh receptors

Electric impulse

Acetyl CoA

Choline acetyl-transferase

ACh

ACh

Na+

K+

ACh attaches to receptors of post-synaptic membrane at apex of junctional folds, causing channels to open for in-flow of Na+ and outflow of K+, which results in depolarization and initiation of electric impulse (action potential)

K+

Na+

ACh

ACh formed in nerve terminal from acetate derived from acetyl CoA of mitochondria plus choline, catalyzed by choline acetyltransferase. ACh enters synaptic vesicles

Choline

Choline

AChE

Acetylcholinesterase (AChE) promptly degrades ACh into acetate and choline, thus terminating its activity

Na+

K+

Choline reenters nerve terminal to be recycled

Acetylcholine (ACh) formed in nerve terminal from acetate derived from acetyl CoA of mitochondria plus choline, catalyzed by choline acetyltransferase. ACh enters synaptic vesicles

Electric impulse traverses sarcolemma to transverse tubules where it causes release of Ca++ from sarcoplasmic reticulum, thus initiating muscle contraction

STRUCTURE	COMMENT
NEUROMUSCULAR JUNCTION	
Neuromuscular junction	• Axon of motor neuron synapses with the muscle (motor end plate). • Acetylcholine (the neurotransmitter) stored in axon crosses the synaptic cleft and binds to receptors on the sarcoplasmic reticulum and depolarizes it.
Motor unit	• All the muscles fibers innervated by a single motor neuron
Electromyography (EMG)	• Evaluates motor units to determine if muscle dysfunction is from the nerve, neuromuscular junction, or the muscle itself. Fibrillation is abnormal.
Disorders	• **Myasthenia gravis:** relative shortage of acetylcholine receptors due to competitive binding to them by thymus-derived antibodies. Treatment involves thymectomy or anti-acetylcholinesterase agents.

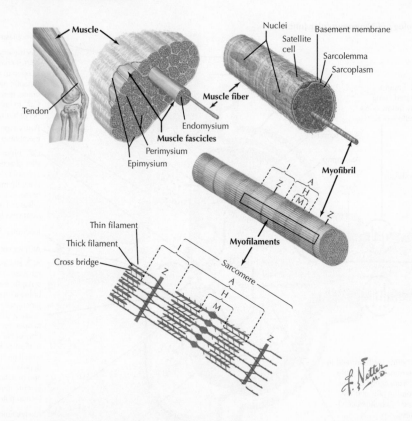

STRUCTURE	COMMENT
MUSCLE ANATOMY	
Types of muscle	• Smooth (e.g., bowel), cardiac, and skeletal • Skeletal muscle: under voluntary control; has an origin and insertion • Types: type 1 "slow twitch" are aerobic; type 2 "fast twitch" are anaerobic
Muscle	• Composed of multiple fascicles (bundles) surrounded by epimysium
Fascicle (bundle)	• Composed of multiple muscle fibers (cells) surrounded by perimysium
Fiber (cell)	• Elongated muscle cell composed of multiple myofibrils surrounded by endomysium
Myofibril	• Composed of multiple myofilaments arranged end to end without a surrounding tissue
Sarcomere	• Composed of interdigitated thick (myosin) and thin (actin) filaments organized into bands • Z line to Z line defines the length of the sarcomere • A band: length of the thick filament, does not change with contraction • I band (actin only), H band (myosin only), and sarcomere length all change with contraction
Myosin	• Thick filament; has "head" that binds ATP and attaches to thin filaments (actin)
Actin	• Thin filament; fixed to Z bands, associated with troponin and tropomyosin
Troponin	• Associated with actin and tropomyosin, binds Ca^{++} ions
Tropomyosin	• Long molecule lies in helical groove of actin and blocks myosin from binding to the actin
Sarcoplasmic reticulum	• Stores intracellular calcium ions (in T tubules), which are stimulated to be released during contraction

Biochemical Mechanics of Muscle Contraction

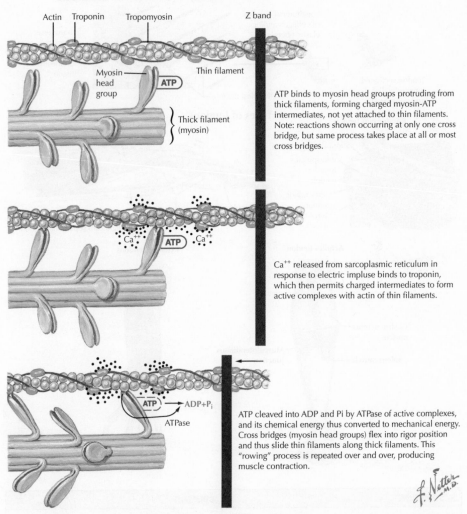

Actin   Troponin   Tropomyosin   Z band

Myosin head group

ATP

Thin filament

Thick filament (myosin)

ATP binds to myosin head groups protruding from thick filaments, forming charged myosin-ATP intermediates, not yet attached to thin filaments. Note: reactions shown occurring at only one cross bridge, but same process takes place at all or most cross bridges.

Ca^{++} ATP Ca^{++}

Ca^{++} released from sarcoplasmic reticulum in response to electric impulse binds to troponin, which then permits charged intermediates to form active complexes with actin of thin filaments.

ATP → ADP+Pi

ATPase

ATP cleaved into ADP and Pi by ATPase of active complexes, and its chemical energy thus converted to mechanical energy. Cross bridges (myosin head groups) flex into rigor position and thus slide thin filaments along thick filaments. This "rowing" process is repeated over and over, producing muscle contraction.

COMMENT
MUSCLE CONTRACTION

Steps	• Contraction initiated when acetylcholine binds to receptors on the sarcoplasmic reticulum, depolarizing it • Depolarization causes release of Ca^{++}, which binds to troponin molecules. This binding causes the tropomyosin to move, allowing the "charged" myosin head (ATP bound) to bind to actin. • Breakdown of the ATP causes contraction of the filament (shortening of the sarcomere) and the release of the filaments (actin and myosin) in preparation to repeat the process.

Types
Isotonic
  Eccentric
  Concentric
Isometric
Isokinetic
	
	• Muscle tension/resistance is the same throughout the contraction
	• Muscle elongates as it contracts. Common injury mechanism (e.g., biceps, quadriceps rupture)
	• Muscle shortens as it contracts
	• Muscle length is constant (resistance changes)
	• Muscle contracts at constant velocity; best for muscle strengthening

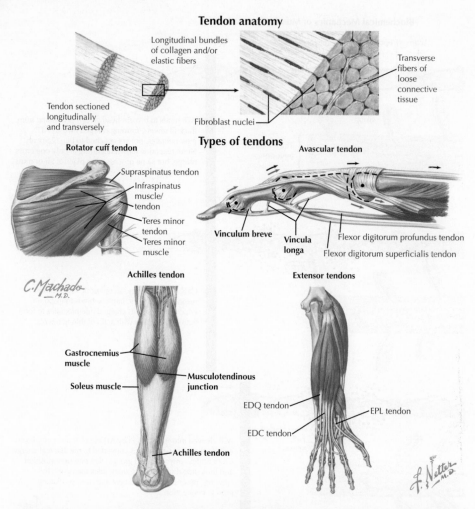

Tendon anatomy

Longitudinal bundles of collagen and/or elastic fibers

Tendon sectioned longitudinally and transversely

Fibroblast nuclei

Transverse fibers of loose connective tissue

Types of tendons

Rotator cuff tendon

Supraspinatus tendon
Infraspinatus muscle/tendon
Teres minor tendon
Teres minor muscle

Avascular tendon

Vinculum breve
Vincula longa
Flexor digitorum profundus tendon
Flexor digitorum superficialis tendon

Achilles tendon

Gastrocnemius muscle
Soleus muscle
Musculotendinous junction
Achilles tendon

Extensor tendons

EDQ tendon
EDC tendon
EPL tendon

STRUCTURE	COMMENT
TENDON	
Function	• Connects muscles to bones so the muscle can exert its effect
Anatomy Fibril Fascicle Tendon	• Various shapes and sizes (long, broad, short, flat, etc) • Type 1 collagen grouped into microfibrils, then subfibrils, then fibrils, surrounded by endotenon • Fibroblasts and fibrils surrounded by a peritenon • Groups of fascicles surrounded by an epitenon
Insertion	• Tendinous tissue (primarily type 1 collagen) attaches to fibrocartilage • Fibrocartilage attaches to calcified fibrocartilage (Sharpey's fibers) • Calcified fibrocartilage (Sharpey's fibers) attaches to bone/periosteum
Blood supply	• Vascular tendons have a paratenon (no sheath) that surrounds them and supplies blood • Avascular tendons (in a sheath) have a vinculum to supply blood
Musculotendinous junction	• Transition from muscle to tendon; weakest portion of the myotendinous complex and site of most injuries

Etiology of Compartment Syndrome

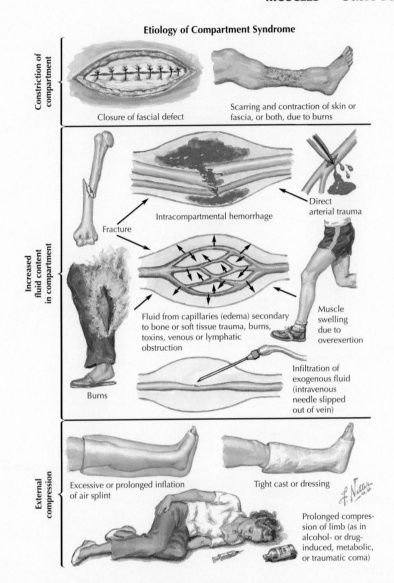

Constriction of compartment

Closure of fascial defect

Scarring and contraction of skin or fascia, or both, due to burns

Increased fluid content in compartment

Fracture

Intracompartmental hemorrhage

Direct arterial trauma

Fluid from capillaries (edema) secondary to bone or soft tissue trauma, burns, toxins, venous or lymphatic obstruction

Muscle swelling due to overexertion

Burns

Infiltration of exogenous fluid (intravenous needle slipped out of vein)

External compression

Excessive or prolonged inflation of air splint

Tight cast or dressing

Prolonged compression of limb (as in alcohol- or drug-induced, metabolic, or traumatic coma)

COMMENT
MUSCLE COMPARTMENTS
Muscles are contained within fibro(fascia)-osseous(bone) spaces known as compartments.

Compartment syndrome	• Results from increased pressure within fibroosseous compartment • Multiple etiologies (fracture/hematoma, edema, burns, compression, etc) • The increased pressure occludes the vascular supply to the compartment muscles • Symptoms: the "5 P's": pain (on passive stretch, most sensitive), paresthesias, pallor, paralysis, pulselessness (a late finding) • Physical exam: firm/tense compartments +/− some or all of the 5 P's; it is a clinical diagnosis • Two methods for intracompartmental pressure tests: 1.absolute value, 2. ΔP from diastolic BP • Compartment release/fasciotomy is a surgical emergency to prevent muscle necrosis/contracture

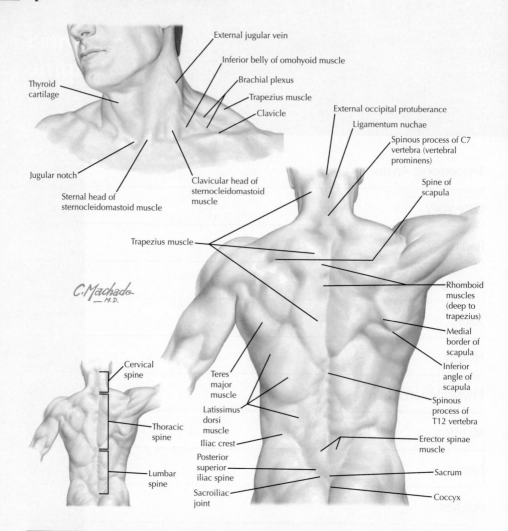

External jugular vein

Inferior belly of omohyoid muscle

Brachial plexus

Trapezius muscle

Clavicle

Thyroid cartilage

External occipital protuberance

Ligamentum nuchae

Spinous process of C7 vertebra (vertebral prominens)

Jugular notch

Clavicular head of sternocleidomastoid muscle

Spine of scapula

Sternal head of sternocleidomastoid muscle

Trapezius muscle

C. Machado —M.D.

Rhomboid muscles (deep to trapezius)

Medial border of scapula

Cervical spine

Teres major muscle

Inferior angle of scapula

Latissimus dorsi muscle

Spinous process of T12 vertebra

Thoracic spine

Iliac crest

Erector spinae muscle

Posterior superior iliac spine

Lumbar spine

Sacrum

Sacroiliac joint

Coccyx

STRUCTURE	CLINICAL APPLICATION
Brachial plexus	Interscalene nerve block commonly used for upper extremity procedures
Sternocleidomastoid	Contracted in torticollis
Trapezius	Large muscle, muscle spasm common cause of neck and upper back pain
Rhomboid muscles	Overuse and spasm common cause of upper back pain
C7 spinous process	"Vertebral prominens" is an easily palpable landmark
Iliac crest	Site for "hip pointers" (contusion of lilac crest) Common site for autologous bone graft harvest
Erector spinae muscles	Overuse and spasm are common causes of lower back pain (LBP)
Posterior superior iliac spine	Site of bone graft harvest in posterior spinal procedures
Sacroiliac joint	Degeneration or injury to joint can cause lower back pain
Coccyx	Distal end of vertebral column (tailbone), can be fractured in a fall (LBP)

GENERAL INFORMATION

- 33 Vertebrae: 7 cervical, 12 thoracic, 5 lumbar, 5 sacral (fused), 4 coccygeal (fused)
- Vertebrae form a functional column
- 3 column theory (Denis): spine is divided into 3 columns
  - Anterior: ALL & anterior ⅔ of vertebral body/annulus
  - Middle: PLL & posterior ⅓ of vertebral body/annulus
  - Posterior: Pedicles, lamina, spinous process, and ligaments
- Spinal curves: normal curves
  - Cervical lordosis
  - Thoracic kyphosis
  - Lumbar lordosis
  - Sacral kyphosis

Spinal Regions

Cervical	C1-C2: unique bones allow stabilization of occiput to spine and rotation of head. Motion: rotation and flexion/extension.
Thoracic	Relatively stiff due to costal articulations. Motion: rotation. Minimal flexion/extension.
Thoraco-lumbar	Facet orientation transitions from semicoronal to sagittal. Segments are mobile. Most common site of lower spine injuries.
Lumbar	Largest vertebrae. Common site for pain. Houses cauda equina. Motion: flexion/extension. Minimal rotation.
Sacrum	No motion. Is center of pelvis.

Vertebrae

- Uniquely shaped bones that support the axial musculature and protect the spinal cord and nerve roots

Body (centrum)	Has articular cartilage on both superior & inferior surfaces. Articulates with intervertebral discs & gets larger distally.
Arch	Made up of pedicles and lamina. Develops from 2 ossifications centers that fuse. Failure to fuse occurs in spina bifida. It forms the vertebral canal for the spinal cord.
Processes	Spinous: ligament attachment site. Transverse: rib (T-spine) and ligament attachment site.
Foramina	Vertebral: spinal cord/cauda equina. Neural: nerve roots exit via here.

LEVEL	CORRESPONDING STRUCTURE
C2-3	Mandible
C3	Hyoid cartilage
C4-5	Thyroid cartilage
C6	Cricoid cartilage
C7	Vertebral prominens
T3	Spine of scapula
T7	Xyphoid, tip of scapula
T10	Umbilicus
L1	Conus medullaris (end of cord)
L3	Aorta bifurcation
L4	Iliac crest

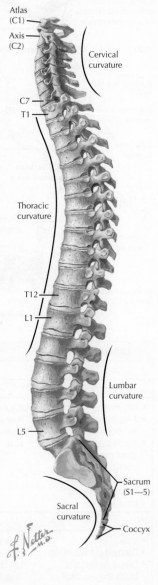

Left lateral view

Atlas (C1)
Axis (C2)
Cervical curvature
C7
T1
Thoracic curvature
T12
L1
Lumbar curvature
L5
Sacrum (S1—5)
Sacral curvature
Coccyx

Atlas

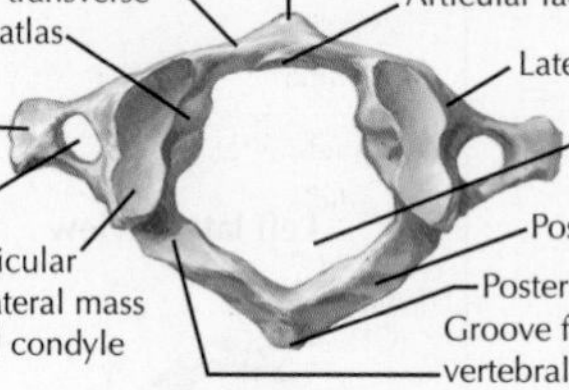

Atlas (C1): superior view

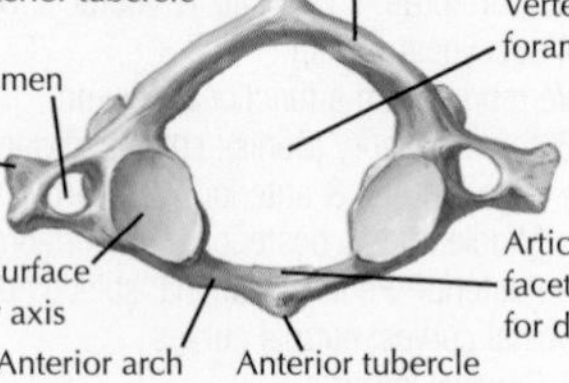

Atlas (C1): inferior view

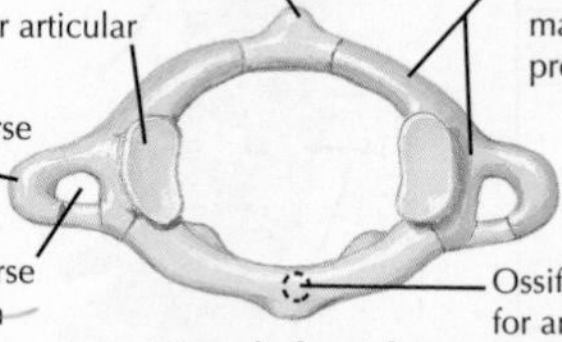

1st cervical vertebra (atlas) (superior view)

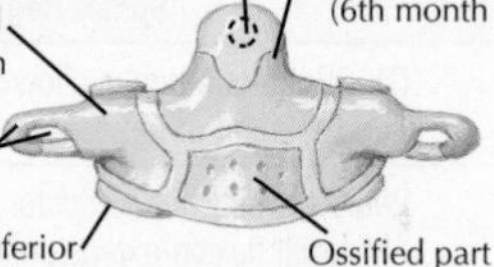

2nd cervical vertebra (axis) (anterior view)

Axis

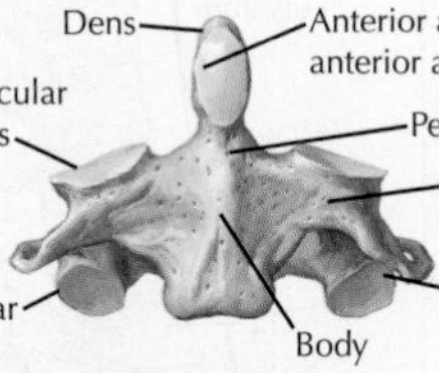

Axis (C2): anterior view

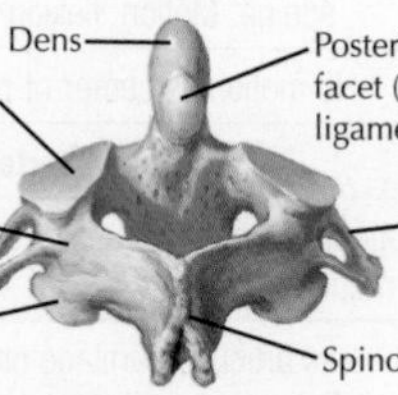

Axis (C2): posterosuperior view

CHARACTERISTICS	OSSIFY	FUSE	COMMENTS
CERVICOCRANIUM			
Atlas (C1)			

• Ring shaped
• 2 lateral masses with facets; facets are concave
• 2 arches connect lateral masses:
  ○ anterior tubercle
  ○ posterior tubercle
• Transverse process has a foramen
	Lateral masses/
	posterior arch
	Body/anterior
	arch
		7mo fetal
		to birth
		6-12mo
			3-4yr
			7yr
				• Ring/arches are susceptible to fracture
				• Superior facets (concave) articulate with occiput; inferior facets articulate with C2
				• Posterior arch has groove for vertebral artery
				• Attachment site of ALL and longus colli
				• Attachment site of ligamentum nuchae
				• Vertebral artery through foramen transversarium

Axis (C2)			
• Body • Odontoid process (dens) • Lateral masses with facets and two small transverse processes • Pedicles (between facets) • Spinous process	**Primary** Body Lateral mass/ neural arch [2] Odontoid—Body Tip	4mo fetal 7mo fetal 6mo fetal 2-3 yr	3-7yr 2-yr 3-6yr 12yr	• Odontoid projects superiorly & allows C1-C2 rotation; primary horizontal stabilizer • Concave superior facets allow for rotation • Vertebral artery through foramen transversarium • Pedicles (isthmus) susceptible to fracture • Bifid, relatively large and palpable
There are two secondary ossification centers in the axis: ossiculum terminale and inferior ring apophysis.			

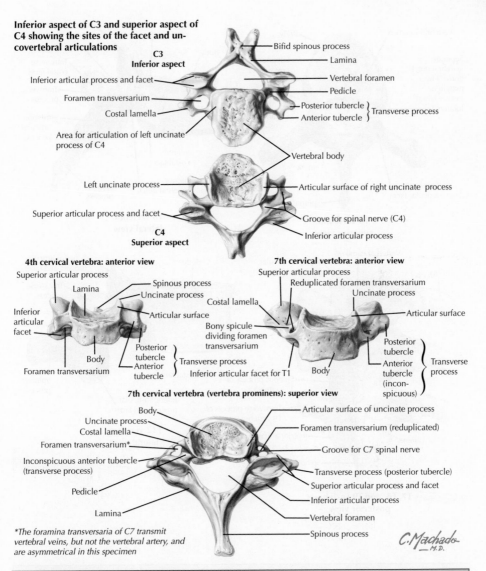

Inferior aspect of C3 and superior aspect of C4 showing the sites of the facet and uncovertebral articulations

C3
Inferior aspect

- Bifid spinous process
- Lamina
- Vertebral foramen
- Pedicle
- Posterior tubercle
- Anterior tubercle } Transverse process

- Inferior articular process and facet
- Foramen transversarium
- Costal lamella
- Area for articulation of left uncinate process of C4

- Vertebral body

- Left uncinate process
- Articular surface of right uncinate process

- Superior articular process and facet
- Groove for spinal nerve (C4)
- Inferior articular process

C4
Superior aspect

4th cervical vertebra: anterior view

- Superior articular process
- Lamina
- Inferior articular facet
- Body
- Foramen transversarium
- Spinous process
- Uncinate process
- Articular surface
- Posterior tubercle
- Anterior tubercle } Transverse process

7th cervical vertebra: anterior view

- Superior articular process
- Reduplicated foramen transversarium
- Uncinate process
- Costal lamella
- Bony spicule dividing foramen transversarium
- Inferior articular facet for T1
- Body
- Articular surface
- Posterior tubercle
- Anterior tubercle (inconspicuous) } Transverse process

7th cervical vertebra (vertebra prominens): superior view

- Body
- Uncinate process
- Costal lamella
- Foramen transversarium*
- Inconspicuous anterior tubercle (transverse process)
- Pedicle
- Lamina

- Articular surface of uncinate process
- Foramen transversarium (reduplicated)
- Groove for C7 spinal nerve
- Transverse process (posterior tubercle)
- Superior articular process and facet
- Inferior articular process
- Vertebral foramen
- Spinous process

*The foramina transversaria of C7 transmit vertebral veins, but not the vertebral artery, and are asymmetrical in this specimen

C.Machado
—M.D.

CHARACTERISTICS	OSSIFY	FUSE		COMMENTS
CERVICAL (C3-7)				
• Body	**Primary**			• Concave superiorly, convex inferiorly
• Uncinate processes [2]	Body/centrum	7-8wk	6yr	• Articulates with adjacent vertebral body
• Small pedicles	Neural arch [2]	fetal	5-8yr	• Angled medial & superior, too small for screws
• Transverse processes	**Secondary**			• Have foramen for vertebral artery except C7
• Lateral masses— 2 facets	Spinous process	12-15yr	25yr	• Can accept screws if angled laterally (artery at risk in foremen)
• Facets (superior & inferior)	Transverse process [2]			• "Semi-coronal" orientation allows for flexion/ extension
• Lamina	Annular (ring) epiphysis [2]			• Connects lateral masses to spinous process
• Spinous process				• Usually bifid (C3-5), C7 is the largest

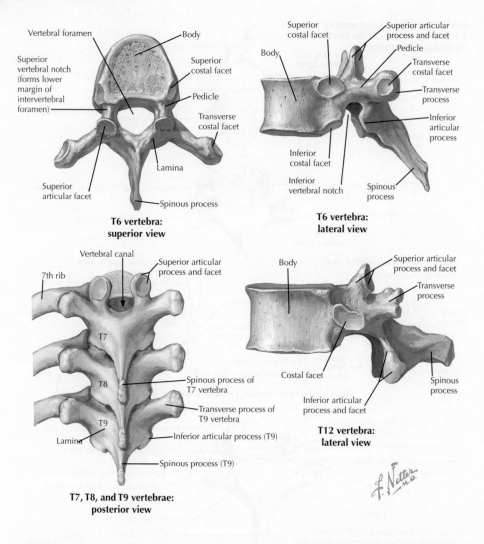

T6 vertebra:
superior view

T6 vertebra:
lateral view

T7, T8, and T9 vertebrae:
posterior view

T12 vertebra:
lateral view

CHARACTERISTICS	OSSIFY		FUSE	COMMENTS
	THORACIC			
• Body: costal facets (articulate w/ ribs)	**Primary**			• Upper thoracic have superior & inferior facets; lower thoracic have a single facet.
	Body/centrum	7-8wk	6yr	
• Pedicles: increase in size in lower T-spine	Neural arch [2]	fetal	5-8yr	• Can accept screws for spinal fixation, have anteromedial orientation.
	Secondary			
• Articular processes/ facets	Spinous process	12-15yr	25yr	• Facets are semicoronal, allow for rotation but minimal flexion/extension
	Transverse process [2]			
• Transverse process	Annular (ring)			• Have costal facet in upper T-spine
• Lamina	epiphysis [2]			• Broad & overlapping (like shingles)
• Spinal process				• Long with steep posterior slope
Landmark for pedicle screw: junction of lines through upper ⅓ transverse process and just lateral to vertical line through facet				

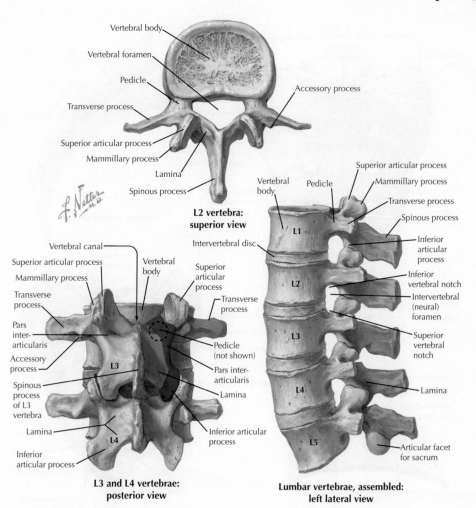

**L2 vertebra:
superior view**

**L3 and L4 vertebrae:
posterior view**

**Lumbar vertebrae, assembled:
left lateral view**

CHARACTERISTICS	OSSIFY		FUSE	COMMENTS
LUMBAR				
• Body: large	**Primary**			• Broad, oval, cylindrical shaped bone
• Pedicles: large, short, but strong	Body/centrum	7-8wk	6yr	• Orientation changes through L-spine; this portion of bone accepts screw fixation
	Neural arch [2]	fetal	5-8yr	
• Articular processes/ facets: has a mammillary process	**Secondary**			• Sagittal orientation allows flexion/extension
	Mammillary proc.	12-15yr	25yr	• Superior facets are lateral to inferior facets/articular processes
	Ring epiphysis [2]			
• Pars interarticularis	Transverse			• Area b/w facets, site of spondylolysis/fx
• Transverse process	process [2]			• Avulsion fracture can occur here.
• Lamina	Spinous process			• Do not overlap adjacent levels
• Spinous process				• Long, palpable posteriorly

Landmark for pedicle screw: junction lines through middle of transverse process and lateral border of facet joint.
Failure of fusion of two neural arch (pedicle/lamina) ossification centers results in spina bifida.

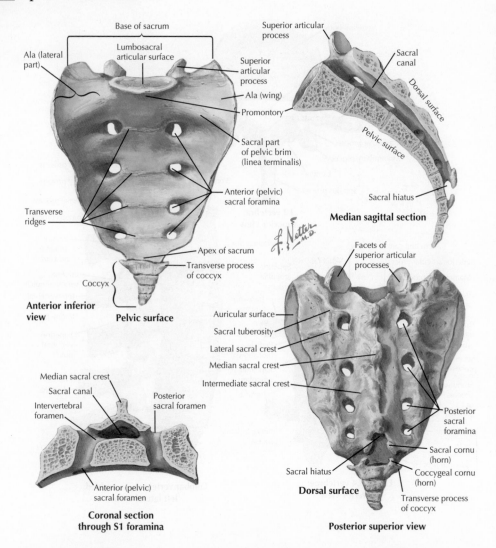

Base of sacrum

Lumbosacral articular surface

Ala (lateral part)

Superior articular process

Ala (wing)

Promontory

Sacral part of pelvic brim (linea terminalis)

Anterior (pelvic) sacral foramina

Transverse ridges

Apex of sacrum

Transverse process of coccyx

Coccyx

Anterior inferior view

Pelvic surface

Superior articular process

Sacral canal

Dorsal surface

Pelvic surface

Sacral hiatus

Median sagittal section

Facets of superior articular processes

Auricular surface

Sacral tuberosity

Lateral sacral crest

Median sacral crest

Intermediate sacral crest

Posterior sacral foramina

Sacral cornu (horn)

Coccygeal cornu (horn)

Transverse process of coccyx

Sacral hiatus

Dorsal surface

Posterior superior view

Median sacral crest

Sacral canal

Intervertebral foramen

Posterior sacral foramen

Anterior (pelvic) sacral foramen

Coronal section through S1 foramina

CHARACTERISTICS	OSSIFY		FUSE	COMMENTS
SACRUM				
• 5 vertebrae are fused • 4 pairs of foramina (left and right) • Ala (wing) expands laterally • Kyphotic (approx 25°), apex at S3 • Sacral canal opens to hiatus distally	**Primary** Body Arches Costal **Secondary**	7-8wk fetal 11-14yr	2-8yr 12-18yr	• Transmits body weight from spine to pelvis • Nerves exit through sacral foramina • Ala is common site for sacral fractures • Sacral canal narrows distally • Segments fuse to each other at puberty
COCCYX				
• 4 vertebrae are fused • Lack features of typical vertebrae • Bones become smaller distally	**Primary** Body Arches	7-8wk fetal	1-2yr 7-10yr	• Attached to gluteus maximus and coccygeal muscle • No neural foramen; distal to sacral hiatus • Common site for "tailbone" fracture

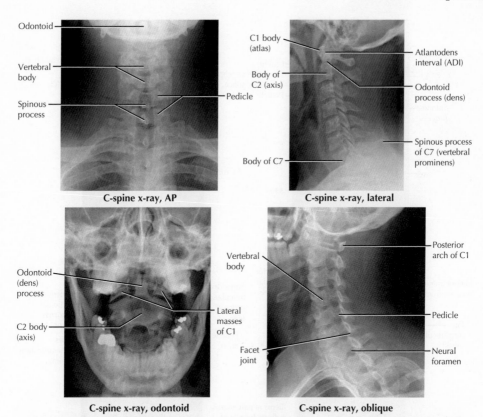

Odontoid

Vertebral body

Spinous process

C-spine x-ray, AP

C1 body (atlas)

Body of C2 (axis)

Pedicle

Body of C7

Atlantodens interval (ADI)

Odontoid process (dens)

Spinous process of C7 (vertebral prominens)

C-spine x-ray, lateral

Odontoid (dens) process

C2 body (axis)

Lateral masses of C1

C-spine x-ray, odontoid

Vertebral body

Facet joint

Posterior arch of C1

Pedicle

Neural foramen

C-spine x-ray, oblique

RADIOGRAPH	TECHNIQUE	FINDINGS	CLINICAL APPLICATION
CERVICAL SPINE			
AP (anteroposterior)	Erect/supine, beam w/slight cephalad tilt at mid C-spine	Vertebral bodies (esp. C3-7), intervertebral disc spaces	Cervical fractures, spondylosis
Lateral (crosstable)	Supine, horizontal beam to mid C-spine (must see C7)	Bodies, disc space, facets 4 lines: 1. Ant. vert. (ALL); 2. Post. vert. (PLL); 3. Spinolaminar (ligamentum flavum); 4. Post. spinous	First x-ray in all trauma cases Fractures & dislocations. Increased retropharyngeal swelling (>6mm at C2 or >22mm at C6) may indicate fx
Odontoid (open mouth)	Beam into open mouth	Odontoid, lateral masses	C1 (Jefferson) or C2/odontoid fx
Swimmer's view	Prone, one arm above head, beam into axilla	C7, T1, and T2	Used if lateral does not show C7 Used to rule out cervical fractures
Obliques	AP, turn body 45°	Neural foramina & facet joints	Foraminal stenosis
Flexion/extension views	Lateral with flexion/extension	Same as lateral	For instability/spondylolisthesis

Multiple measurements can be made from the lateral C-spine radiograph
1. ADI (atlantodens interval): Posterior aspect of C1 anterior arch to anterior border of odontoid. Normal is ≤3mm
2. SAC (space available for cord): Posterior odontoid to anterior aspect of posterior arch: Normal = 17mm
3. Power ratio: Basion (B) to C1 post. arch (C), opisthion (O) to C1 ant. arch (A). Ratio BC/OA >1 = occipitoatlantal dx
4. Chamberlain's line: Opisthion to hard palate. Odontoid tip ≤5mm above line. >5mm is basilar invagination

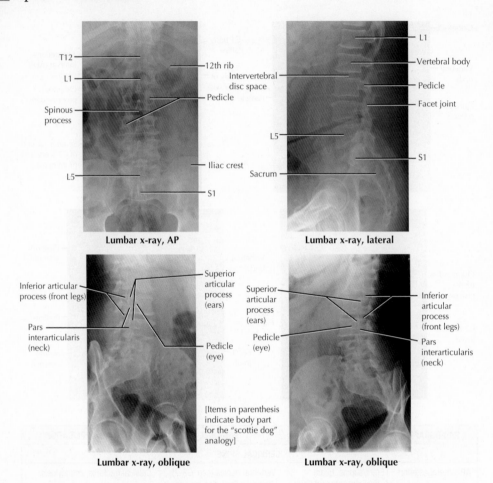

Lumbar x-ray, AP

Lumbar x-ray, lateral

Lumbar x-ray, oblique

Lumbar x-ray, oblique

[Items in parenthesis indicate body part for the "scottie dog" analogy]

RADIOGRAPH	TECHNIQUE	FINDINGS	CLINICAL APPLICATION
THORACIC SPINE			
AP (anteroposterior)	Supine, beam to mid T-spine	Vertebral bodies	Alignment, scoliosis (Cobb angle)
Lateral	Lateral, beam to T-spine	Bodies & posterior elements	Alignment, kyphosis, scoliosis, fx
Bending films	AP or lateral w/ bending	Thoracic vertebrae	Access flexibility of scoliosis curves
LUMBAR SPINE			
AP (anteroposterior)	Supine, flex hips, beam @L3	Bodies, disc spaces, pedicle position, transverse process	Fracture (body-pedicle widening, transverse process), dislocation
Lateral	Lateral, flex hips, beam @L3	Bodies, pars, disc spaces	Fractures, spondylolisthesis
Obliques	AP, turn body 45°	Neural foramina, pars interarticularis, facet joints	Foraminal stenosis, spondylosis, facet hypertrophy (DJD)
Flexion/extension views	Lateral with flexion/ extension	Same as lateral	Instability/spondylolisthesis

Jefferson fracture of atlas (C1)
Each arch may be broken in one or more places

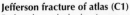
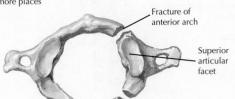

Fracture of anterior arch

Superior articular facet

Fracture of posterior arch

Fracture of odontoid process

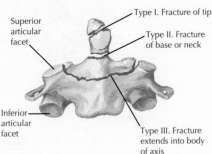

Type I. Fracture of tip

Superior articular facet

Type II. Fracture of base or neck

Inferior articular facet

Type III. Fracture extends into body of axis

Traumatic spondylolisthesis

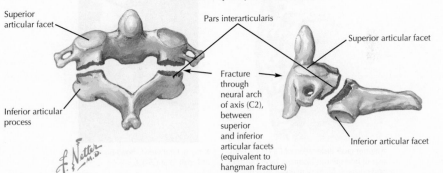

Superior articular facet

Inferior articular process

Pars interarticularis

Superior articular facet

Fracture through neural arch of axis (C2), between superior and inferior articular facets (equivalent to hangman fracture)

Inferior articular facet

DESCRIPTION	EVALUATION	CLASSIFICATION	TREATMENT
CERVICOCRANIUM INJURIES			

• Injuries to this region can be both subtle and devastating
• ATLS protocols warranted
• Occipital/cervical dx: high mortality, increased incidence in pediatric patients
• Atlantoaxial instability: disruption of transverse ligament [TAL] +/– alar & apical ligaments determine degree of instability
• Type 2 odontoid fractures have high nonunion rate
• Traumatic spondylolisthesis is bilateral pars fracture (similar to hangman's fx, but different mechanism)
	Hx: High-energy trauma, (e.g., MVA, fall, diving), +/– pain, numbness, tingling, weakness
	PE: Stabilize head & neck Inspect & palpate neck Neuro exam: CN's, UE & LE motor/sensory/ reflexes
	XR: Lateral, odontoid, AP basion to dens ≤5mm Power's ratio <1 is normal; ADI ≤3mm is normal; flexion/extension views: to evaluate dynamic instability
	CT: Best for all fractures
	MR: Ligaments, cord, roots
		Occipitocervical dissociation
		Atlantoaxial instability:
		1. midsubstance, 2. avulsion
		C1 (atlas) (7 types): burst (3-4 fx, Jefferson)[1], post. arch [2], comminuted [3], ant. arch [4], lat. mass [5], transv. proc.[6], inf. tubercle [7]
		C2 (axis):
		  ○ **Odontoid fx:** type 1: tip, type 2: base (jxn dens/ body), type 3: C2 body
		  ○ **Traumatic spondylolisthesis:** 1. nondisplaced, 2. displaced & angulated, 2a. angulated, 3. fx w/ C2-3 facet dx
			• O-C dx: halo vs fusion
			• C1-C2: ADI <5mm: collar
			• ADI >5mm: C1-2 fusion
			• C1 fracture:
			  ○ Unstable/wide: C1-2 fusion
			  ○ Stable: halo vs collar immobilization 3mo
			• Avulsion: soft collar 6wk
			• C2 fracture:
			• Odontoid:
			  ○ Collar
			  ○ ORIF(displaced) vs halo (nondisplaced)
			  ○ Halo vest
			• Traumatic spondylolisthesis
			  ○ Collar immobilization
			  ○ CR/halo vs ORIF
			  ○ ORIF (C2 screws)

COMPLICATIONS: Nonunion (esp. odontoid type 2); neurologic (cord trauma); persistent pain, instability, or stiffness			

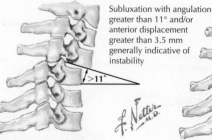

Subluxation with angulation greater than 11° and/or anterior displacement greater than 3.5 mm generally indicative of instability

>11°

>3.5 mm

Subluxation with angulation greater than 11°

Anterior displacement greater than 3.5 mm

Facet dislocation

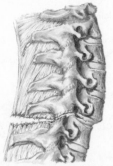

Anterior facet dislocation of C5 on C6 with tear of interspinous ligament, facet capsules, and posterior fibers of intervertebral disc

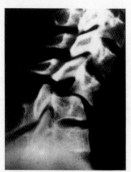

X-ray (lateral view) shows bilateral facet dislocation at C5–C6

DESCRIPTION	EVALUATION	CLASSIFICATION	TREATMENT
	**SUBAXIAL CERVICAL FRACTURES**		
• Compression fx: involve ant. half of vertebral body • Burst fx: involve whole vertebral body & have retropulsion into spinal canal • Instability (White & Panjabi) ○ >3.5mm of translation ○ >11° kyphotic angulation ○ + stretch test ○ Neuro (cord or root) injury ○ Ant. elements destroyed ○ Post. elements destroyed ○ Narrow spinal canal ○ Disc space narrowing • Heavy loads anticipated	**Hx:** High-energy trauma, (e.g., MVA, fall, diving), +/− pain, numbness, tingling or weakness **PE:** Stabilize head & neck Palpate neck for "step off." Neuro exam: CN's, UE & LE motor/sensory/ reflexes **XR:** Lateral, odontoid, AP Evaluate for stability criteria Flexion/extension views: to evaluate dynamic instability **CT:** Best study for all fractures **MR:** Assess posterior ligaments & for disc herniation on cord	**By mechanism** (each class is subclassified by severity) 1. Flexion-compression [#1] 2. Vertical compression 3. Flexion-distraction [#2] 4. Extension-compression 5. Extension-distraction 6. Lateral flexion **Descriptive** Compression Burst Facet dislocation Unilateral Bilateral	• Compression fx: collar • Burst fx: ACDF (anterior corpectomy, diskectomy, and fusion [ant. plate]) vs decompression/post. fusion • Flexion-compression: ○ Stable: collar or halo; ○ Unstable: ant. or post. fusion • Flexion-distraction/ facet dx: Closed (acute, awake pt) vs open (unconscious or late presentation) reduction with anterior (ACDF) or posterior spinal fusion
	COMPLICATIONS: Neurologic: quadriplegia, paraplegia, radiculopathy. Vascular: vertebral artery. Immobilization: halo.		

Three-Column Concept of Spinal Stability

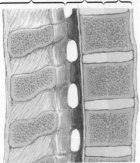

Posterior column   Middle column   Anterior column

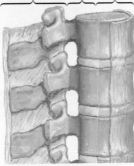

Posterior column   Middle column   Anterior column

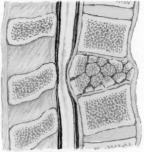

Burst fracture

Three-column concept. If more than one column involved in fracture, then instability of spine usually results

Lateral view. Note that lateral facet (zygapophyseal) joints in posterior column, with intervertebral foramina in middle column

Burst fracture of unstable vertebral body involving both anterior and middle columns resulted in instability and spinal cord compression

Chance fracture

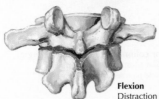

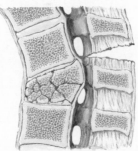

Flexion
Distraction results in complete transverse fracture through entire vertebra. Note hinge effect of anterior longitudinal ligament

Fracture/Dislocation:
All 3 columns are involved

DESCRIPTION	EVALUATION	CLASSIFICATION	TREATMENT
THORACOLUMBAR FRACTURES			
• Mechanism: MVA or fall (lap belt can be fulcrum to cause flexion-distraction fx) • Thoracolumbar junction is most common site of fracture/injury • Determining stability is key to treatment • 3-column theory (Denis): >1 column injured = unstable • Burst fx: caused by 1. flexion and 2. axial compression • Chance fx: flexion-distraction fx, all 3 columns fail in tension	**Hx:** High-energy trauma, pain +/– numbness or weakness **PE:** Palpate for "step off" Neuro exam: LE motor/sensory/reflexes (including anal wink & bulbocavernosus) **XR:** Lateral (body ht, kyphosis) AP (pedicle widening) Flexion/extension views: to evaluate dynamic instability **CT:** Best study for all fractures Evaluate for retropulsion **MR:** Discs & post. ligaments	**Compression:** 1 (anterior) column only, stable fx **Stable burst:** 2 columns 1. <25° kyphosis 2. <50% body ht loss 3. <50% canal retropulsion **Unstable burst:** 2-3 columns fail above criteria or have neurologic compromise **Flexion-distraction:** 2-3 columns; columns fail posterior to anterior **Translation** (fx/dx): All 3 columns fail: unstable	• Compression: observation or orthosis 12wk • Stable burst: TLSO or hyperextension brace for 12wk (f/u x-rays to confirm stability) • Unstable burst: decompression & posterior spinal fusion • Flexion-distraction: most require posterior fusion • Translation: needs reduction and stabilization/fusion
COMPLICATIONS: Neurologic: Spinal cord/cauda equina injury. Immobilization: DVT, PE. Surgical: Infection, dural tears.			

Central cord syndrome
Central cord hemorrhage and edema. Parts of 3 main tracts involved on both sides. Upper limbs more affected than lower limbs ▷

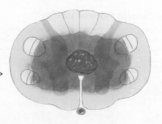

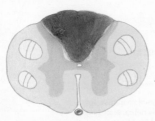

Anterior spinal artery syndrome
Artery damaged by bone or cartilage spicules (shaded area affected). Bilateral loss of motor function and pain sensation below injured ◁ segment; position sense preserved

Brown-Sequard syndrome
One side of cord affected. Loss of motor function and position sense on same side and of pain sensation on opposite side ▷

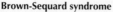

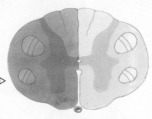

Posterior column syndrome (uncommon)
Position sense lost below lesion; motor ◁ function and pain sensation preserved

DESCRIPTION	EVALUATION	CLASSIFICATION	TREATMENT
SPINAL CORD TRAUMA			

• Young males most common
• High association w/C-spine fractures (easily missed)
• Central: #1, hyperextension mechanism, seen in elderly, with cervical spondylosis
• Anterior: #2, worst prognosis
• Brown-Sequard: usually penetrating trauma, rare injury, best prognosis
• Posterior: very rare; this pattern may not exist
	Hx: High-energy trauma (MVA, fall), +/− numbness or weakness
	PE: Find lowest functional neurologic level
	Central: UE>LE motor loss
	Anterior: LE>UE motor and sensory, proprioception intact
	B-S: Ipsilateral motor loss, contralateral pain/temp loss
	XR: r/o C-spine fx
	CT: r/o or evaluate C-spine fx
	MR: Shows cord, disc herniation (on cord), posterior ligaments
		• **Complete:** no function below the injured level (spinal shock must be resolved to diagnose)
		• **Incomplete:** partial sparing of distal function
		  ◦ **Central:** central gray matter
		  ◦ **Anterior:** Spinothalamic & corticospinal tracts out, posterior columns spared
		  ◦ **Brown-Sequard:** lateral half of spinal cord ("hemisection")
		  ◦ **Posterior:** posterior columns
			• Methylprednisolone IV given within 8hr of injury may improve functional level
			• Most patients recover 1 (or 2) levels of function in complete injuries
			• Decompression of cord (reduce dislocations or remove bone fragments) with internal or external (e.g., collar or halo) immobilization

COMPLICATIONS: Neurologic; autonomic dysreflexia (treat with urinary catheter/rectal disimpaction); spinal instability.			
• Spinal shock: Paralysis/areflexia from physiologic cord injury. Return of bulbocavernosus reflex is end of spinal shock. • Neurogenic shock: Hypotension with bradycardia. Decreased sympathetic (unopposed vagal) tone. Treat with vasopressors. • Hypovolemic shock: Hypotension with tachycardia. Treat with fluid/volume resuscitation.			

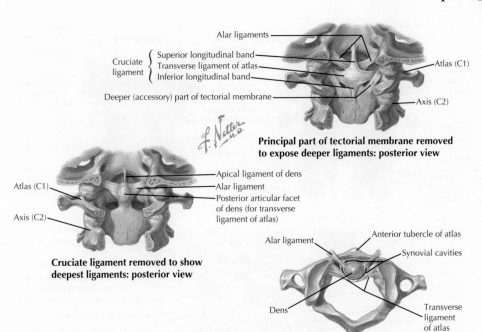

Alar ligaments

Cruciate ligament {
Superior longitudinal band
Transverse ligament of atlas
Inferior longitudinal band
}

Deeper (accessory) part of tectorial membrane

Atlas (C1)

Axis (C2)

Principal part of tectorial membrane removed to expose deeper ligaments: posterior view

Atlas (C1)

Axis (C2)

Apical ligament of dens
Alar ligament
Posterior articular facet of dens (for transverse ligament of atlas)

Cruciate ligament removed to show deepest ligaments: posterior view

Alar ligament

Anterior tubercle of atlas
Synovial cavities

Dens

Transverse ligament of atlas

Median atlantoaxial joint: superior view

LIGAMENT	ATTACHMENTS	COMMENTS
OCCIPITOATLANTAL JOINT		
• Articulation between convex occipital condyles and concave superior facets of atlas (C1). This articulation is horizontal (especially in pediatrics) allowing for rotation, but is inherently horizontally unstable. ROM: flexion/extension 25°; lateral bending 5° (each side); rotation 5° (each side).		
Capsule	Surrounds joints (condyle & facet)	Loose tissue provides minimal stability
Ant. atlantooccipital	Ant. atlas arch to ant. foramen mag.	Continuation of ALL
Tectorial membrane	Post. axis to ant. foramen magnum	Primary stabilizer. Continuation of PLL, limits extension
Post. atlantooccipital	Post. arch to post. foramen magnum	Homologous to ligamentum flavum
ATLANTOAXIAL JOINT (C1-2)		
• Made up of 3 articulations: Central (median) atlantoaxial joint (pivot type): between the odontoid and anterior arch. Lateral atlantoaxial joints [2] (plane type): between the articulating facets of atlas and axis, allow for rotation. ROM: flex/extend 20°; lateral bending 5° (each side); rotation 40° (each side). Supplies 50% of cervical rotation.		
Capsule	Surrounds lateral facet joints	Loose capsule allows for rotation
Cruciate **Transverse atlantal** (TAL) Superior longitudinal Inferior longitudinal	Posterior odontoid to anterior arch Odontoid to ant. foramen magnum Odontoid to body of axis	Has 3 components, is anterior to tectorial membrane Strongest ligament, holds odontoid to atlas. ADI <3mm. Injury results in C1-2 instability. Posterior to apical ligament, secondary stabilizer. Secondary stabilizer
Alar	Odontoid to occipital condyles	Strong, stabilizing ligaments, limit rotation & lateral bending. Injury results in C1-2 instability.
Apical	Odontoid to ant. foramen magnum	Thin ligament provides minimal stability
Accessory	Axis body to occipital condyles	Secondary stabilizers

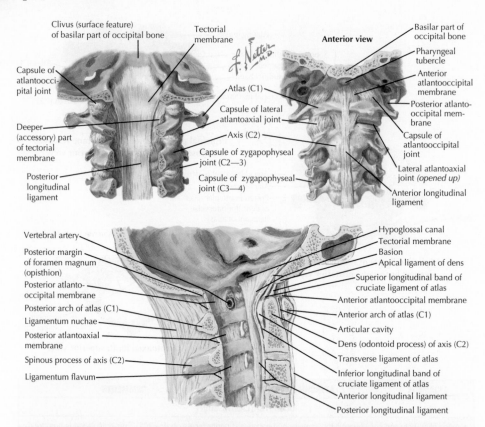

LIGAMENT	ATTACHMENTS	COMMENTS
INTERVERTEBRAL ARTICULATION		
Adjacent vertebrae are joined by a complex of smaller joints/articulations, ligaments, muscles, & connecting structures. • An intervertebral disc lies between the vertebral bodies (except b/w C1-2 and b/w the fused sacral segments). • Paired facet (apophyseal) joints connect the posterior elements. Their orientation dictates that intervertebral motion. • Uncovertebral joints (of Luschka) add stability between vertebral bodies in the cervical spine.		
Intervertebral disc	To adjacent vertebral bodies	Annulus gives strong connection b/w adjacent bodies
Anterior longitudinal ligament (ALL)	Adjacent anterior vertebral bodies and discs	Strong, thick ligament. Resists hyperextension.
Posterior longitudinal ligament (PLL)	Adjacent posterior vertebral bodies & discs (full length of spine)	Weak, limits hyperflexion. Disc herniates around ligament. Tectorial membrane is the superior continuation.
Ligamentum flavum	Anterior lamina (superior vert.) to posterior lamina (inferior vert.)	Strong, yellow, not a long continuous structure. Hypertrophy may contribute to nerve root impingement.
Ligamentum nuchae	Occipital protuberance to C1 post. arch & C2-C6 spinous processes	Continuation of supraspinous ligament
Supraspinous	Dorsal spinous processes to C7	Strong. Ligamentum nuchae is its superior continuation.
Interspinous	Between spinous processes	Weak. Torn in ligamentous flexion-distraction injuries.
Intertransverse	Between transverse processes	Weak ligament, adds little support.
Iliolumbar	L5 transverse process to ilium	May avulse in pelvic fracture (e.g., vertical shear fx).

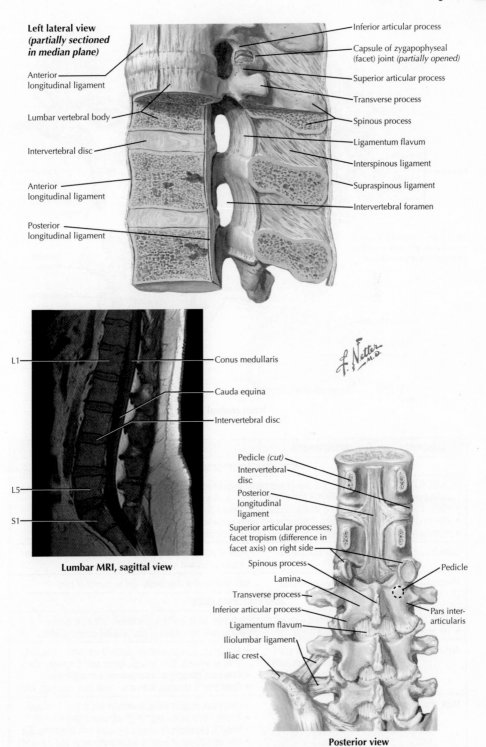

Left lateral view (partially sectioned in median plane)

Anterior longitudinal ligament

Lumbar vertebral body

Intervertebral disc

Anterior longitudinal ligament

Posterior longitudinal ligament

Inferior articular process

Capsule of zygapophyseal (facet) joint *(partially opened)*

Superior articular process

Transverse process

Spinous process

Ligamentum flavum

Interspinous ligament

Supraspinous ligament

Intervertebral foramen

L1

L5

S1

Conus medullaris

Cauda equina

Intervertebral disc

Lumbar MRI, sagittal view

Pedicle *(cut)*
Intervertebral disc
Posterior longitudinal ligament
Superior articular processes; facet tropism (difference in facet axis) on right side
Spinous process
Lamina
Transverse process
Inferior articular process
Ligamentum flavum
Iliolumbar ligament
Iliac crest

Pedicle

Pars inter-articularis

Posterior view

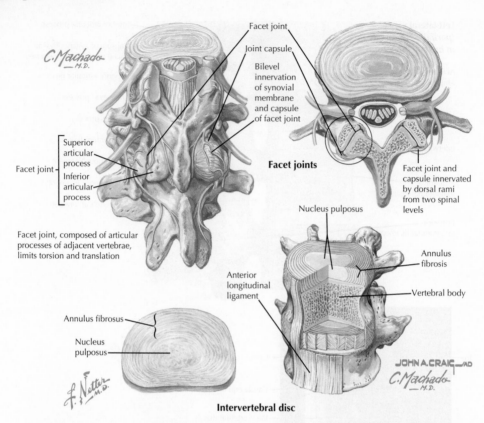

Facet joint

Joint capsule

Bilevel innervation of synovial membrane and capsule of facet joint

Superior articular process

Facet joint — Inferior articular process

Facet joint, composed of articular processes of adjacent vertebrae, limits torsion and translation

Facet joints

Facet joint and capsule innervated by dorsal rami from two spinal levels

Nucleus pulposus

Annulus fibrosis

Anterior longitudinal ligament

Vertebral body

Annulus fibrosus

Nucleus pulposus

Intervertebral disc

LIGAMENT	ATTACHMENTS	COMMENTS
FACET ([ZYG]APOPHYSEAL) JOINT		
Paired (L & R) articulations between the inferior & superior articular processes of adjacent vertebrae. • Orientation changes from semi-coronal (cervical) to sagittal (lumbar) and allows/dictates motion of that segment. • Inferior articular process is anterior & inferior (C-spine) and anterior & lateral (L-spine) to the superior articular process. • Joint innervation is from dorsal rami of two adjacent nerve root levels. • Hypertrophic changes in degenerative disease can cause/contribute to nerve root impingement.		
Capsule	Surrounds the articular processes	Weak structure, adds little support. May hypertrophy in degenerative joints and narrow neural foramen.
Meniscus/disc	Within joint b/w processes	Can be injured or degenerate and be source of pain
INTERVERTEBRAL DISCS		
Stabilize and maintain spine by anchoring adjacent vertebral bodies. Allow flexibility and absorb/distribute energy. • The discs make up 25% of the spine height. Disc degeneration with age results in loss of spinal column height.		
Annulus fibrosus	Strong attachments to end plates of adjacent vertebral bodies (via "outer annulus")	• Two layers: 1. outer annulus: dense fibers (type 1 collagen); 2. inner annulus: fibrocartilage, looser type 2 collagen fibers • Fibers are obliquely oriented and resist tensile loads • Outer layer innervated, tears can cause back pain (esp. LBP)
Nucleus pulposus	Contained within the annulus	• Gelatinous mass of water, proteoglycans, & type 2 collagen • Resists compressive loads (highest when sitting forward) • Water & proteoglycan content decrease with advancing age • Can herniate out of annulus & compress nerve root (L4-5 #1)

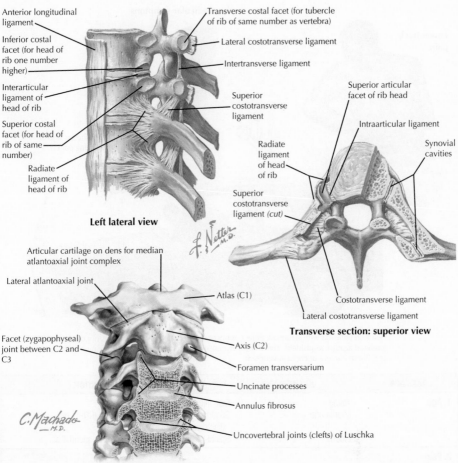

Anterior longitudinal ligament

Inferior costal facet (for head of rib one number higher)

Interarticular ligament of head of rib

Superior costal facet (for head of rib of same number)

Radiate ligament of head of rib

Transverse costal facet (for tubercle of rib of same number as vertebra)

Lateral costotransverse ligament

Intertransverse ligament

Superior costotransverse ligament

Radiate ligament of head of rib

Superior costotransverse ligament *(cut)*

Superior articular facet of rib head

Intraarticular ligament

Synovial cavities

Left lateral view

Articular cartilage on dens for median atlantoaxial joint complex

Lateral atlantoaxial joint

Facet (zygapophyseal) joint between C2 and C3

Atlas (C1)

Axis (C2)

Foramen transversarium

Uncinate processes

Annulus fibrosus

Uncovertebral joints (clefts) of Luschka

Costotransverse ligament

Lateral costotransverse ligament

Transverse section: superior view

LIGAMENT	ATTACHMENTS	COMMENTS
UNCOVERTEBRAL JOINTS		
• "Joints of Luschka": articulation in cervical spine b/w the uncinate process on the concave superior end plates of the inferior vertebral body & the articulating portion of the convex inferior end plate of the superior adjacent vertebral body. • Articular cartilage at this joint can degenerate and contribute to cervical spondylosis.		
COSTOVERTEBRAL JOINTS		
Articulation between the head of the rib and the thoracic vertebra (body and transverse process)		
Capsule	Surround head of rib/joint	Weak support of joint
Intraarticular	Head of rib to body/disc	Deep to radiate
Radiate	Head of rib to bodies & disc	Fan shaped, reinforces joint anteriorly
Costotransverse	Transverse process to rib	Superior costotransverse attaches to TP of superior vertebrae
OTHER		
Neural foramen: Boundaries: *superior & inferior:* pedicles; *anterior:* body & disc (uncinate process in C-spine); *posterior:* facet joint & capsule. Osteophytes, discs, facet hypertrophy, and ligamentum flavum can all narow foramen.		

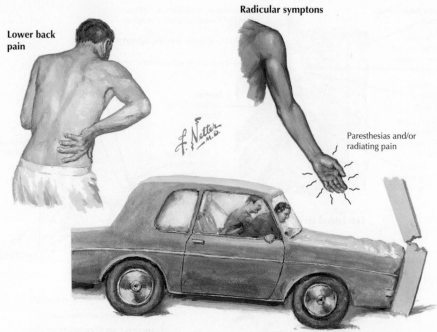

Head-on collision with stationary object or oncoming vehicle may, if seat belts not used, drive forehead against windshield. This sharply hyperextends neck, resulting in dislocation with or without fracture of cervical vertebrae

QUESTION	ANSWER	CLINICAL APPLICATION
1. Age	Young	Disc injuries, spondylolisthesis
	Middle age	Sprain/strain, nucleus pulposis/disc (HNP), degenerative disc disease (DDD)
	Elderly	Spinal stenosis, herniated disc, DDD, spondylosis
2. Pain **a. Character**	Radiating (shooting)	Radiculopathy (herniated nucleus pulposis [HNP])
	Diffuse, dull, non radiating	Cervical or lumbar strain
b. Location	Unilateral vs bilateral	Unilateral: herniated nucleus pulposis; Bilateral: systemic or metabolic disease, space-occupying lesion
	Neck	Cervical spondylosis, neck sprain or muscle strain
	Arms (+/− radiating)	Cervical spondylosis (+/− myelopathy), HNP
	Lower back	DDD, back sprain/muscle strain, spondylolisthesis
	Legs (+/− radiating)	Herniated nucleus pulposis, spinal stenosis
c. Occurrence	Night pain	Infection, tumor
	With activity	Usually mechanical etiology
d. Alleviating	Arms elevated	Herniated cervical disc (HNP)
	Sit down	Spinal stenosis (stenosis relieved)
e. Exacerbating	Back extension	Spinal stenosis (going down stairs), DJD/facet hypertrophy
3. Trauma	MVA (seatbelt?)	Cervical strain (whiplash), cervical fractures, ligamentous injury
4. Activity	Sports (stretching injury)	"Burners/stingers"(esp. in football), fractures
5. Neurologic symptoms	Pain, numbness, tingling	Radiculopathy, neuropathy, cauda equina syndrome
	Spasticity, clumsiness	Myelopathy
	Bowel/bladder symptoms	Cauda equina syndrome
6. Systemic complaints	Fever, weight loss, night sweats	Infection, tumor

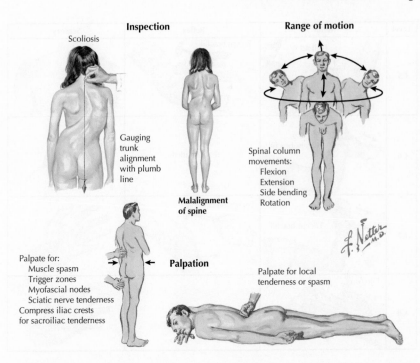

Inspection

Scoliosis

Gauging
trunk
alignment
with plumb
line

**Malalignment
of spine**

Range of motion

Spinal column
movements:
　Flexion
　Extension
　Side bending
　Rotation

Palpate for:
　Muscle spasm
　Trigger zones
　Myofascial nodes
　Sciatic nerve tenderness
Compress iliac crests
for sacroiliac tenderness

Palpation

Palpate for local
tenderness or spasm

EXAM	TECHNIQUE	CLINICAL APPLICATION
INSPECTION		
Gait	Leaning forward Wide-based	Spinal stenosis Myelopathy
Alignment	Malalignment	Dislocation, scoliosis, lordosis, kyphosis
Posture	Head tilted Pelvis tilted	Dislocation, spasm, spondylosis, torticollis Loss of lordosis: spasm
Skin	Disrobe patient	Cafe-au-lait spots, growths: possibly neurofibromatosis Port wine spots, soft masses: possibly spina bifida
PALPATION		
Bony structures	Spinous processes	Focal/point tenderness: fracture; step-off: dislocation/ spondylolisthesis
Soft tissues	Cervical facet joints Coccyx, via rectal exam Paraspinal muscles	Tenderness: osteoarthritis, dislocation Tenderness: fracture or contusion Diffuse tenderness: sprain/muscle strain; trigger point: spasm
RANGE OF MOTION		
Flexion/extension: cervical Flexion/extension: lumbar	Chin to chest/occiput back Touch toes with legs straight	Normal: Flexion: chin within 3-4cm of chest; ext. 70° Normal: 45-60° in flexion, 20-30° in extension
Lateral flexion: cervical Lateral flexion: lumbar	Ear to shoulder Bend to each side	Normal: 30-40° in each direction Normal: 10-20° in each direction
Rotation: cervical Rotation: lumbar	Stabilize shoulders: rotate Stabilize hip: rotate	Normal: 75° in each direction Normal: 5-15° in each direction

Level	Motor	Reflex	Sensory
C5	Deltoid	Biceps brachii	
C6	Biceps brachii	Brachioradialis	
C7	Triceps brachii	Triceps brachii	
C8	Interossei	None	

EXAM	TECHNIQUE	CLINICAL APPLICATION
		NEUROVASCULAR
		Cervical
		Sensory
C5	Lateral shoulder	Deficit indicates a corresponding cervical root compression/lesion
C6	Thumb	Deficit indicates a corresponding cervical root compression/lesion
C7	Middle finger	Deficit indicates a corresponding cervical root compression/lesion
C8	Ring & small fingers	Deficit indicates a corresponding cervical root compression/lesion
T1	Ulnar forearm & hand	Deficit indicates a corresponding cervical root compression/lesion
		Motor
C5	Deltoid: resisted abduction	Weakness indicates corresponding cervical root compression/lesion
C6	Biceps: resisted elbow flexion	Weakness indicates corresponding cervical root compression/lesion
C7	Triceps: resisted elbow ext.	Weakness indicates corresponding cervical root compression/lesion
C8	Intrinsics: resisted finger	Weakness indicates corresponding cervical root compression/lesion
T1	abduction	Weakness indicates corresponding cervical root compression/lesion
		Reflexes
C5	Biceps	Hypoactive/absent indicates C5 radiculopathy
C6	Brachioradialis (BR)	Hypoactive/absent indicates C6 radiculopathy
C7	Triceps	Hypoactive/absent indicates C7 radiculopathy
Inverted radial	Tap BR tendon in distal forearm	Hypoactive brachioradialis & hyperactive finger flexion: myelopathy
Hoffman's	Flick MF DIPJ into flexion	Pathologic if thumb IPJ flexes: myelopathy
		Pulses
	Brachial, radial, ulnar	Diminished/absent = vascular injury or compromise

Level	Motor	Reflex	Sensory
L4	Quadriceps / Tibialis anterior / L4	Patella tendon ("knee jerk")	Medial calf/ankle
L5	Extensor hallucis longus	None	Dorsal foot and 1st web space
S1	S1 / Gastroc-nemius	Achilles tendon ("ankle jerk")	Plantar and lateral foot

EXAM	TECHNIQUE	CLINICAL APPLICATION
NEUROVASCULAR		
Lumbar		
Sensory		
L3	Anterior & medial thigh	Deficit indicates corresponding lumbar root compression/lesion
L4	Medial leg & ankle	Deficit indicates corresponding lumbar root compression/lesion
L5	Dorsal foot & 1st web space	Deficit indicates corresponding lumbar root compression/lesion
S1	Lateral & plantar foot	Deficit indicates corresponding lumbar root compression/lesion
S2-4	Perianal sensation	Deficit indicates corresponding lumbar root compression/lesion
Motor		
L3-4	Quadriceps: knee extension	Weakness indicates corresponding lumbar root compression/lesion
L4	Tibialis anterior: ankle DF	Weakness indicates corresponding lumbar root compression/lesion
L5	Extensor hallucis longus: toe DF	Weakness indicates corresponding lumbar root compression/lesion
S1	Gastrocnemius: ankle PF	Weakness indicates corresponding lumbar root compression/lesion
S2-4	Anal sphincter: anal squeeze	Weakness indicates corresponding lumbar root compression/lesion
Reflexes		
L4	Patellar tendon ("knee jerk")	Hypoactive/absent indicates L4 radiculopathy
S1	Achilles tendon ("ankle jerk")	Hypoactive/absent indicates S1 radiculopathy
S2-3	Bulbocavernosus	Hypoactive/absent indicates S2-3 radiculopathy or spinal shock
Babinski	Run stick along plantar foot	Upgoing great toe: upper motor neuron/myelopathy
Ankle clonus	Rapidly flex & extend ankle	Multiple beats of clonus: upper motor neuron/myelopathy
Pulses		
	Posterior tibial, dorsalis pedis	Diminished/absent = vascular injury or compromise

Forward bending test

Estimation of rib hump and evaluation of curve unwinding as patient turns trunk from side to side

Spurling maneuver

Hyperextension and flexion of neck ipsilateral to the side of lesion cause radicular pain in neck and down the affected arm

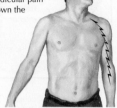

Straight leg test

Passively flex hip. Stop when pain occurs. Lower leg until pain resolves, then dorsiflex foot.

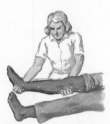

Extend knee, hip relaxed

EXAM	TECHNIQUE	CLINICAL APPLICATION
SPECIAL TESTS		
Cervical		
Spurling	Axial load, then laterally flex & rotate neck	Radiating pain indicates nerve root compression
Distraction	Upward distracting force	Relief of symptoms indicates foraminal compression of nerve root
Kernig	Supine: flex neck	Pain in or radiating to legs indicates meningeal irritation/infection
Brudzinski	Supine: flex neck, hip flex	Pain reduction with knee flexion indicates meningeal irritation
Lumbar		
Straight leg	Flex hip to pain, dorsiflex foot	Symptoms reproduced (pain radiating below knee) indicative of radiculopathy
Straight leg 90/90	Supine: flex hip & knee 90°, extend knee	>20° of flexion = tight hamstrings: source of pain
Bowstring	Raise leg, flex knee, popliteal press	Radicular pain with popliteal pressure indicates sciatic nerve cause
Sitting root (flip sign)	Seated: distract patient, passively extend knee	Patient with sciatic pain will arch/flip backward when knee extended
Forward bending	Standing, bend at waist	Asymmetry of back (scapula/ribs) is indicative of scoliosis
Hoover	Supine: hands under heels, patient then raises one leg	Pressure should be felt under opposite heel. No pressure indicates lack of effort, not true weakness
Waddell signs	Presence indicates nonorganic pathology: 1. Exaggerated response/overreaction, 2. Pain to light touch, 3. Nonanatomic pain localization, 4. Negative flip sign with positive straight leg test	

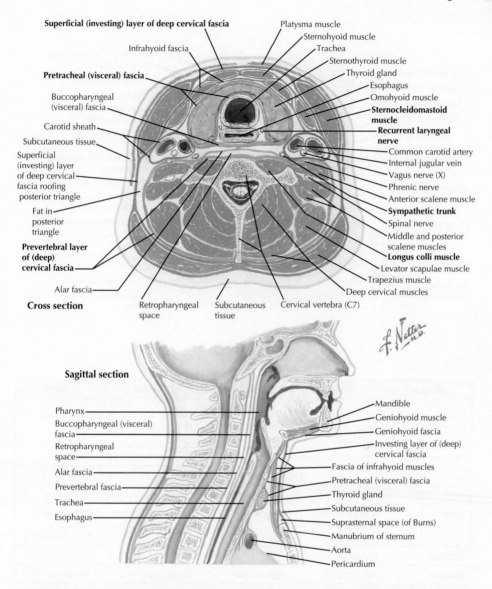

Superficial (investing) layer of deep cervical fascia
Infrahyoid fascia
Pretracheal (visceral) fascia
Buccopharyngeal (visceral) fascia
Carotid sheath
Subcutaneous tissue
Superficial (investing) layer of deep cervical fascia roofing posterior triangle
Fat in posterior triangle
Prevertebral layer of (deep) cervical fascia
Alar fascia
Cross section

Platysma muscle
Sternohyoid muscle
Trachea
Sternothyroid muscle
Thyroid gland
Esophagus
Omohyoid muscle
Sternocleidomastoid muscle
Recurrent laryngeal nerve
Common carotid artery
Internal jugular vein
Vagus nerve (X)
Phrenic nerve
Anterior scalene muscle
Sympathetic trunk
Spinal nerve
Middle and posterior scalene muscles
Longus colli muscle
Levator scapulae muscle
Trapezius muscle
Deep cervical muscles
Cervical vertebra (C7)

Retropharyngeal space
Subcutaneous tissue

Sagittal section

Pharynx
Buccopharyngeal (visceral) fascia
Retropharyngeal space
Alar fascia
Prevertebral fascia
Trachea
Esophagus

Mandible
Geniohyoid muscle
Geniohyoid fascia
Investing layer of (deep) cervical fascia
Fascia of infrahyoid muscles
Pretracheal (visceral) fascia
Thyroid gland
Subcutaneous tissue
Suprasternal space (of Burns)
Manubrium of sternum
Aorta
Pericardium

LAYER	CONTENTS	COMMENT
FASCIA LAYERS		
Platysma	Thin superficial muscle	Highly vascular, must be split to access cervical spine
Deep cervical fascia	Invests sternocleidomastoid	Incised in anterior cervical approach
Pretracheal fascia	Invests thyroid, trachea	Incised off of carotid sheath to access cervical spine
Carotid sheath	Carotid artery, internal jugular vein, vagus nerve (CN 10)	Left intact and used to retract structures laterally unless access to contents of sheath is needed
Prevertebral fascia	Covers A.L.L. & longus colli	Deepest fascial layer, incised to access vertebral body and disc

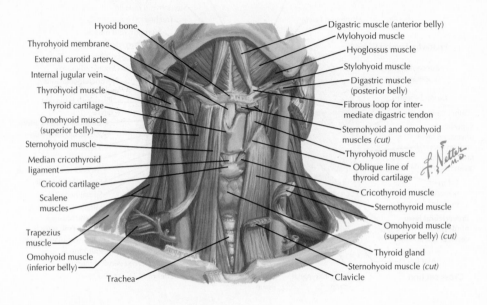

Hyoid bone
Thyrohyoid membrane
External carotid artery
Internal jugular vein
Thyrohyoid muscle
Thyroid cartilage
Omohyoid muscle (superior belly)
Sternohyoid muscle
Median cricothyroid ligament
Cricoid cartilage
Scalene muscles
Trapezius muscle
Omohyoid muscle (inferior belly)
Trachea

Digastric muscle (anterior belly)
Mylohyoid muscle
Hyoglossus muscle
Stylohyoid muscle
Digastric muscle (posterior belly)
Fibrous loop for intermediate digastric tendon
Sternohyoid and omohyoid muscles (cut)
Thyrohyoid muscle
Oblique line of thyroid cartilage
Cricothyroid muscle
Sternothyroid muscle
Omohyoid muscle (superior belly) (cut)
Thyroid gland
Sternohyoid muscle (cut)
Clavicle

MUSCLE	ORIGIN	INSERTION	ACTION	NERVE
ANTERIOR NECK				
Platysma	Fascia: deltoid/pectoralis major	Mandible; skin	Depress jaw	CN 7
Sternocleidomastoid	Manubrium & clavicle	Mastoid process	Turn head opposite side	CN 11
ANTERIOR CERVICAL TRIANGLE				
Suprahyoid Muscles				
Digastric	Anterior: mandible Posterior: mastoid notch	Hyoid body	Elevate hyoid, depress mandible	Anterior: mylohyoid (CN 5) Post: facial (CN 7)
Mylohyoid	Mandible	Raphe on hyoid	Same as above	Mylohyoid (CN 5)
Stylohyoid	Styloid process	Body of hyoid	Elevate hyoid	Facial nerve (CN 7)
Geniohyoid	Genial tubercle of mandible	Body of hyoid	Elevate hyoid	C1 via CN 12
Infrahyoid Muscles				
Superficial				
Sternohyoid	Manubrium & clavicle	Body of hyoid	Depress hyoid	Ansa cervicalis
Omohyoid	Suprascapular notch	Body of hyoid	Depress hyoid	Ansa cervicalis
Deep				
Thyrohyoid	Thyroid cartilage	Greater horn of hyoid	Depress hyoid/larynx	C1 via CN 12
Sternothyroid	Manubrium	Thyroid cartilage	Depress/retract hyoid/larynx	Ansa cervicalis (C1-3)

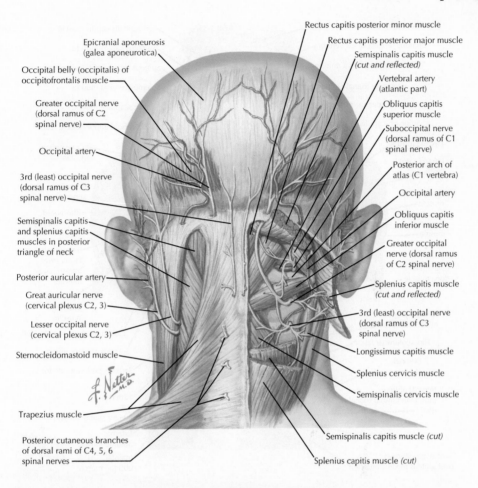

Rectus capitis posterior minor muscle

Rectus capitis posterior major muscle

Semispinalis capitis muscle *(cut and reflected)*

Vertebral artery (atlantic part)

Obliquus capitis superior muscle

Suboccipital nerve (dorsal ramus of C1 spinal nerve)

Posterior arch of atlas (C1 vertebra)

Occipital artery

Obliquus capitis inferior muscle

Greater occipital nerve (dorsal ramus of C2 spinal nerve)

Splenius capitis muscle *(cut and reflected)*

3rd (least) occipital nerve (dorsal ramus of C3 spinal nerve)

Longissimus capitis muscle

Splenius cervicis muscle

Semispinalis cervicis muscle

Semispinalis capitis muscle *(cut)*

Splenius capitis muscle *(cut)*

Epicranial aponeurosis (galea aponeurotica)

Occipital belly (occipitalis) of occipitofrontalis muscle

Greater occipital nerve (dorsal ramus of C2 spinal nerve)

Occipital artery

3rd (least) occipital nerve (dorsal ramus of C3 spinal nerve)

Semispinalis capitis and splenius capitis muscles in posterior triangle of neck

Posterior auricular artery

Great auricular nerve (cervical plexus C2, 3)

Lesser occipital nerve (cervical plexus C2, 3)

Sternocleidomastoid muscle

Trapezius muscle

Posterior cutaneous branches of dorsal rami of C4, 5, 6 spinal nerves

F. Netter M.D.

MUSCLE	ORIGIN	INSERTION	ACTION	NERVE
POSTERIOR NECK				
Scalene muscles				
Anterior	C3-6 transverse process	1st rib	Laterally flexes neck and elevates 1st or 2nd rib	C5-C8 nerve roots
Middle	C2-7 transverse process	1st rib		
Posterior	C4-6 transverse process	2nd rib		
Suboccipital Triangle				
Rectus capitis posterior major	Spine of axis	Inferior nuchal line	Extend, rotate, laterally flex head	Suboccipital nerve
Rectus capitis posterior minor	Posterior tubercle of atlas	Occipital bone	Extend, laterally flex	Suboccipital nerve
Obliquus capitis superior	Atlas transverse process	Occipital bone	Extend, rotate, laterally flex	Suboccipital nerve
Obliquus capitis inferior	Spine of axis	Atlas transverse process	Extend, laterally rotate	Suboccipital nerve
Semispinalis, see page 58; Splenius, see page 57.				

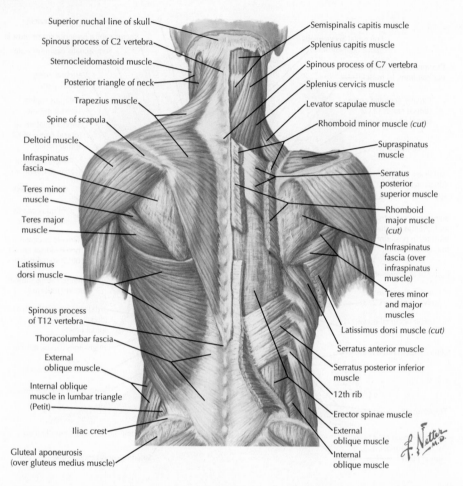

MUSCLE	ORIGIN	INSERTION	ACTION	NERVE
SUPERFICIAL (EXTRINSIC)				
Trapezius	Spinous process C7-T12	Clavicle; scapula (spine, acromion)	Rotate scapula	CN 11
Latissimus dorsi	Spinous process T6-S5	Humerus	Extend, adduct, IR arm	Thoracodorsal
Levator scapulae	Transverse process C1-4	Scapula (medial)	Elevate scapula	Dorsal scapular, C3, C4 (dorsal rami)
Rhomboid minor	Spinous process C7-T1	Scapula (spine)	Adduct scapula	Dorsal scapular
Rhomboid major	Spinous process T2-T5	Scapula (medial border)	Adduct scapula	Dorsal scapular
Serratus posterior superior	Spinous process C7-T3	Ribs 2-5 (upper border)	Elevate ribs	Intercostal n. (T1-4)
Serratus posterior inferior	Spinous process T11-L3	Ribs 9-12 (lower border)	Depress ribs	Intercostal n. (T9-12)

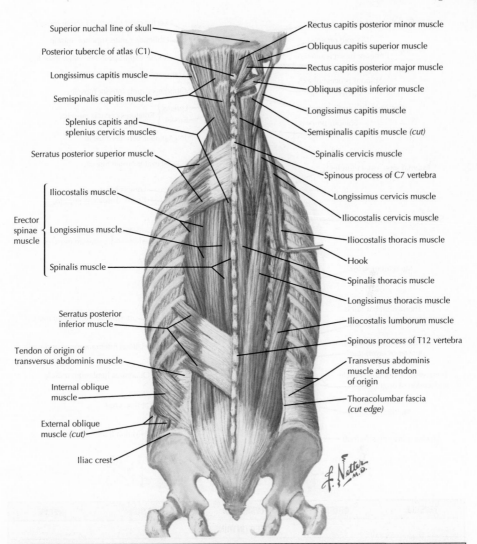

Superior nuchal line of skull

Posterior tubercle of atlas (C1)

Longissimus capitis muscle

Semispinalis capitis muscle

Splenius capitis and splenius cervicis muscles

Serratus posterior superior muscle

Erector spine muscle
- Iliocostalis muscle
- Longissimus muscle
- Spinalis muscle

Serratus posterior inferior muscle

Tendon of origin of transversus abdominis muscle

Internal oblique muscle

External oblique muscle (cut)

Iliac crest

Rectus capitis posterior minor muscle

Obliquus capitis superior muscle

Rectus capitis posterior major muscle

Obliquus capitis inferior muscle

Longissimus capitis muscle

Semispinalis capitis muscle (cut)

Spinalis cervicis muscle

Spinous process of C7 vertebra

Longissimus cervicis muscle

Iliocostalis cervicis muscle

Iliocostalis thoracis muscle

Hook

Spinalis thoracis muscle

Longissimus thoracis muscle

Iliocostalis lumborum muscle

Spinous process of T12 vertebra

Transversus abdominis muscle and tendon of origin

Thoracolumbar fascia (cut edge)

MUSCLE	ORIGIN	INSERTION	ACTION	NERVE
DEEP (INTRINSIC)				
Superficial Layer: Spinotransverse Group				
Splenius capitis Splenius cervicis	Ligamentum nuchae Spinous process T1-6	Mastoid & nuchal line Transverse process C1-4	Both: laterally flex & rotate neck to same side	Dorsal rami of inferior cervical nerves
Intermediate Layer: Sacrospinalis Group (Erector Spinae)				
Iliocostalis Longissimus Spinalis	Common origin: sacrum, iliac crest, and lumbar spinous process	Ribs T & C spinous process, mastoid process T-spine: spinous process	Laterally flex, extend, and rotate head (to same side) and vertebral column	Dorsal rami of spinal nerves
All have three parts: thoracis, cervicis, and capitus				

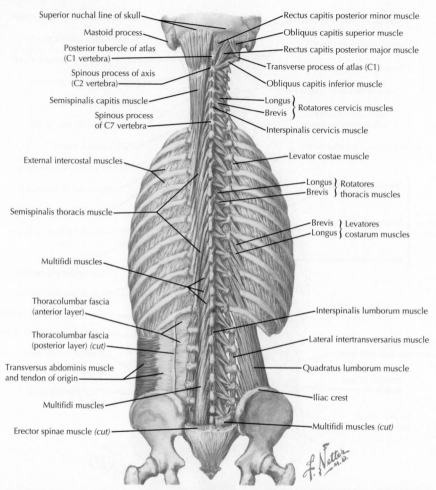

Superior nuchal line of skull
Mastoid process
Posterior tubercle of atlas (C1 vertebra)
Spinous process of axis (C2 vertebra)
Semispinalis capitis muscle
Spinous process of C7 vertebra
External intercostal muscles
Semispinalis thoracis muscle
Multifidi muscles
Thoracolumbar fascia (anterior layer)
Thoracolumbar fascia (posterior layer) *(cut)*
Transversus abdominis muscle and tendon of origin
Multifidi muscles
Erector spinae muscle *(cut)*

Rectus capitis posterior minor muscle
Obliquus capitis superior muscle
Rectus capitis posterior major muscle
Transverse process of atlas (C1)
Obliquus capitis inferior muscle
Longus / Brevis } Rotatores cervicis muscles
Interspinalis cervicis muscle
Levator costae muscle
Longus } Rotatores
Brevis } thoracis muscles
Brevis } Levatores
Longus } costarum muscles
Interspinalis lumborum muscle
Lateral intertransversarius muscle
Quadratus lumborum muscle
Iliac crest
Multifidi muscles *(cut)*

MUSCLE	ORIGIN	INSERTION	ACTION	NERVE
DEEP (INTRINSIC)				
Deep Layers: Transversospinalis Group				
Semispinalis capitus	Transverse process T1-6	Nuchal ridge	Extend head	Dorsal primary rami
Semispinalis (C&T)	Transverse process	Spinous process	Extend, rotate opposite side	Dorsal primary rami
Multifidus (C2-S4)	Transverse process	Spinous process	Flex laterally, rotate opposite	Dorsal primary rami
Rotatores	Transverse process	Spinous process +1	Rotate superior vertebrae opposite	Dorsal primary rami
Levator costarum	Transverse process	Brevis: rib −1 Longus: rib −2	Elevate rib during inspiration	Dorsal primary rami
Interspinales	Spinous process	Spinous process +1	Extend column	Dorsal primary rami
Intertransversarii	Tranverse process	Transverse process +1	Laterally flex column	Dorsal primary rami

Cervical Spine Injury: Incomplete Spinal Syndromes

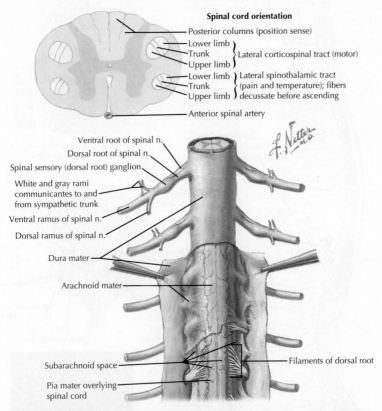

Spinal cord orientation

Posterior columns (position sense)

Lower limb
Trunk — Lateral corticospinal tract (motor)
Upper limb

Lower limb — Lateral spinothalamic tract
Trunk — (pain and temperature); fibers
Upper limb — decussate before ascending

Anterior spinal artery

Ventral root of spinal n.
Dorsal root of spinal n.
Spinal sensory (dorsal root) ganglion
White and gray rami communicantes to and from sympathetic trunk
Ventral ramus of spinal n.
Dorsal ramus of spinal n.
Dura mater
Arachnoid mater
Subarachnoid space — Filaments of dorsal root
Pia mater overlying spinal cord

TRACT	FUNCTION	COMMENT
SPINAL CORD		
• Runs from brain stem to conus medullaris (termination at L1) within the spinal canal where it is protected. • Terminale filum and cauda equina (lumbar and sacral nerve roots) continue in the spinal canal. • It has a layered covering (membranes): dura mater, arachnoid mater, pia mater. • It is made up of multiple ascending (sensory) and descending (motor) tracts and columns. • It is wider in the cervical and lumbar spines, where the roots form plexus to innervate the upper and lower extremities. • Paired (R & L) nerve roots emerge from each level. Nerve roots made up of ventral (motor) and dorsal (sensory) roots. • Injury can be either complete or incomplete (see page 42 for spinal cord injuries).		
Descending (Motor)		
Anterior corticospinal	Innervates motor neurons—voluntary motor	Minor motor pathway, injured in anterior cord syndrome
Lateral corticospinal	Innervates motor neurons—voluntary motor	Major motor pathway, injured in Brown-Sequard syndrome
Ascending (Sensory)		
Anterior spinothalamic	Light touch sensation	Injured in anterior cord syndrome
Lateral spinothalamic	Pain and temperature sensation	Injured in Brown-Sequard syndrome
Dorsal columns	Proprioception and vibratory sensation	Usually preserved, injured in posterior cord syndrome

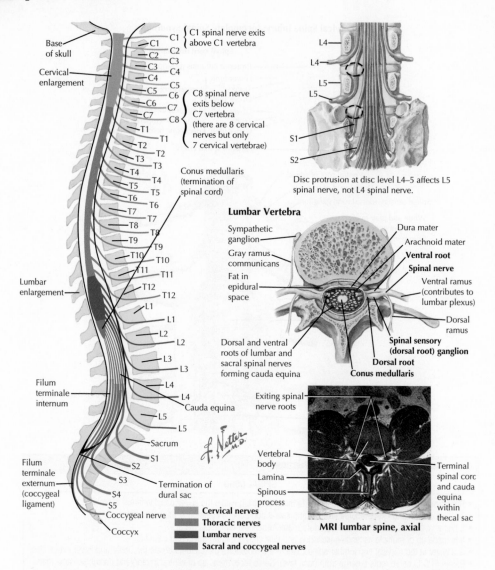

C1 spinal nerve exits above C1 vertebra

C8 spinal nerve exits below C7 vertebra (there are 8 cervical nerves but only 7 cervical vertebrae)

Base of skull

Cervical enlargement

Conus medullaris (termination of spinal cord)

Lumbar enlargement

Filum terminale internum

Filum terminale externum (coccygeal ligament)

Cauda equina

Termination of dural sac

Coccygeal nerve

Coccyx

Disc protrusion at disc level L4–5 affects L5 spinal nerve, not L4 spinal nerve.

Lumbar Vertebra

Sympathetic ganglion

Gray ramus communicans

Fat in epidural space

Dorsal and ventral roots of lumbar and sacral spinal nerves forming cauda equina

Dura mater

Arachnoid mater

Ventral root

Spinal nerve

Ventral ramus (contributes to lumbar plexus)

Dorsal ramus

Spinal sensory (dorsal root) ganglion

Dorsal root

Conus medullaris

Exiting spinal nerve roots

Vertebral body

Lamina

Spinous process

Terminal spinal cord and cauda equina within thecal sac

MRI lumbar spine, axial

Cervical nerves
Thoracic nerves
Lumbar nerves
Sacral and coccygeal nerves

SPINAL NERVES

- Spinal nerves are made up of a ventral (motor) root and a dorsal (sensory) root. There are 31 pairs (L & R).
- Cell bodies for sensory nerves are in dorsal root ganglia. Motor nerve cell bodies are in ventral horn of spinal cord.
- Roots exit spinal column via the intervertebral (neural) foramen (under pedicle); (C1-7 exit above their vertebrae, C8-L5 exit below their vertebrae [C7 exits above and C8 exits below C7 vertebra]).
- They can be compressed by herniated discs, osteophytes, and hypertrophied soft tissues (ligamentum flavum, facet capsule). In lumbar spine the traversing nerve is usually affected, and exiting root is not (except in far lateral compression).
- The lumbar and sacral nerves form the cauda equina ("horse's tail") in the spinal canal before exiting.
- Spinal nerve divides into dorsal and ventral rami. Dorsal rami innervate local structures (neck and back musculature, overlying skin, facet capsules, etc). Ventral rami contribute to plexus (e.g., cervical, brachial, lumbosacral) and become peripheral nerves to the extremities.
- Ventral rami of spinal nerve commonly referred to as a spinal "roots." The roots combine to form the various plexus.

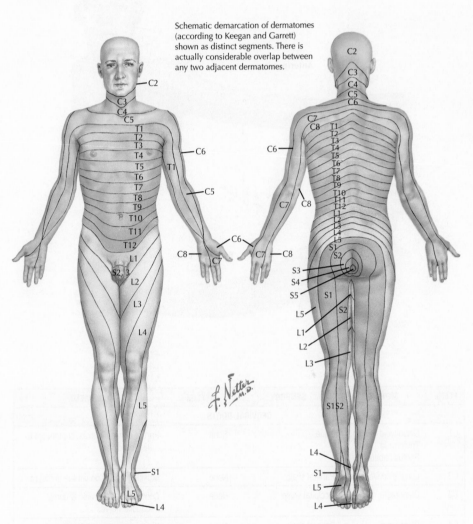

Schematic demarcation of dermatomes (according to Keegan and Garrett) shown as distinct segments. There is actually considerable overlap between any two adjacent dermatomes.

Levels of principal dermatomes

C5	Clavicles
C5, 6, 7	Lateral parts of upper limbs
C8, T1	Medial sides of upper limbs
C6	Thumb
C6, 7, 8	Hand
C8	Ring and little fingers
T4	Level of nipples

T10	Level of umbilicus
L1	Inguinal or groin regions
L1, 2, 3, 4	Anterior and inner surfaces of lower limbs
L4, 5, S1	Foot
L4	Medial side of great toe
S1, 2, L5	Posterior and outer surfaces of lower limbs
S1	Lateral margin of foot and little toe
S2, 3, 4	Perineum

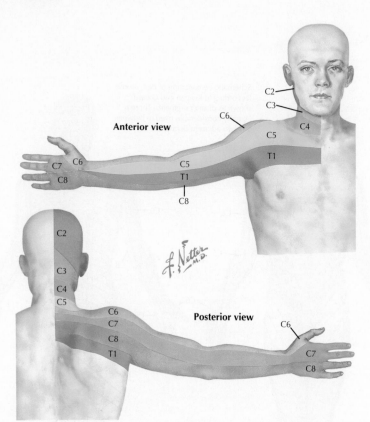

Anterior view

Posterior view

LEVEL	MOTOR	SENSORY	REFLEX	COMMENT
CERVICAL ROOTS				
C1	Geniohyoid Thyrohyoid Rectus capitus	None	None	Part of cervical plexus, contributes to ansa cervicalis
C2	Longus colli/capitis	Parietal scalp	None	Muscle innervation via the dorsal rami
C3	Diaphragm	Occipital scalp	None	Contributes to phrenic & dorsal scapular nerves
C4	Diaphragm	Base of neck	None	Branches to phrenic and dorsal scapular nerves & levator scapula muscle
C5	Deltoid	Lateral shoulder and arm	Biceps	Dorsal scapular n. branches from C5 root
C6	Biceps brachii ECRL, ECRB	Lateral forearm and thumb	Brachioradialis	Most commonly compressed cervical nerve root
C7	Triceps brachii FCR, FCU	Posterior forearm, central hand, and middle finger	Triceps	Exits above C7 vertebra
C8	FDS, FDP	Medial forearm, ulnar fingers	None	Exits below C7 vertebra
T1	Interosseous	Medial arm	None	Only thoracic root in brachial plexus

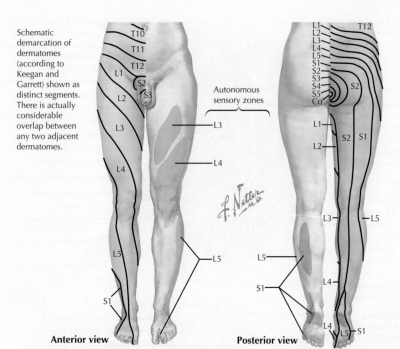

Schematic demarcation of dermatomes (according to Keegan and Garrett) shown as distinct segments. There is actually considerable overlap between any two adjacent dermatomes.

Autonomous sensory zones

Anterior view   **Posterior view**

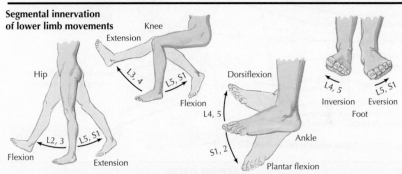

Segmental innervation of lower limb movements

LEVEL	MOTOR	SENSORY	REFLEX	COMMENT
LUMBOSACRAL ROOTS				
L1	Transversus abdominis Internal oblique	Inguinal region	None	Rarely injured nerve root
L2	Psoas	Upper thigh	None	Test with hip flexion
L3	Quadriceps	Anterior and medial thigh	None	L3 & L4 tested with quadriceps
L4	Tibialis anterior	Medial leg, ankle, foot	Patellar	Test with ankle dorsiflexion
L5	Extensor hallux longus	Dorsal/plantar foot, 1st web space, lateral leg	Hamstring	Most commonly compressed lumbar root; test with hallux dorsiflexion
S1	Gastrocnemius	Lateral foot, posterior leg	Achilles	Test with ankle plantar flexion/toe walking
S2-4	Sphincter	Perianal sensation	Anal wink	Test tone to evaluate for cauda equina syndrome

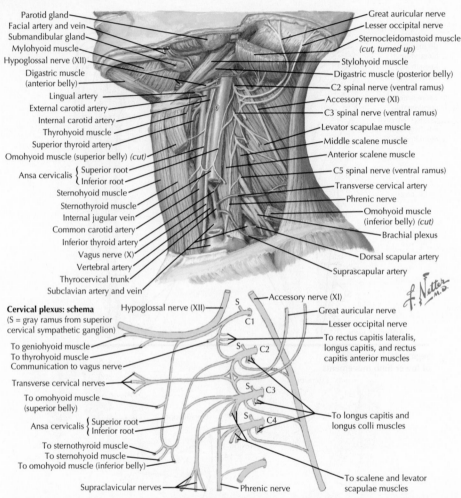

Parotid gland
Facial artery and vein
Submandibular gland
Mylohyoid muscle
Hypoglossal nerve (XII)
Digastric muscle (anterior belly)
Lingual artery
External carotid artery
Internal carotid artery
Thyrohyoid muscle
Superior thyroid artery
Omohyoid muscle (superior belly) *(cut)*
Ansa cervicalis { Superior root
Inferior root
Sternohyoid muscle
Sternothyroid muscle
Internal jugular vein
Common carotid artery
Inferior thyroid artery
Vagus nerve (X)
Vertebral artery
Thyrocervical trunk
Subclavian artery and vein

Great auricular nerve
Lesser occipital nerve
Sternocleidomastoid muscle *(cut, turned up)*
Stylohyoid muscle
Digastric muscle (posterior belly)
C2 spinal nerve (ventral ramus)
Accessory nerve (XI)
C3 spinal nerve (ventral ramus)
Levator scapulae muscle
Middle scalene muscle
Anterior scalene muscle
C5 spinal nerve (ventral ramus)
Transverse cervical artery
Phrenic nerve
Omohyoid muscle (inferior belly) *(cut)*
Brachial plexus
Dorsal scapular artery
Suprascapular artery

Cervical plexus: schema
(S = gray ramus from superior
cervical sympathetic ganglion)

Hypoglossal nerve (XII)

Accessory nerve (XI)
Great auricular nerve
Lesser occipital nerve

C1

To geniohyoid muscle
To thyrohyoid muscle
Communication to vagus nerve

C2

To rectus capitis lateralis,
longus capitis, and rectus
capitis anterior muscles

Transverse cervical nerves

C3

To omohyoid muscle
(superior belly)
Ansa cervicalis { Superior root
Inferior root

C4

To longus capitis and
longus colli muscles

To sternothyroid muscle
To sternohyoid muscle
To omohyoid muscle (inferior belly)

Supraclavicular nerves

Phrenic nerve

To scalene and levator
scapulae muscles

CERVICAL PLEXUS	
C1-C4 ventral rami (behind IJ and SCM)	
Lesser Occipital Nerve (C2-3): arises from posterior border of sternocleidomastoid	**Supraclavicular** (C3-4): splits into 3 branches: anterior, middle, posterior
Sensory: Superior region behind auricle *Motor:* None	*Sensory:* Over clavicle, outer trapezius and deltoid *Motor:* None
Great Auricular Nerve (C2-3): exits inferior to lesser occipital nerve, ascends on SCM	**Ansa Cervicalis** (C1-3): superior (C1-2) & inferior (C2-3) roots form loop
Sensory: Over parotid gland and behind ear *Motor:* None	*Sensory:* None *Motor:* Omohyoid Sternohyoid Sternothyroid
Tranverse Cervical Nerve (C2-3): exits inferior to greater auricular nerve, then to anterior neck	**Phrenic Nerve** (C3-5):On anterior scalene, into thorax between subclavian artery and vein
Sensory: Anterior triangle of the neck *Motor:* None	*Sensory:* Pericardium and mediastinal pleura *Motor:* Diaphragm

Right anterior dissection

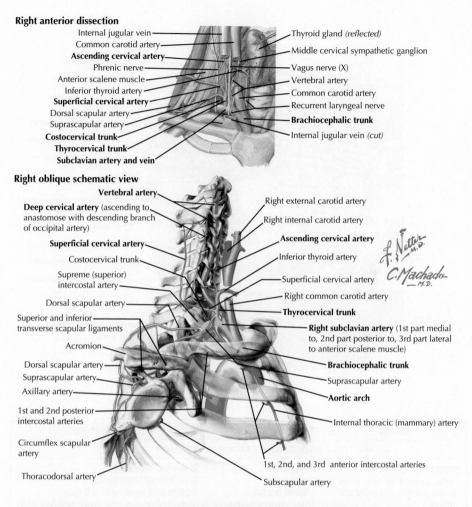

Right anterior dissection labels:
- Internal jugular vein
- Common carotid artery
- **Ascending cervical artery**
- Phrenic nerve
- Anterior scalene muscle
- Inferior thyroid artery
- **Superficial cervical artery**
- Dorsal scapular artery
- Suprascapular artery
- **Costocervical trunk**
- **Thyrocervical trunk**
- **Subclavian artery and vein**
- Thyroid gland *(reflected)*
- Middle cervical sympathetic ganglion
- Vagus nerve (X)
- Vertebral artery
- Common carotid artery
- Recurrent laryngeal nerve
- **Brachiocephalic trunk**
- Internal jugular vein *(cut)*

Right oblique schematic view

Right oblique schematic view labels:
- **Vertebral artery**
- **Deep cervical artery** (ascending to anastomose with descending branch of occipital artery)
- **Superficial cervical artery**
- Costocervical trunk
- Supreme (superior) intercostal artery
- Dorsal scapular artery
- Superior and inferior transverse scapular ligaments
- Acromion
- Dorsal scapular artery
- Suprascapular artery
- Axillary artery
- 1st and 2nd posterior intercostal arteries
- Circumflex scapular artery
- Thoracodorsal artery
- Right external carotid artery
- Right internal carotid artery
- **Ascending cervical artery**
- Inferior thyroid artery
- Superficial cervical artery
- Right common carotid artery
- **Thyrocervical trunk**
- **Right subclavian artery** (1st part medial to, 2nd part posterior to, 3rd part lateral to anterior scalene muscle)
- **Brachiocephalic trunk**
- Suprascapular artery
- **Aortic arch**
- Internal thoracic (mammary) artery
- 1st, 2nd, and 3rd anterior intercostal arteries
- Subscapular artery

COURSE	BRANCHES	COMMENT/SUPPLY
SUBCLAVIAN ARTERY		

Branches off aorta (L) or brachiocephalic trunk (R) b/w anterior and middle scalene muscles	**Vertebral arteries** (R & L)
	Thyrocervical trunk
	  Ascending cervical
	  Superficial cervical
	  Deep cervical
		Main arterial supply to the cervical spine and cord
		Has 4 primary branches
		Runs with phrenic nerve on anterior scalene muscles
		Crosses posterior triangle of neck (scalenes, etc)
		Off costocervical trunk, anastomoses w/ occipital artery

VERTEBRAL ARTERY		
Enters foramen transversarium from C6 through C1 then runs in a groove on the atlas, then to brain stem to form basilar artery	**Anterior spinal artery** **Posterior spinal arteries** Anterior ascending Posterior ascending Ant. segmental medullary Post. segmental medullary	Single midline artery supplies anterior ⅔ of spinal cord 2 paired arteries supply posterior ⅓ of spinal cord Give primary supply to odontoid Give primary supply to odontoid Contribute to anterior spinal artery Contribute to posterior spinal arteries
Injury or infarct of the anterior or posterior spinal arteries can result in an anterior/central or posterior cord syndrome.		

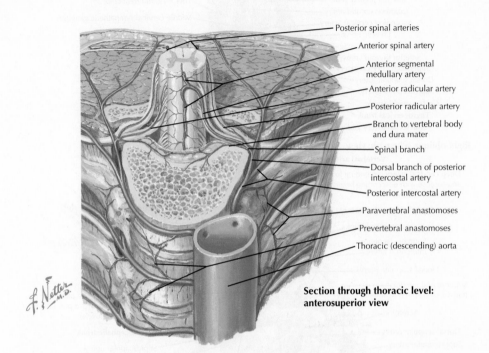

Posterior spinal arteries
Anterior spinal artery
Anterior segmental medullary artery
Anterior radicular artery
Posterior radicular artery
Branch to vertebral body and dura mater
Spinal branch
Dorsal branch of posterior intercostal artery
Posterior intercostal artery
Paravertebral anastomoses
Prevertebral anastomoses
Thoracic (descending) aorta

Section through thoracic level: anterosuperior view

COURSE	BRANCHES	COMMENT/SUPPLY
INTERCOSTAL(THORACIC)/LUMBAR ARTERY		
Paired arteries (R & L) branch off aorta, run posterior along vertebral bodies (between ribs in thoracic region)	Ventral branch	To vertebral bodies
	Dorsal branch	To posterior elements and cord
	Spinal branch	Supplies cord, nerve roots, and body
	Major anterior segmental medullary (radicular)	"Artery of Adamkiewicz"—single medullary artery (usually left T10-T12) to ant. spinal artery is primary supply to thoracolumbar cord. Injury can cause cord ischemia/paralysis.
SPINAL BRANCH		
Branches off dorsal branch and enters intervertebral foramen	**Anterior radicular**	Runs on ventral root, anastomoses with anterior spinal artery
	Posterior radicular	Runs on dorsal root, anastomoses with posterior spinal artery
	Postcentral branch	Supplies vertebral body and dura
	Prelaminar branch	Supplies lamina/posterior elements
ANTERIOR SPINAL		
Single midline artery supplies anterior ⅔ of spinal cord	Central (sulcal) branches	Supplies central cord region
	Pial arterial plexus	Supplies peripheral ⅔ of spinal cord
POSTERIOR SPINAL		
Paired (R & L) arteries supply posterior ⅓ of spinal cord		Supplied by posterior medullary/radicular arteries

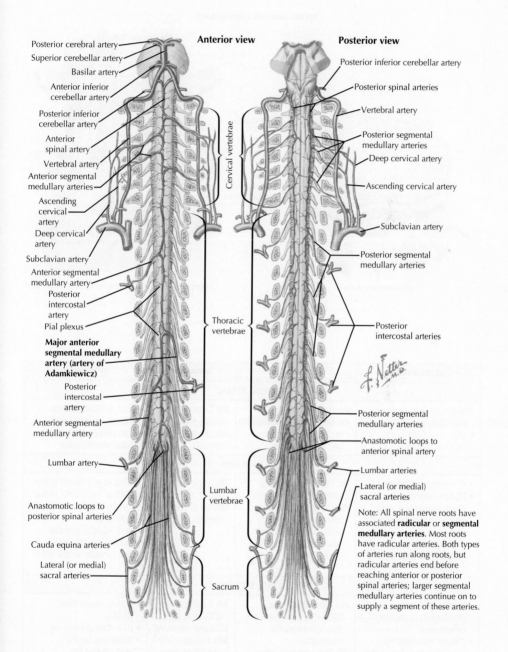

Anterior view

Posterior cerebral artery

Superior cerebellar artery

Basilar artery

Anterior inferior cerebellar artery

Posterior inferior cerebellar artery

Anterior spinal artery

Vertebral artery

Anterior segmental medullary arteries

Ascending cervical artery

Deep cervical artery

Subclavian artery

Anterior segmental medullary artery

Posterior intercostal artery

Pial plexus

Major anterior segmental medullary artery (artery of Adamkiewicz)

Posterior intercostal artery

Anterior segmental medullary artery

Lumbar artery

Anastomotic loops to posterior spinal arteries

Cauda equina arteries

Lateral (or medial) sacral arteries

Cervical vertebrae

Thoracic vertebrae

Lumbar vertebrae

Sacrum

Posterior view

Posterior inferior cerebellar artery

Posterior spinal arteries

Vertebral artery

Posterior segmental medullary arteries

Deep cervical artery

Ascending cervical artery

Subclavian artery

Posterior segmental medullary arteries

Posterior intercostal arteries

Posterior segmental medullary arteries

Anastomotic loops to anterior spinal artery

Lumbar arteries

Lateral (or medial) sacral arteries

Note: All spinal nerve roots have associated **radicular** or **segmental medullary arteries**. Most roots have radicular arteries. Both types of arteries run along roots, but radicular arteries end before reaching anterior or posterior spinal arteries; larger segmental medullary arteries continue on to supply a segment of these arteries.

Spinal stenosis: Laminectomy

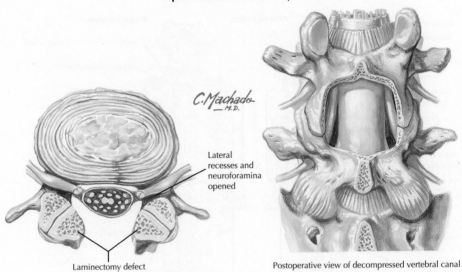

Lateral recesses and neuroforamina opened

Laminectomy defect

Postoperative view of decompressed vertebral canal

DESCRIPTION	Hx & PE	WORKUP	TREATMENT
CERVICAL STRAIN			
• Strain or spasm of cervical musculature • Often from MVA ("whiplash") or overuse	**Hx:** Pain (nonradiating) **PE:** Decreased ROM, muscle tenderness, normal neurologic exam	**XR:** C-spine series: usually normal **MR:** Usually not needed	• Rest, NSAIDs, physical therapy, usually 2-6wk • Can consider limited soft collar immobilization
LOW BACK PAIN			
• #2 medical complaint in U.S. • Multiple etiologies: muscle strain, annular tear, early spondylosis, or degenerative disc disease • Common workman compensation/disability complaint	**Hx:** Pain (may radiate to buttocks, not below knee) **PE:** Limited ROM, muscle (erector spinae) spasm/tenderness, normal neurologic exam; test for Waddell's signs	**XR:** L-spine series: usually normal **MR:** Usually not needed	• "Red flags" indicate further workup: fever/chills, radiculopathy, abnormal neurologic exam • Rest, NSAIDs, physical therapy, usually 2-6wk • Can consider lumbar brace
SPINAL STENOSIS			
• Narrowing of spinal canal results in cord/root compression • Causes: hypertrophy of facet capsule or ligamentum flavum, bulging disc, DDD/osteophytes	**Hx:** Pain, paresthesias relieved by sitting/forward leaning (neurogenic claudication) **PE:** Pain with back extension, do good neurologic exam	**XR:** L-spine series: DDD, facet DJD **CT:** Canal narrowing **MR:** Evaluate cord/root compression	• Activity modification, NSAIDs • PT— flexion exercises • Nerve root blocks/epidural injection • Decompression (laminectomy +/– partial facetectomy)

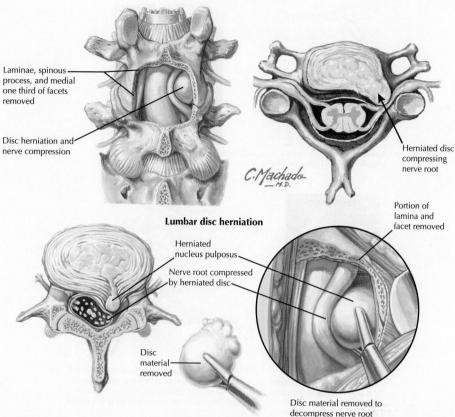

Cervical disc herniation

Laminae, spinous process, and medial one third of facets removed

Disc herniation and nerve compression

Herniated disc compressing nerve root

Portion of lamina and facet removed

Lumbar disc herniation

Herniated nucleus pulposus

Nerve root compressed by herniated disc

Disc material removed

C. Machado — M.D.

Disc material removed to decompress nerve root

DESCRIPTION	Hx & PE	WORKUP	TREATMENT
HERNIATED NUCLEUS PULPOSUS (HNP)			

• Protrusion of nucleus pulposus through torn annulus fibers
• Lumbar: L4-5 #1, traversing root affected except in far lateral herniation (exiting root)
• Thoracic: rare
• Cervical: associated with spondylosis
• Can compress cord or roots
	Hx: Neck/back pain, +/− extremity (radiating) pain, paresthesias, and weakness
	PE: Variable: decreased ROM, spinal tenderness
	Cervical: +/− Spurling's
	Lumbar: +/− straight leg raise
	Neuro: Radicular findings
		XR: Often normal +/− disc space narrowing or spondylosis
		MR: Best study to show protruding disc and nerve or cord compression
			• Rest, activity modification
			• NSAIDs (limit narcotic use)
			• Physical therapy
			• Epidural steroid injections
			• Diskectomy +/− fusion:
			  ○ Failed conservative treatment
			  ○ Progressive neurologic deficit
			  ○ Cauda equina syndrome

CAUDA EQUINA SYNDROME			
• Compression of cauda equina • Usually from large midline disc herniation or extrusion • Bowel & bladder dysfunction • Surgical emergency	**Hx/PE:** "Saddle" (perianal) anesthesia, lower extremity numbness/ weakness, decreased rectal tone	**XR:** Normal or disc space narrowing **MR:** Study of choice: compression of cauda equina	• Emergency surgical decompression-laminectomy/ diskectomy • (Prognosis is still guarded even with prompt diagnosis and treatment.)

Spine Involvement in Osteoarthritis

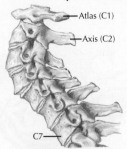

- Atlas (C1)
- Axis (C2)
- C7

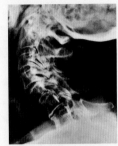

Extensive thinning of cervical discs and hyperextension deformity with narrowing of intervertebral foramina. Lateral radiograph reveals similar changes

Degenerative Disc Disease

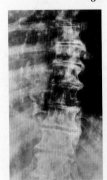

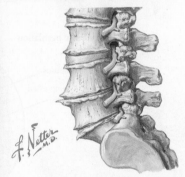

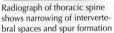

Radiograph of thoracic spine shows narrowing of intervertebral spaces and spur formation

Degeneration of lumbar intervertebral discs and hypertrophic changes at vertebral margins with spur formation. Osteophytic encroachment on intervertebral foramina compresses spinal nerves

DESCRIPTION	Hx & PE	WORKUP	TREATMENT
CERVICAL SPONDYLOSIS			

• Degenerative changes in discs, facets, and unco-vertebral joints
• C5-6 #1, C6-7 #2; men>women
• Causes axial/neck pain
• Can result in cord or root compression: myelo/radiculopathy
	Hx: Neck pain, +/− UE pain, paresthesias, and/or weakness
	PE: Decreased ROM, + Spurling's test, +/− neurologic symptoms
		XR: Loss of lordosis/ cervical straightening, loss of disc space
		MR: Shows disc degeneration or herniation
			• NSAIDs, activity modification
			• Physical therapy, +/− traction
			• Epidural or facet injections
			• Surgical
			  ○ Anterior diskectomy and fusion (ACDF)
			  ○ Posterior decompression/ fusion

DEGENERATIVE DISC DISEASE			
• Disc properties change (decr. H_2O, proteins altered, etc) leads to decr. mechanical properties • Ligaments/facets assume greater load, can be source of pain • Natural process: unclear why only some have pain	**Hx:** Back pain without radiculopathy **PE:** +/− decreased ROM or painful ROM, normal tension signs (straight leg/bowstring tests)	**XR:** Can be normal or disc height loss **MR:** Low signal (black disc), decreased height **Discography:** confirms disc as pain source (used for preop. eval.)	• Rest, activity modification, NSAIDs, +/− muscle relaxers • Physical therapy: stretching, strengthening, weight control • Consider lumbar bracing • Surgical: lumbar fusion or disc replacement are options

Spondylolysis and Spondylolisthesis

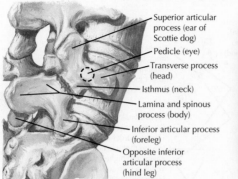

- Superior articular process (ear of Scottie dog)
- Pedicle (eye)
- Transverse process (head)
- Isthmus (neck)
- Lamina and spinous process (body)
- Inferior articular process (foreleg)
- Opposite inferior articular process (hind leg)

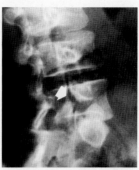

Spondylolysis without spondylolisthesis. Posterolateral view demonstrates formation of radiographic Scottie dog. On lateral radiograph, dog appears to be wearing a collar

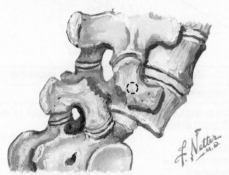

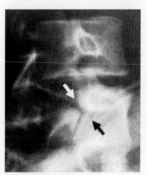

Isthmic type spondylolisthesis. Anterior subluxation of L5 on sacrum due to fracture of isthmus. Note that gap is wider and dog appears decapitated

DESCRIPTION	Hx & PE	WORKUP	TREATMENT
SPONDYLOLYSIS			
• Defect or fracture of pars interarticularis (without slip) • Assoc. w/ hyperextension sports (gymnasts, linemen) • Common in pediatrics • L5 most common site	**Hx:** Insidious onset of low back pain, worse with activities **PE:** Decreased lumbar lordosis, +/− tight hamstrings	**XR:** L-spine obliques "Scottie dog has a collar/neck" **CT:** For subtle lesions **SPECT:** Indicates if lesion has healing capacity	• Rest, activity modification • Physical therapy: esp. stretching, flexion exercises • Lumbar brace • Surgery uncommon without advanced spondylolisthesis
SPONDYLOLISTHESIS			

• Slippage of one vertebra on adjacent vertebrae
 • Six types:
  ○ Dysplastic (congenital)
  ○ Isthmic (#1, L5-S1, hyperextension)
  ○ Degenerative (elderly)
  ○ Traumatic (acute pars fx)
  ○ Pathologic
  ○ Post-surgical
	Hx: Insidious onset of low back pain, worse with activities +/− radicular symptoms
	 PE: Decreased ROM, often painful (esp. extension) +/− sensory or motor findings
		XR: Lateral view used to determine grade (% of vertebral body slipped)
		  Grade 1: 0-25%
		  Grade 2: 25-50%
		  Grade 3: 50-75%
		  Grade 4: >75%
		 CT/SPECT: For subtle defects and healing potential
			Low grade (1-2):
			 • Rest, activity modification
			 • Physical therapy
			 • Lumbar bracing
			 High grade (3-4):
			 • Peds: prophylactic posterolateral (PL) fusion
			 • Adults: decompression and PL fusion

Scoliosis

Measurement of curvature (Cobb method)

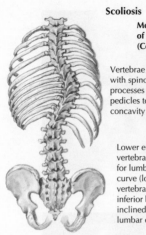

Vertebrae rotated with spinous processes and pedicles toward concavity

Lower end vertebrae for lumbar curve (lowest vertebra with inferior border inclined toward lumbar concavity)

Upper end vertebrae for thoracic curve (highest vertebra with superior border inclined toward thoracic concavity)

Transitional vertebra (lowest vertebra with inferior border inclined toward thoracic concavity and highest vertebra with superior border inclined toward lumbar concavity)

Torticollis (Wryneck)

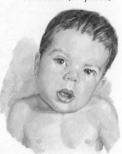

DESCRIPTION	EVALUATION	TREATMENT
MYELODYSPLASIA		

• Incomplete spinal cord development (neural tube closure defect)
• 4 types depending on severity
• Associated w/elevated maternal AFP
• Prenatal folic acid decreases incidence
• Associated with multiple deformities (spine, hips, knees, and feet)
• Often associated with latex allergy
	Hx: Can be diagnosed intrauterine
	PE/XR: Based on type of defect:
	  1. Spina bifida
	  2. Meningocele
	  3. Myelomeningocele
	  4. Rachischisis
	Symptoms/exam based on lowest functional level (intact L4 allows for ambulation)
		• Must individualize for each patient
		• Most need ambulation aids and/or orthoses
		• Muscle balancing (releases)
		• Individual deformities
		  ○ Scoliosis: most need fusion
		  ○ Hips: keep them contained
		  ○ Feet: release or arthrodesis

SCOLIOSIS		

• Lateral bending & rotation of the spine
• Types:
  ○ I. Congenital (abnormal vertebrae)
  ○ II. Idiopathic: #1, often +fam hx;
  ○ Infantile: <3y.o., M>F;
  ○ Juvenile: 3-10y.o.;
  ○ Adolescent: #1, F>M, R>L;
  ○ III. Neuromuscular: associated with neuromuscular disease
• Curve progression evaluated by:
  ○ Curve magnitude: x-ray/Cobb angle
  ○ Skeletal maturity: use Risser stage
• Classifications: King & Moe, Lenke
	Hx: Patient or parents may notice asymmetry of back; found on school screening; +/− pain; neuro sx rare
	PE: Gross or subtle spinal deformity, + forward bending test; neurologic findings rare (increased with left-sided curves)
	XR: Full length spinal films: use Cobb technique to determine angle
	Bending films used to determine flexibility of the curve/deformity
		• School screening is effective
		• Congenital: progression & need for surgery depend on severity/type
		• Idiopathic: depends on curve & age
		  ○ <25°: observation
		  ○ 25-40°: bracing
		  ○ >40°: spinal fusion
		• Juvenile type often needs fusion
		• Neuromuscular: often require longer fusions, both anterior & posterior

TORTICOLLIS		
• Head tilted, chin rotated opposite side • Sternocleidomastoid (SCM) contracture • Etiology unknown • Associated with intrauterine position • Associated with other disorders	**Hx:** Parents notice deformity, +/− lump in the neck (on sternocleido-mastoid) **PE:** Head tilted/rotated, +/− SCM lump. +/− cranial and/or facial asymmetry **XR:** Spine/hips: r/o other deformities	• Rule out any associated disorders • Physical therapy/stretching (SCM) • Helmet may be needed for cranium • Surgical release if persistent • Poor eye development is concern

Anterior Approach to Cervical Spine

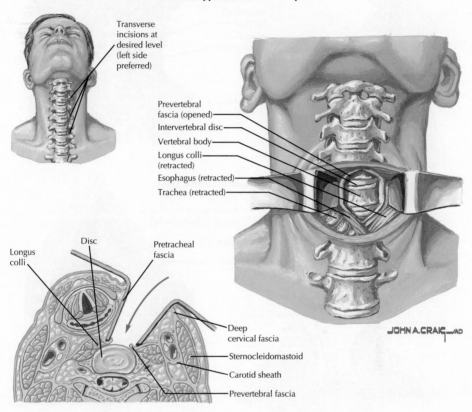

Transverse incisions at desired level (left side preferred)

Prevertebral fascia (opened)
Intervertebral disc
Vertebral body
Longus colli (retracted)
Esophagus (retracted)
Trachea (retracted)

Longus colli
Disc
Pretracheal fascia

Deep cervical fascia
Sternocleidomastoid
Carotid sheath
Prevertebral fascia

JOHN A.CRAIG—AD

USES	INTERNERVOUS PLANE	DANGERS	COMMENT
ANTERIOR APPROACH			
• Anterior cervical diskectomy & fusion (ACDF) for cervical spondylosis and/or HNP • Tumor or biopsy	**Superficial** Deep cervical fascia: SCM goes lateral Pretracheal fascia: carotid sheath goes lateral **Deep** Prevertebral fascia between longus collis muscles (right & left)	• Recurrent laryngeal n. • Sympathetic n. • Carotid artery • Internal jugular • Vagus nerve • Inferior thyroid artery	• Access C3 to T1 • Right recurrent laryngeal nerve more susceptible to injury; many surgeons approach on left side • Thyroid arteries limit extension of the approach

Posterior Approach to Cervical Spine

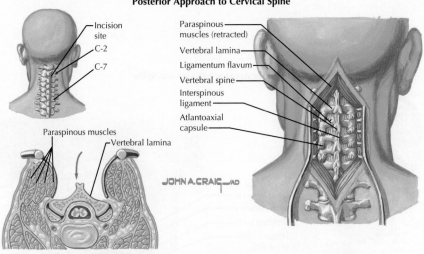

Incision site
C-2
C-7

Paraspinous muscles (retracted)
Vertebral lamina
Ligamentum flavum
Vertebral spine
Interspinous ligament
Atlantoaxial capsule

Paraspinous muscles
Vertebral lamina

JOHN A.CRAIG—AD

Posterior Approach to Lumbar Spine

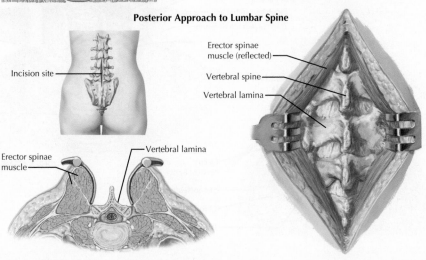

Incision site

Erector spinae muscle (reflected)
Vertebral spine
Vertebral lamina

Erector spinae muscle
Vertebral lamina

USES	INTERNERVOUS PLANE	DANGERS	COMMENT
POSTERIOR APPROACH			
Cervical			
• Posterior fusion/spondylosis • Facet dislocation	Left and right paracervical muscles (posterior cervical rami)	• Spinal cord • Nerve roots • Posterior rami • Vertebral artery • Segmental vessels	• Most common C-spine approach • Mark level of pathology with radiopaque marker preop to assist finding the appropriate level intraoperatively
Lumbar			
• Herniated disc (HNP)/nerve compression & diskectomy • Lumbar fusion	Left and right paraspinal muscles (dorsal rami)	• Segmental vessels to paraspinals	• Incision is along the spinous processes

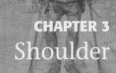

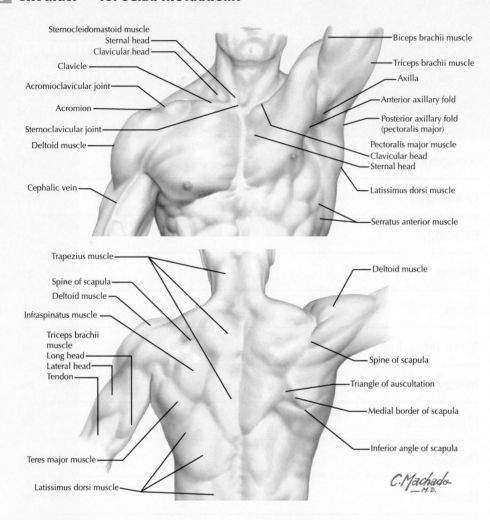

Sternocleidomastoid muscle
Sternal head
Clavicular head
Clavicle
Acromioclavicular joint
Acromion
Sternoclavicular joint
Deltoid muscle
Cephalic vein

Biceps brachii muscle
Triceps brachii muscle
Axilla
Anterior axillary fold
Posterior axillary fold
(pectoralis major)
Pectoralis major muscle
Clavicular head
Sternal head
Latissimus dorsi muscle
Serratus anterior muscle

Trapezius muscle
Spine of scapula
Deltoid muscle
Infraspinatus muscle
Triceps brachii
muscle
Long head
Lateral head
Tendon

Deltoid muscle
Spine of scapula
Triangle of auscultation
Medial border of scapula
Inferior angle of scapula

Teres major muscle
Latissimus dorsi muscle

C. Machado
_M.D.

STRUCTURE	CLINICAL APPLICATION
Sternoclavicular (SC) joint	Uncommon site of infection or dislocation
Clavicle	Subcutaneous bone: most common bone to fracture
Acromioclavicular (AC) joint	Common site of "shoulder separation" or degenerative joint disease/pain
Acromion	Landmark of shoulder (especially for injections, e.g., subacromial)
Deltoid muscle	Can test muscle function for axillary nerve motor function
Trapezius	Common site of pain; weakness results in lateral scapular winging
Serratus anterior	Weakness/palsy results in medial scapular winging
Pectoralis major	Can rupture off humeral insertion, results in a defect in the axillary fold
Cephalic vein	Lies in the deltopectoral interval
Spine of scapula	More prominent with supra/infraspinatus muscle wasting (suprascapular nerve palsy)
Inferior angle of scapula	May "wing" medially or laterally if muscles are weak (nerve palsies)

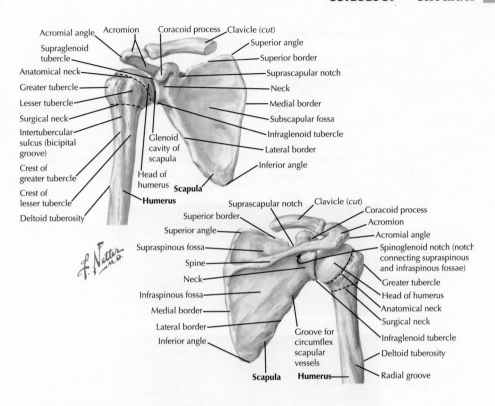

CHARACTERISTICS	OSSIFY		FUSE	COMMENTS
SCAPULA				
• Flat, triangular bone	**Primary**			• Suprascapular nerve can be compressed
• Spine posteriorly	Body	8wk fetal	15-20yr	in suprascapular notch (denervates SS &
separates two fossae				IS) or in the spinoglenoid notch (dener-
(supra/infraspinatus)				vates IS only)
• Two notches	**Secondary**			• Suprascapular & spinoglenoid notches
• Coracoid process	Coracoid	1yr	All fuse	• Coracoid is the "lighthouse" to the
anteriorly	Glenoid	15-18yr	between	shoulder
• Glenoid: pear shaped	Acromion	15-18yr	15-20yr	• Glenoid: 5-7° retroverted, 5° superior tilt
• Acromion: hook-shaped	Inferior angle	15-18yr		• Unfused acromion results in os acromiale
lateral prominence				• Body of scapula is very thin, angle is
				thicker
PROXIMAL HUMERUS				
• Head is retroverted: 35°	**Primary**		Birth	• Anatomic neck fxs: risk for osteonecrosis
• Anatomic and surgical	Shaft	8-9wk		• Surgical neck: common fx site (especially
necks		fetal		in the elderly)
• Head/neck angle: 130°	**Secondary**			• 80% of bone growth from proximal
• Two tuberosities:	Proximal (3):		17-20yr	physis; proximal fxs in children have
Greater is lateral	Head	Birth		great remodeling potential
Lesser is anterior	Gtr tuberosity	1-2yr		• Greater tuberosity: insertion site of su-
• Bicipital groove between	Lsr tuberosity	3-4yr		praspinatus, infraspinatus, teres minor
gtr and lsr tuberosities:				• Lesser tuberosity: insertion site of
bicep tendon				subscapularis

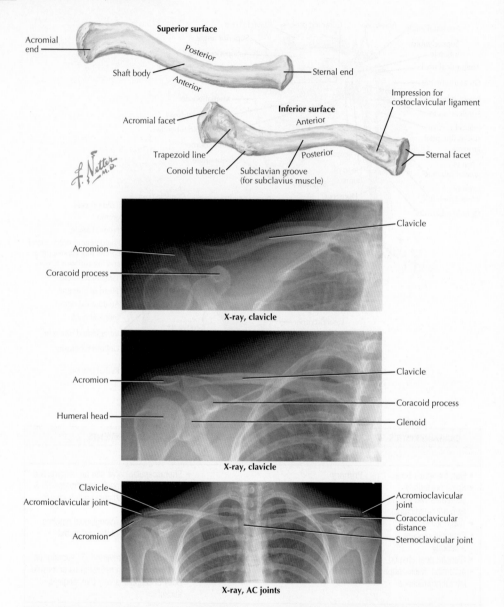

Superior surface

Acromial end

Posterior

Shaft body

Anterior

Sternal end

Impression for costoclavicular ligament

Acromial facet

Inferior surface

Anterior

Trapezoid line

Conoid tubercle

Subclavian groove (for subclavius muscle)

Posterior

Sternal facet

Clavicle

Acromion

Coracoid process

X-ray, clavicle

Acromion

Clavicle

Humeral head

Coracoid process

Glenoid

X-ray, clavicle

Clavicle

Acromioclavicular joint

Acromion

Acromioclavicular joint

Coracoclavicular distance

Sternoclavicular joint

X-ray, AC joints

CHARACTERISTICS	OSSIFY	FUSE	COMMENTS
CLAVICLE			
• S-shaped cylindrical bone • Middle ⅓ is narrowest, no muscle insertions • Clavicle widens laterally • No true medullary canal	**Primary** (2) Medial & lateral	7wk fetal	9wk fetal	• Only link from upper extremity to axial skeleton • Most commonly fractured bone in body; middle ⅓ is most common location of fracture (80%) • First bone to ossify, last to fuse • Starts as intramembranous, then finishes as membranous ossification

	Secondary
	  Sternal
	  Acromial
		18-20yr
		18-20yr
			19-25yr
			19-22yr	

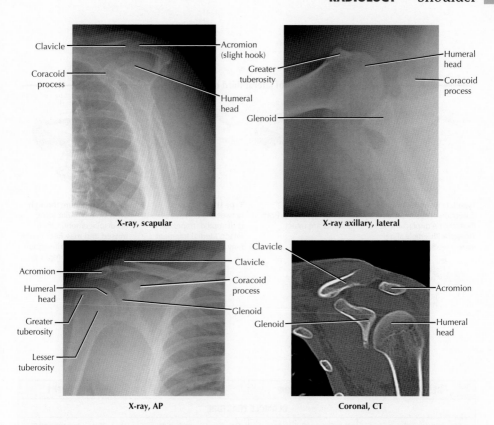

X-ray, scapular

X-ray axillary, lateral

X-ray, AP

Coronal, CT

RADIOGRAPH	TECHNIQUE	FINDINGS	CLINICAL APPLICATION
CLAVICLE			
Clavicle (2 view)	AP w/caudal & cephalic tilt	Clavicle	Fracture, DJD of ACJ
Zanca	AP (of ACJ) w/10° cephalic tilt	Acromioclavicular joint	ACJ pathology (DJD, fx)
Stress views	Both ACJs w/w-out weights	Acromioclavicular joints	ACJ separation/instability
Serendipity	40° cephalic tilt manubrium	Sternoclavicular joint	Sternoclavicular pathology
SHOULDER			
AP	Plate perpendicular to scapula	Glenohumeral joint space	Trauma (fx/dx), arthritis
Axillary lateral	Abduct arm, beam into axilla	Glenoid/humeral head position	Dislocations, Hill-Sachs lesion
Scapular Y	Beam parallel to scapula	Humeral head position	Trauma, acromion type
Supraspinatus outlet	Scapular Y w/10° caudal tilt	Acromion morphology	Hooked acromion (type 3) is assoc. w/ impingement synd.
Stryker notch	Hand on head, 10° cephalic tilt	Humeral head	Hill-Sachs lesion
West point	Prone, beam into axilla	Anterior inferior glenoid	Bony Bankart lesion
OTHER STUDIES			
CT	Axial, coronal, sagittal	Articular congruity, fx fragment position	Fractures (esp. proximal humerus, glenoid/intraarticular)
MRI	Sequence protocols vary	Soft tissues (tendons, labrum)	Rotator cuff or labral tears

─────── **Fractures of lateral third of clavicle** ───────►

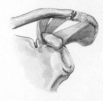 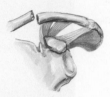 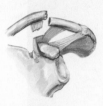 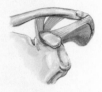

Type I. Fracture with no disruption of ligaments and therefore no displacement. Treated with simple sling for few weeks

Type IIA. Fracture is medial to ligaments. Both ligaments are intact.

Type IIB. Fracture is between ligaments; coroid is disrupted, trapezoid is intact. Medial fragment may elevate.

Type III. Fracture through acromioclavicular joint; no displacement. Often missed and may later cause painful osteoarthritis requiring resection arthroplasty

DESCRIPTION	EVALUATION	CLASSIFICATION	TREATMENT
CLAVICLE FRACTURE			
• Most common fx • 80% in middle third (group 1) • 15% group 2, 5% group 3 • Mechanism: fall onto shoulder (e.g., football, hockey) • Clavicle is unfused until early 20's, periosteal sleeve avulsion fx can result distally	**Hx:** Trauma/fall, pain **PE:** Swelling, tenderness. +/− tenting of skin/clinical deformity; do thorough neurovascular exam **XR:** 2 views of clavicle (evaluate for shortening) **CT:** Rarely needed	• Group 1: middle 1/3 • Group 2: distal 1/3 ○ Type 1: lateral to CC ligaments ○ Type 2a: medial to CC ligaments ○ Type 2b: between CC ligaments (conoid torn, trapezoid intact) ○ Type 3: fx into ACJ • Group 3: proximal 1/3	• Closed treatment/sling for most groups 1& 3 fxs • ORIF for fxs severely shortened, tented, open, associated with vascular injuries • ORIF for most group 2/type 2 distal fxs
COMPLICATIONS: Nonunion (esp. distal/group 2 fx); vascular or nerve injury			
SCAPULA FRACTURE			
• Mechanism: high-energy trauma • Uncommon injury • Young males most common • >85% have associated injuries: pulmonary contusion, pneumothorax • Good healing potential provided by surrounding muscles	**Hx:** Trauma (e.g., MVA), pain in back and/or shoulder **PE:** Swelling, tenderness to palpation, decreased ROM **XR:** AP/axillary lateral/scapular Y; CXR **CT:** Intraarticular/glenoid fractures, displaced body fractures	• Anatomic classification: A-G • Ideberg (glenoid fx) ○ Type I: anterior avulsion fx ○ Type II: transverse/oblique fx through glenoid; exits inferiorly ○ Type III: oblique fx through glenoid, exits superiorly ○ Type IV: transverse fx exits through the scapula body ○ Type V: types II + IV	• Closed treatment with sling for 2wk for most fxs, then early ROM • ORIF for displaced, unstable, or large (>25%) intraarticular or angulated neck fxs
COMPLICATIONS: Associated injuries: Rib fracture #1, pulmonary contusion, pneumothorax, vascular or brachial plexus			

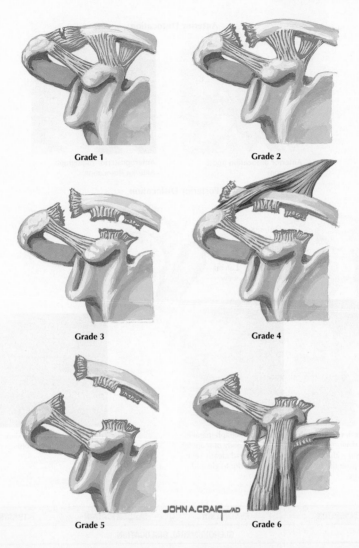

Grade 1

Grade 2

Grade 3

Grade 4

Grade 5

Grade 6

JOHN A.CRAIG—MD

DESCRIPTION	EVALUATION	CLASSIFICATION	TREATMENT
ACROMIOCLAVICULAR SEPARATION			
• Mechanism: fall onto shoulder (e.g., football, bicycles, etc) • Progression from isolated AC ligament injury to combined AC and CC (coracoclavicular) ligament disruption with varying clavicle displacement • Aka "shoulder separation"	**Hx:** Fall/direct blow, pain, swelling, +/− popping **PE:** AC tenderness, +/− instability & deformity **XR:** AC joint (+/− stress views, esp. grade II) (measure CC distance) **MR:** Evaluate CC ligaments	Rockwood grade: I. AC ligament sprain II. AC tear, CC intact III. AC & CC ligament tears ≤ 100% superior displacement IV: Grade III w /posterior displacement V: Grade III ≤ 300% superior displacement VI: Grade III w/ inferior displacement	• Grades I & II: sling, rest, physical therapy • Grade III: controversial. Nonoperative for most, CC reconstruction for high-level athletes & laborers • Grades IV-VI: CC ligament reconstruction
COMPLICATIONS: AC arthrosis/DJD; stiffness; associated injuries (pneumothorax, fracture, neurapraxia)			

Anterior Dislocation

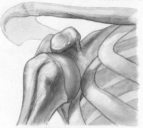

Anterior dislocation (most common)

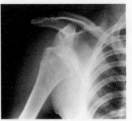

Anteroposterior radiograph
Anterior dislocation

Posterior Dislocation

Posterior
(subacromial)
← dislocation →

Antero-   Lateral
posterior   view
view

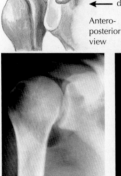

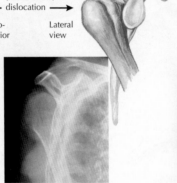

Anteroposterior radiograph.
Difficult to determine if
humeral head within,
anterior, or posterior to
glenoid cavity.

Lateral radiograph (parallel
to plane of body of scapula).
Humeral head clearly seen
to be posterior to glenoid
cavity.

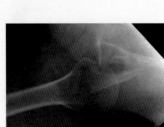

True axillary view. Also shows humeral
head posterior to glenoid cavity.

DESCRIPTION	EVALUATION	CLASSIFICATION	TREATMENT
GLENOHUMERAL DISLOCATION			

• Most common dislocation
• Common in young/athletic patients (recurrence >90% if <25y.o.)
• Associated w/ labral tears (<40y.o.) and rotator cuff tears (>40y.o.)
• Associated w/ fxs: tuberosity or glenoid rim ("bony Bankart")
• Posterior dislocations associated w/ seizures
• Humeral head impression fracture (Hill-Sachs lesion) can occur
	Hx: Trauma/fall, pain, inability to move arm
	PE: "Flattened" shoulder, no ROM, test axillary nerve function
	XR: 3-view shoulder; must have axillary lateral for posterior dislocation
	CT: To evaluate fxs: tuberosity or glenoid
		Anatomic (based on location of humeral head):
		• Anterior (>90%)
		• Posterior (often missed)
		• Inferior (luxatio erecta: abducted arm cannot be lowered [rare])
		• Superior (extremely rare)
			• Acute: reduce dislocation
			• Methods (with sedation):
			  ○ Hippocratic/traction
			  ○ Stimson
			  ○ Milch
			  ○ Scapular retraction
			• Immobilize: sling for 2wk
			• Physical therapy
			• ORIF of displaced fxs
			• Consider early labral repair in young patients

COMPLICATIONS: Recurrent dislocation/instability (esp. in young/<25y.o.); nerve injury (axillary, musculocutaneous)			

Reduction of Anterior Dislocation of Glenohumeral Joint

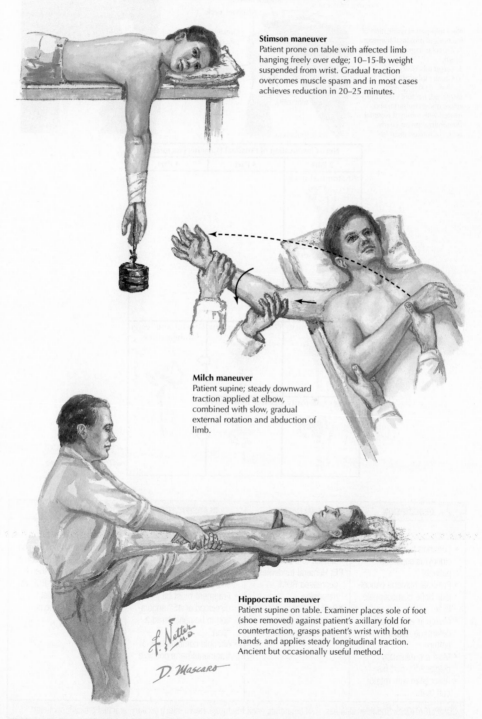

Stimson maneuver
Patient prone on table with affected limb hanging freely over edge; 10–15-lb weight suspended from wrist. Gradual traction overcomes muscle spasm and in most cases achieves reduction in 20–25 minutes.

Milch maneuver
Patient supine; steady downward traction applied at elbow, combined with slow, gradual external rotation and abduction of limb.

Hippocratic maneuver
Patient supine on table. Examiner places sole of foot (shoe removed) against patient's axillary fold for countertraction, grasps patient's wrist with both hands, and applies steady longitudinal traction. Ancient but occasionally useful method.

Neer four-part classification of fractures of proximal humerus.
1. Articular fragment (humeral head).
2. Lesser tuberosity.
3. Greater tuberosity.
4. Shaft. If no fragments displaced, fracture considered stable (most common) and treated with minimal external immobilization and early range-of-motion exercise.

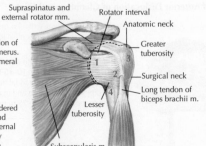

Supraspinatus and external rotator mm.
Rotator interval
Anatomic neck
Greater tuberosity
Surgical neck
Long tendon of biceps brachii m.
Lesser tuberosity
Subscapularis m.

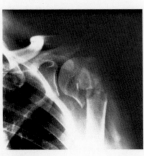

Neer Classification of Proximal Humerus Fractures		
2 Part	**3 Part**	**4 Part**
Anatomical neck		
Surgical neck		
Greater tuberosity	Greater tuberosity	Greater and lesser tuberosities
Lesser tuberosity	Lesser tuberosity	

JOHN A.CRAIG—AD

DESCRIPTION	EVALUATION	CLASSIFICATION	TREATMENT
PROXIMAL HUMERUS FRACTURE			
• Common fx, esp. in elderly/osteoporotic patients • Proximal humeral cancellous bone is susceptible to fx • Muscular attachments determine displacement pattern • Most are minimally displaced/1-part fxs • Associated with rotator cuff tears	**Hx:** Trauma/fall, pain, difficult to move arm **PE:** Humeral tenderness, decreased ROM, +/− deformity **XR:** 3-view shoulder **CT:** Identify fragments and displacement	• Neer: based on number of parts (fragments) • Parts (4): head, GT, LT, shaft • Fragment must be >1cm displaced or 45° angulation to be considered a "part" • Multiple combinations of fragments/parts possible	• 1 part: sling, early motion • 2 part: closed reduction & coaptation splint, then PT • 3 part: operative: PCP vs ORIF (locking plate) • 4 part: ORIF vs hemiarthroplasty
COMPLICATIONS: Shoulder stiffness, AVN (anatomic neck fractures), nerve injury (axillary, brachial plexus), nonunion			

Sternoclavicular Joint

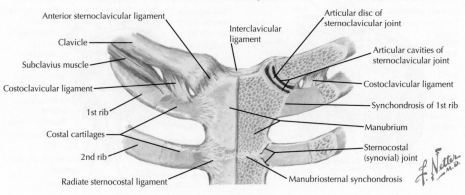

LIGAMENT	ATTACHMENTS	COMMENTS
SHOULDER JOINTS		
General		

- The shoulder is made up of 4 separate articulations. Shoulder motion is a combined movement from all 4 articulations: 1. Sternoclavicular joint, 2. Glenohumeral joint, 3. Acromioclavicular joint, 4. Scapulothoracic articulation
- The shoulder joint has the most range of motion in the body.
  - Forward flexion: 0-170°
  - Extension: 0-60°
  - Abduction: 0-170/180°
  - Internal rotation: to thoracic spine
  - External rotation: up to 70°
- 2:1 ratio of glenohumeral joint to scapulothoracic articulation motion during shoulder abduction
- Inherently unstable joint with huge ROM potential. Static and dynamic stabilizers give joint stability.
  - Static: glenoid, labrum, articular congruity, glenohumeral ligaments & capsule, negative intraarticular pressure
  - Dynamic: rotator cuff muscles/tendons, biceps tendon, scapular stabilizers (periscapular muscles), proprioception
- Shallow glenoid "socket" gives minimal bony stability, but is deepened/stabilized by the fibrocartilaginous labrum.
- Labrum serves as a "bumper"/stop to humeral subluxation, as well attachment site for capsuloligamentous structures. Joint instability can result from labral tear/detachment with loss of "bumper" and resultant ligamentous laxity.
- Rotator cuff: confluent "horseshoe-" shaped insertion of 4 stabilizing muscle tendons inserting on the proximal humerus (greater & lesser tuberosities). RC muscles actively keep humeral head seated into glenoid during all motions.

STERNOCLAVICULAR JOINT		

Diarthrodial/double gliding joint. Only true attachment of upper extremity to axial skeleton. ROM: clavicle rotates in joint up to 50° on the fixed sternum.

Capsule	Surrounds joint	Secondary stabilizer
Sternoclavicular	Medial clavicle to sternum Anterior and posterior ligaments	Primary stabilizer of sternoclavicular joint Posterior stronger, anterior dislocation more common
Costoclavicular	Inferior clavicle to costal cartilage	Strongest sternoclavicular ligament
Interclavicular	Between medial ends of clavicle	Secondary stabilizer
Disc	Intraarticular disc	Fibrocartilage disc within the joint

SCAPULOTHORACIC ARTICULATION		

The articulation is not an actual joint. Scapula slides/rotates along posterior ribs (2-7). Multiple muscles (including serratus anterior and trapezius) are involved. 2:1 ratio of GHJ to scapulothoracic motion during flexion & abduction

Coronal section through joint

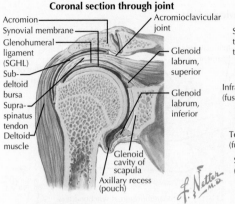

Acromion
Synovial membrane
Glenohumeral ligament (SGHL)
Sub-deltoid bursa
Supra-spinatus tendon
Deltoid muscle
Glenoid cavity of scapula
Axillary recess (pouch)
Acromioclavicular joint
Glenoid labrum, superior
Glenoid labrum, inferior

Joint opened: lateral view

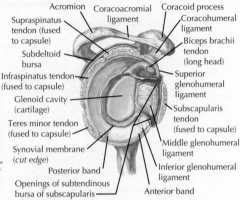

Acromion
Coracoacromial ligament
Coracoid process
Coracohumeral ligament
Supraspinatus tendon (fused to capsule)
Subdeltoid bursa
Infraspinatus tendon (fused to capsule)
Glenoid cavity (cartilage)
Teres minor tendon (fused to capsule)
Synovial membrane (cut edge)
Posterior band
Openings of subtendinous bursa of subscapularis
Biceps brachii tendon (long head)
Superior glenohumeral ligament
Subscapularis tendon (fused to capsule)
Middle glenohumeral ligament
Inferior glenohumeral ligament
Anterior band

MRI axial, shoulder

Key	
G	Greater tuberosity
L	Lesser tuberosity
h	Humeral head
^	Biceps tendon
#	Subscapularis tendon
s	Subscapularis
g	Glenoid
*	Anterior labrum
+	Posterior labrum

MRI coronal, shoulder

Key	
D	Deltoid
s	Supraspinatus
+	Supraspinatus tendon
a	Acromion
G	Greater tuberosity
*	Superior labrum
g	Glenoid

LIGAMENT	ATTACHMENTS	COMMENTS
GLENOHUMERAL JOINT		
Spheroidal ("ball & socket") joint. Inherently unstable joint stabilized by dynamic and static restraints		
Glenohumeral Ligaments		
Superior (SGHL)	Anterosuperior glenoid rim/labrum to proximal lesser tuberosity	Resists inferior translation & ER in shoulder adduction Resists posterior translation in 90° of forward flexion
Middle (MGHL)	Anterosuperior glenoid rim/labrum (inferior to SGHL) to just medial to lesser tuberosity	Resists anteroposterior translation in 45° of abduction Secondary restraint to translation & ER in adduction Buford complex: thickened MGHL & absent anterior/superior labrum
Inferior (IGHL)	Most important ligament, forms sling that tightens in abduction & ER (ant. band)/IR (post. band)	
• Anterior band (AIGHL)	Anterior glenoid/labrum (3 o'clock) to inferior humeral neck	Resists anterior & inferior translation in abduction & ER; must be tightened/"shifted" in anterior instability or MDI
• Posterior band (PIGHL)	Posterior glenoid/labrum (9 o'clock) to inferior humeral neck	Resists posterior translation in IR & 90° flexion
Other		
Coracohumeral (CHL)	Coracoid base to both LT and GT (either side of bicipital groove)	With SGHL, resists inferior translation in adduction; part of pulley to stabilize biceps tendon in joint and groove
Labrum	Circumferentially attached to glenoid	Fibrocartilage: deepens glenoid, provides more contact area, adds stability; insertion site for some GH ligaments
Capsule	Surrounds joint	Maintains intraarticular negative pressure, thin posteriorly

- Glenohumeral ligaments: Discrete thickenings of anterior and inferior capsule that provide stability to the joint. There are no ligaments posteriorly or superiorly.
- Rotator interval: Triangular space between anterior border of supraspinatus and superior border of subscapularis
  ○ Contents: SGHL, CHL, and biceps tendon, anterosuperior glenohumeral capsule
  ○ Tightening of this interval can decrease the inferior translation in adduction/"sulcus sign" in the unstable shoulder
- Biceps pulley: SGHL, CHL, subscapularis form an anterior pulley to keep biceps tendon located in joint/bicipital groove

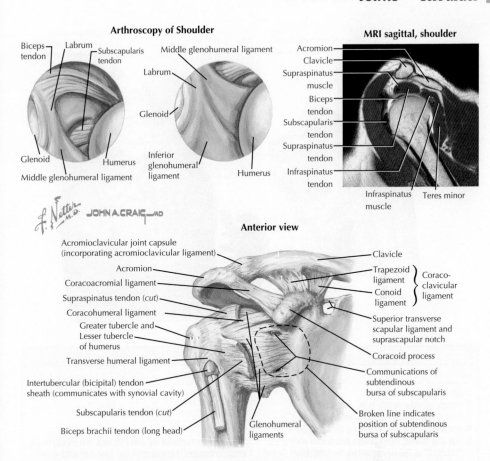

Arthroscopy of Shoulder

Biceps tendon • Labrum • Subscapularis tendon • Middle glenohumeral ligament

Labrum

Glenoid

Glenoid • Humerus • Middle glenohumeral ligament • Inferior glenohumeral ligament • Humerus

JOHN A.CRAIG—AD

MRI sagittal, shoulder

Acromion • Clavicle • Supraspinatus muscle • Biceps tendon • Subscapularis tendon • Supraspinatus tendon • Infraspinatus tendon

Infraspinatus muscle • Teres minor

Anterior view

Acromioclavicular joint capsule (incorporating acromioclavicular ligament)

Acromion

Coracoacromial ligament

Supraspinatus tendon (*cut*)

Coracohumeral ligament

Greater tubercle and Lesser tubercle of humerus

Transverse humeral ligament

Intertubercular (bicipital) tendon sheath (communicates with synovial cavity)

Subscapularis tendon (*cut*)

Biceps brachii tendon (long head)

Clavicle

Trapezoid ligament } Coraco-clavicular ligament
Conoid ligament }

Superior transverse scapular ligament and suprascapular notch

Coracoid process

Communications of subtendinous bursa of subscapularis

Broken line indicates position of subtendinous bursa of subscapularis

Glenohumeral ligaments

LIGAMENT	ATTACHMENTS	COMMENTS
ACROMIOCLAVICULAR JOINT		
Diarthrodial (plane/gliding) joint. Very limited motion (5° rotation). Common site of injury and/or painful degeneration.		
Capsule	Surrounds joints	Weak stabilizer, but sufficient under routine loads
Acromioclavicular	Thickening of superior capsule	Provides anterior to posterior stability and axial stability Injured (to some degree) in all AC separations
Coracoclavicular ∘ Conoid ∘ Trapezoid	Coracoid base to inferior clavicle Posteromedial insertion on clavicle Anterolateral insertion on clavicle	Provides vertical stability to the clavicle at the AC joint Stronger resistance to vertical load than trapezoid Resists axial load to shoulder (more oblique fibers)
Disc	In joint, between clavicle & acromion	Interposed to cushion partially incongruent joint
OTHER STRUCTURES		
Coracoacromial	Coracoid tip to anterior and inferior acromion	Key component of the coracoacromial arch; prevents humerus migration in rotator cuff–deficient shoulder
Superior transverse scapular	Crosses suprascapular notch	Suprascapular nerve travels under ligament, suprascapular artery crosses over it.
Transverse humeral	Lesser tuberosity to greater tuberosity (crosses bicipital groove)	Stabilizes biceps tendon within the bicipital groove Lateral aspect of rotator interval

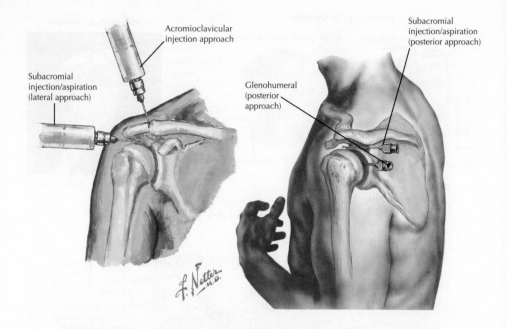

Acromioclavicular
injection approach

Subacromial
injection/aspiration
(lateral approach)

Subacromial
injection/aspiration
(posterior approach)

Glenohumeral
(posterior
approach)

STEPS
INJECTION OF ACROMIOCLAVICULAR JOINT
1. Ask patient about allergies
2. Palpate clavicle distally to AC joint (sulcus)
3. Prep skin (iodine/antiseptic soap) over AC joint
4. Anesthetize skin with local (quarter size spot)
5. Use 25g needle, insert needle into sulcus vertically (or with slight lateral to medial tilt) and into joint. You should feel a "pop/give" as the needle enters the joint. Inject 2ml of 1:1 local/corticosteroid preparation (the joint may hold <2ml of fluid). A subcutaneous wheal indicates that the needle tip is superficial to the AC capsule.
6. Dress injection site
INJECTION OF THE SUBACROMIAL SPACE
1. Ask patient about allergies
2. Palpate the acromion: define its borders (esp. lateral border & posterolateral corner)
3. Prep skin (iodine/antiseptic soap) over acromial edge
4. Anesthetize skin with local (quarter size spot)
5. Hold finger (sterile glove) on acromion, insert needle under acromion (lateral or posterior) w/ slight cephalad tilt. Aspirate to ensure not in a vessel, then inject 5ml of preparation; will flow easily if in joint. Use: a. diagnostic injection: local only; b. therapeutic injection: local/corticosteroid
6. Dress injection site
GLENOHUMERAL INJECTION
1. Ask patient about allergies
2. Palpate the posterior shoulder for the "soft spot" (usually 2cm down, 1cm medial to posterolateral corner of the acromion). Also palpate the coracoid process on the anterior aspect of the shoulder.
3. Prepare skin (iodine/antiseptic soap) over the "soft spot" on posterior shoulder
4. Anesthetize the skin overlying the "soft spot" (quarter size spot)
5. With sterile gloves, palpate the "soft spot" and the coracoid process. Then insert the needle into the soft spot and aim it toward the coracoid process. If the needle hits bone it should be redirected (glenoid: move lateral; humerus: move medial). Aspirate to ensure not in a vessel. Inject preparation (local +/− corticosteroid) into joint (should flow easily if in the joint space)
6. Dress injection site

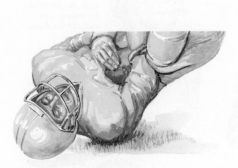

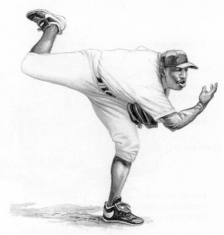

Injury to acromioclavicular joint. Usually caused by fall on tip of shoulder, depressing acromion (shoulder separation)

Throwing athletes can develop rotator cuff tears, internal impingement, and motion abnormalities

Shoulder instability is common in swimmers

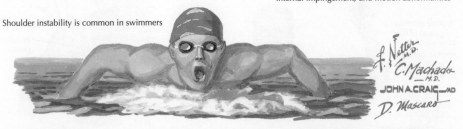

QUESTION	ANSWER	CLINICAL APPLICATION
1. Age	Old	Rotator cuff tear, impingement, arthritis (OA), adhesive capsulitis (frozen shoulder), humerus fracture (after fall)
	Young	Instability, labral tear, AC injury, distal clavicle osteolysis, impingement in athletes
2. Pain		
a. Onset	Acute	Fracture, dislocation, rotator cuff tear, acromioclavicular injury
	Chronic	Impingement, arthritis/DJD, rotator cuff tear
b. Location	On top/AC joint	AC joint arthrosis/separation
c. Occurrence	Night pain	Classic for RC tear, tumor (rare)
d. Exacerbating/	Overhead worse	Rotator cuff tear, impingement
relieving	Overhead better	Cervical radiculopathy
3. Stiffness	Yes	Osteoarthritis (OA), adhesive capsulitis
4. Instability	"Slips in and out"	Dislocation (>90% anterior, esp. in abduction & ER (e.g., throwing), subluxation, labral tear
5. Trauma	Direct blow	Acromioclavicular (AC) injury
	Fall on outstretched hand	Glenohumeral dislocation (subluxation; fracture)
6. Work/activity	Overhead usage	Rotator cuff tear
	Weight lifting	Osteolysis (distal clavicle)
	Athlete: throwing type	RC tear/impingement (internal), instability (swimmer's)
	Long-term manual labor	Arthritis (OA)
7. Neurologic sx	Numbness/tingling/"heavy"	Thoracic outlet syndrome, brachial plexus injury
8. PMHx	Cardiopulmonary/GI	Referred pain to shoulder

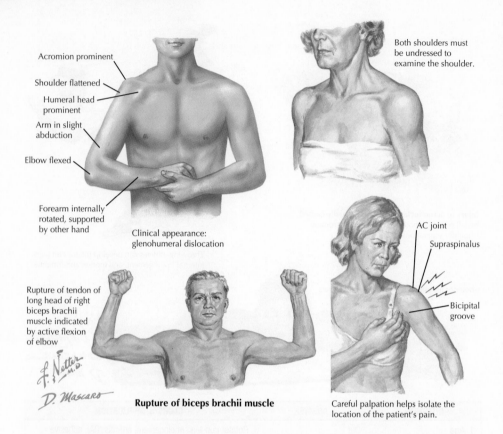

Acromion prominent

Shoulder flattened

Humeral head prominent

Arm in slight abduction

Elbow flexed

Forearm internally rotated, supported by other hand

Clinical appearance: glenohumeral dislocation

Both shoulders must be undressed to examine the shoulder.

AC joint

Supraspinalus

Bicipital groove

Careful palpation helps isolate the location of the patient's pain.

Rupture of tendon of long head of right biceps brachii muscle indicated by active flexion of elbow

Rupture of biceps brachii muscle

EXAM/OBSERVATION	TECHNIQUE	CLINICAL APPLICATION
INSPECTION		
Both shoulders must be undressed for proper inspection and examination of the shoulder.		
Symmetry	Compare both sides	Acromioclavicular separation, dislocation, muscle atrophy
Wasting	Loss of contour/muscle mass	RC tear, nerve compression (e.g., suprascapular)
Gross deformity	Superior displacement	Acromioclavicular injury (separation)
Gross deformity	Anterior displacement	Anterior dislocation (glenohumeral joint)
Gross deformity	"Popeye" arm	Biceps tendon rupture (usually proximal end of long head)
PALPATION		
AC joint	Feel for end of clavicle	Pain indicates acromioclavicular pathology, instability of distal clavicle, AC separation
Supraspinatus tendon	Feel acromion, down to acromio-humeral sulcus	Pain indicates bursitis and/or supraspinatus tendon (rotator cuff) tear
Greater tuberosity	Prominence on lateral humeral head	Pain indicates rotator cuff tendinitis, tear, or fx
Biceps tendon/bicipital groove	Feel tendon in groove on humerus	Pain indicates biceps tendinitis

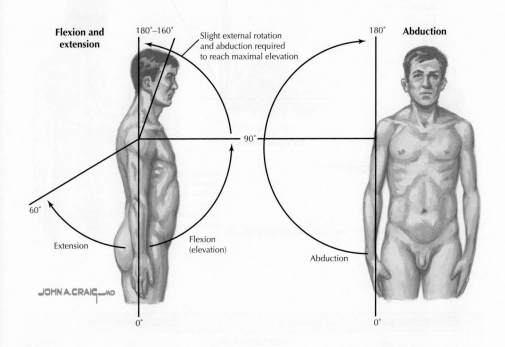

EXAM/OBSERVATION	TECHNIQUE	CLINICAL APPLICATION
RANGE OF MOTION		
Forward flexion	Arms from sides forward	0-160°/180° normal
Extension	Arms from sides backward	0-60° normal
Abduction	Arms from sides outward	0-160°/180 normal
Internal rotation	Reach thumb up back, note level	Mid thoracic (T7) normal, compare sides
External rotation	1. Elbow at side, rotate forearms laterally 2. Abduct arm to 90°, externally rotate up	30-60° normal ER decreased in adhesive capsulitis

• Rotator cuff tear: AROM decreased, PROM ok. Adhesive capsulitis: AROM and PROM are both decreased.
• Increased ER may indicate a subscapularis tear

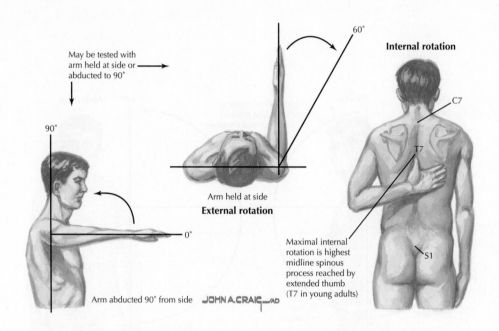

May be tested with
arm held at side or ⟶
abducted to 90°

90°

External rotation
Arm held at side

0°

Arm abducted 90° from side JOHN A.CRAIG—AD

60°

Internal rotation

C7

T7

S1

Maximal internal
rotation is highest
midline spinous
process reached by
extended thumb
(T7 in young adults)

EXAM/OBSERVATION	TECHNIQUE	CLINICAL APPLICATION
NEUROVASCULAR		
Sensory		
Supraclavicular nerve (C4)	Superior shoulder/clavicular area	Deficit indicates corresponding nerve/root lesion
Axillary nerve (C5)	Lateral shoulder	Deficit indicates corresponding nerve/root lesion
T2 segmental nerve	Axilla	Deficit indicates corresponding nerve/root lesion
Motor		
Spinal accessory (CN11)	Resisted shoulder shrug	Weakness = Trapezius or corresponding nerve lesion
Suprascapular (C5-6)	Resisted abduction Resisted external rotation	Weakness = Supraspinatus or nerve/root lesion Weakness = Infraspinatus or nerve/root lesion
Axillary (C5)	Resisted abduction Resisted external rotation	Weakness = Deltoid or corresponding nerve/root lesion Weakness = Teres minor or nerve/root lesion
Dorsal scapular nerve (C5)	Shoulder shrug	Weakness = Levator scapulae/rhomboid or corresponding nerve/root lesion
Thoracodorsal nerve (C7-8)	Resisted adduction	Weakness = Latissimus dorsi or nerve/root lesion
Lateral pectoral nerve (C5-7)	Resisted adduction	Weakness = Pect. major or nerve/root lesion
U/L subscapular nerve (C5-6)	Resisted internal rotation	Weakness = Subscapularis or nerve/root lesion
Long thoracic nerve (C5-7)	Scapular protraction/reach	Weakness = Serratus anterior or nerve/root lesion

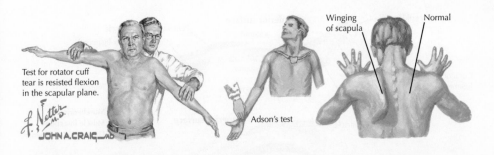

Test for rotator cuff tear is resisted flexion in the scapular plane.

Adson's test

Winging of scapula

Normal

EXAM	TECHNIQUE	CLINICAL APPLICATION/DDX
SPECIAL TESTS		
Impingement/Rotator Cuff		
Impingement sign	Forward flexion >90°	Pain indicates impingement syndrome
Hawkins test	FF 90°, then IR	Pain indicates impingement syndrome
Supraspinatus/ Jobe empty can	Pronate arm, resisted FF in scapular plane	Pain or weakness indicates rotator cuff (supraspinatus) tear (partial or full thickness)
Drop arm	FF >90°, try to maintain it	Inability to hold flexion (arm drops) indicates supraspinatus tear
ER lag sign	ER shoulder, patient holds it	Inability to maintain ER indicates infraspinatus tear
Horn blower's	Resisted ER in slight abduction	Weakness indicates rotator cuff tear involving infraspinatus
Lift off	Hand behind back, push backward	Weakness indicates subscapularis tear
Lift off lag sign	Lift hand off back, patient holds it	Inability to hold hand off of low back indicates subscapularis tear
Belly press	Hand on belly, push toward belly	Weakness indicates subscapularis tear
Biceps/Superior Labrum		
Active compres- sion (O'Brien's)	FF 90°, adduct 10°, resisted flex- ion; in pronation, *then* supination	Pain with resisted flexion, greater in pronation indicates SLAP tear; may also suggest AC joint pathology
Crank	Abduct 90°, axial load, rotate	Pain indicates a SLAP tear
Speed's test	Resisted flexion in scapular plane	Pain indicates biceps lesion or tendinitis
Yergason's test	Elbow 90°, resisted supination	Pain indicates biceps tendinitis
Instability		
Apprehension test	Abduct, externally rotate	Pain or apprehension of indicates anterior instability
Relocation	Abduct, ER, posterior force to arm	Relief of pain/apprehension indicates anterior instability
Load & shift	Axial load, ant/post translation	Increased translation indicates anterior OR posterior instability
Jerk test	Supine, adduct, FF 90°, push posterior	Pain/apprehension/translation indicates posterior instability
Sulcus	Pull down on adducted arm	Sulcus under lateral acromion indicates inferior instability
Other		
X-body adduction	Adduct arm across body	Pain at AC joint indicates AC joint pathology (e.g., arthrosis)
Scapular winging	Push against a wall	Winging of scapula indicates nerve palsy or muscle weakness
Adson's test	Palpate pulse, rotate neck	Numbness or tingling suggestive of thoracic outlet syndrome
Wright's test	Extend arm, rotate neck away	Numbness or tingling suggestive of thoracic outlet syndrome
Spurling's test	Lateral flex/axially compress neck	Reproduction of symptoms indicates cervical neck pathology

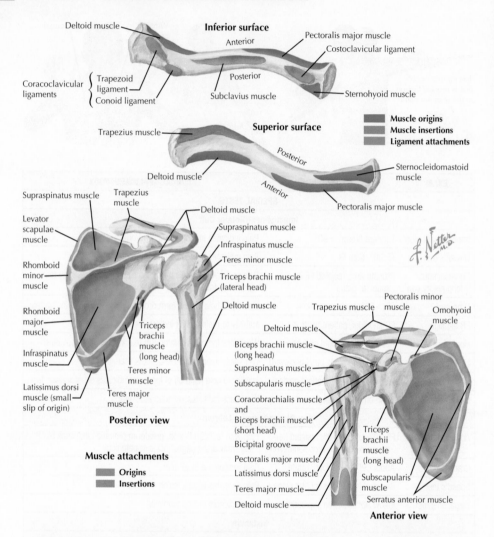

CORACOID PROCESS	GREATER TUBEROSITY	PROXIMAL HUMERUS	SCAPULA (ANTERIOR)	SCAPULA (POSTERIOR)
ORIGINS				
Biceps (SH)			Subscapularis	Supraspinatus
			Triceps brachii	Infraspinatus
Coracobrachialis			Omohyoid	Deltoid (spine/acromion)
				Teres major & minor
				Latissimus dorsi
INSERTIONS				
Pectoralis minor	Supraspinatus	Pectoralis major	Serratus anterior	Trapezius (spine/acromion)
	Infraspinatus	Latissimus dorsi		Levator scapulae
	Teres minor	Teres major		Rhomboid major & minor

- The scapula has 17 muscles that either originate or insert on it.
- Mnemonic for proximal humerus insertions (from lateral to medial): "PLT sandwich" (Pect., Lat., Teres major)

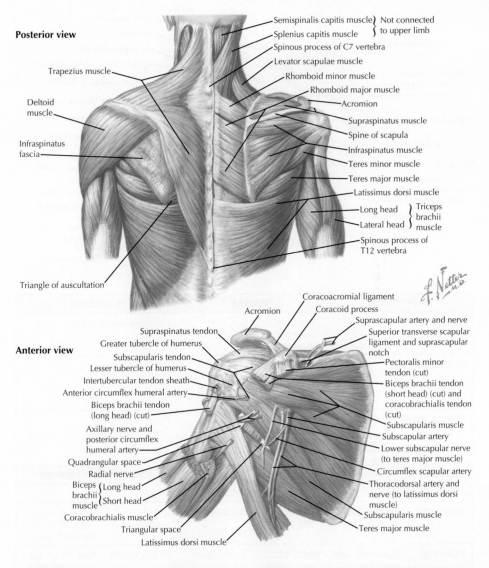

Posterior view

Semispinalis capitis muscle ⎫ Not connected
Splenius capitis muscle ⎭ to upper limb
Spinous process of C7 vertebra
Levator scapulae muscle
Rhomboid minor muscle
Rhomboid major muscle
Acromion
Supraspinatus muscle
Spine of scapula
Infraspinatus muscle
Teres minor muscle
Teres major muscle
Latissimus dorsi muscle
Long head ⎫ Triceps
Lateral head ⎭ brachii muscle
Spinous process of T12 vertebra

Trapezius muscle
Deltoid muscle
Infraspinatus fascia
Triangle of auscultation

Anterior view

Coracoacromial ligament
Acromion
Coracoid process
Suprascapular artery and nerve
Superior transverse scapular ligament and suprascapular notch
Pectoralis minor tendon (cut)
Biceps brachii tendon (short head) (cut) and coracobrachialis tendon (cut)
Subscapularis muscle
Subscapular artery
Lower subscapular nerve (to teres major muscle)
Circumflex scapular artery
Thoracodorsal artery and nerve (to latissimus dorsi muscle)
Subscapularis muscle
Teres major muscle

Supraspinatus tendon
Greater tubercle of humerus
Subscapularis tendon
Lesser tubercle of humerus
Intertubercular tendon sheath
Anterior circumflex humeral artery
Biceps brachii tendon (long head) (cut)
Axillary nerve and posterior circumflex humeral artery
Quadrangular space
Radial nerve
Biceps brachii muscle ⎰ Long head
⎱ Short head
Coracobrachialis muscle
Triangular space
Latissimus dorsi muscle

MUSCLE	ORIGIN	INSERTION	NERVE	ACTION	COMMENT
Trapezius	C7-T12 spinous process	Clavicle, acromion spine of scapula	Cranial nerve XI	Elevate & rotate scapula	Weakness results in lateral winging
Latissimus dorsi	T7-T12, iliac crest	Humerus (intertubercular groove)	*Thoracodorsal*	Adduct, extend arm, IR humerus	Used for large free flap
Levator scapulae	C1-C4 transverse process	Superior medial scapula	*Dorsal scapular, C3-4*	Elevate scapula	Connects UE to spine
Rhomboid minor	C7-T1 spinous process	Medial scapula (at the spine)	*Dorsal scapular*	Adduct scapula	Connects UE to spine
Rhomboid major	T2-T5 spinous process	Medial scapula	*Dorsal scapular*	Adduct scapula	Connects UE to spine

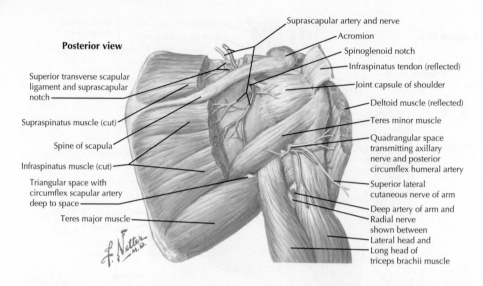

Posterior view

Suprascapular artery and nerve
Acromion
Spinoglenoid notch
Infraspinatus tendon (reflected)
Joint capsule of shoulder
Deltoid muscle (reflected)
Teres minor muscle
Quadrangular space transmitting axillary nerve and posterior circumflex humeral artery
Superior lateral cutaneous nerve of arm
Deep artery of arm and Radial nerve shown between
Lateral head and
Long head of triceps brachii muscle

Superior transverse scapular ligament and suprascapular notch
Supraspinatus muscle (cut)
Spine of scapula
Infraspinatus muscle (cut)
Triangular space with circumflex scapular artery deep to space
Teres major muscle

SPACE/INTERVAL	BORDERS	STRUCTURES
Triangular space	Teres minor Teres major Triceps (long head)	Circumflex scapular artery
Quadrangular space	Teres minor Teres major Triceps (long head) Humerus (medial border)	Axillary nerve Posterior circumflex artery Humeral artery
Triangular interval	Teres major Triceps (long head) Triceps (lateral head)	Radial nerve Deep artery of arm

MUSCLE	ORIGIN	INSERTION	NERVE	ACTION	COMMENT
ROTATOR CUFF					
Supraspinatus	Supraspinatus fossa (scapula)	Greater tuberosity (superior)	*Suprascapular*	Abduct FF arm stability	Trapped in impingement, #1 torn rotator cuff tendon
Infraspinatus	Infraspinatus fossa (scapula)	Greater tuberosity (middle)	*Suprascapular*	ER arm, stability	Weak ER: cuff tear or ss nerve lesion in notch
Teres minor	Lateral scapula	Greater tuberosity (inferior)	*Axillary*	ER arm, stability	Rarely torn rotator cuff tendon
Subscapularis	Subscapular fossa (scapula)	Lesser tuberosity	Upper and lower *subscapular*	IR, adduct arm, stability	At risk from anterior approach
OTHER					
Deltoid	Clavicle, acromion spine of scapula	Humerus (deltoid tuberosity)	*Axillary*	Abduct arm	Atrophy: axillary nerve damage
Teres major	Inferior angle of the scapula	Humerus (intertubercular groove)	Low *subscapular*	IR, adduct arm	Protects radial nerve in posterior approach

Oblique parasagittal section of axilla

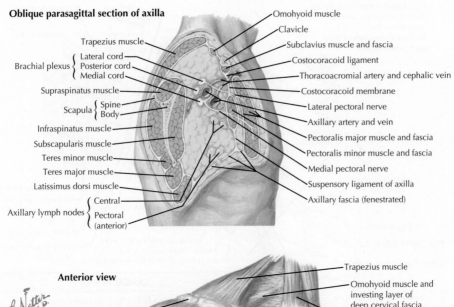

Omohyoid muscle
Clavicle
Subclavius muscle and fascia
Costocoracoid ligament
Thoracoacromial artery and cephalic vein
Costocoracoid membrane
Lateral pectoral nerve
Axillary artery and vein
Pectoralis major muscle and fascia
Pectoralis minor muscle and fascia
Medial pectoral nerve
Suspensory ligament of axilla
Axillary fascia (fenestrated)

Trapezius muscle
Brachial plexus { Lateral cord / Posterior cord / Medial cord
Supraspinatus muscle
Scapula { Spine / Body
Infraspinatus muscle
Subscapularis muscle
Teres minor muscle
Teres major muscle
Latissimus dorsi muscle
Axillary lymph nodes { Central / Pectoral (anterior)

Anterior view

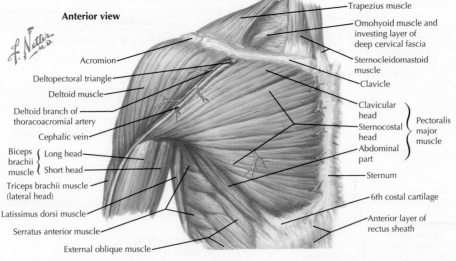

Acromion
Deltopectoral triangle
Deltoid muscle
Deltoid branch of thoracoacromial artery
Cephalic vein
Biceps brachii muscle { Long head / Short head
Triceps brachii muscle (lateral head)
Latissimus dorsi muscle
Serratus anterior muscle
External oblique muscle

Trapezius muscle
Omohyoid muscle and investing layer of deep cervical fascia
Sternocleidomastoid muscle
Clavicle
Clavicular head / Sternocostal head / Abdominal part } Pectoralis major muscle
Sternum
6th costal cartilage
Anterior layer of rectus sheath

MUSCLE	ORIGIN	INSERTION	NERVE	ACTION	COMMENT
Deltoid	Clavicle, acromion spine of scapula	Humerus (deltoid tuberosity)	*Axillary*	Abducts arm	Atrophy: axillary nerve damage
Pectoralis major	1. Clavicle 2. Sternal	Humerus (intertu-bercular groove)	Lateral *pectoral* Medial *pectoral*	Adducts arm, IR humerus	Can rupture during weight lifting
Pectoralis minor	Ribs 3-5	Coracoid process (scapula)	Medial *pectoral*	Stabilizes scapula	Divides axillary artery into 3 parts
Serratus anterior	Ribs 1-8 (lateral)	Scapula (antero-medial border)	Long *thoracic*	Holds scapula to chest wall	Paralysis results in medial winging
Subclavius	Rib 1 (and costal cartilage)	Clavicle (inferior border/mid 3rd)	Nerve to sub-clavius	Depresses clavicle	Cushions subcla-vian vessels

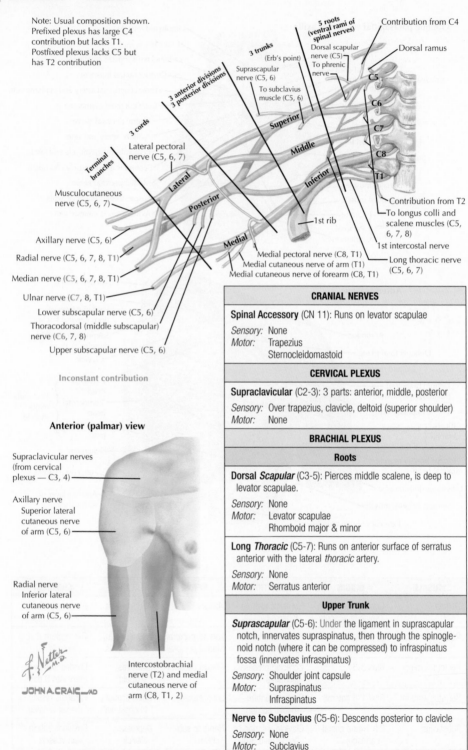

Note: Usual composition shown. Prefixed plexus has large C4 contribution but lacks T1. Postfixed plexus lacks C5 but has T2 contribution

5 roots (ventral rami of spinal nerves)

Contribution from C4

3 trunks

Dorsal scapular nerve (C5)

Dorsal ramus

(Erb's point)

To phrenic nerve

Suprascapular nerve (C5, 6)

3 anterior divisions
3 posterior divisions

To subclavius muscle (C5, 6)

C5

C6

Superior

C7

3 cords

Middle

C8

Lateral pectoral nerve (C5, 6, 7)

Inferior

T1

Terminal branches

Lateral

Contribution from T2

Musculocutaneous nerve (C5, 6, 7)

Posterior

1st rib

To longus colli and scalene muscles (C5, 6, 7, 8)

Axillary nerve (C5, 6)

Medial

Radial nerve (C5, 6, 7, 8, T1)

Medial pectoral nerve (C8, T1)

1st intercostal nerve

Median nerve (C5, 6, 7, 8, T1)

Medial cutaneous nerve of arm (T1)

Long thoracic nerve (C5, 6, 7)

Ulnar nerve (C7, 8, T1)

Medial cutaneous nerve of forearm (C8, T1)

Lower subscapular nerve (C5, 6)

Thoracodorsal (middle subscapular) nerve (C6, 7, 8)

Upper subscapular nerve (C5, 6)

Inconstant contribution

Anterior (palmar) view

Supraclavicular nerves (from cervical plexus — C3, 4)

Axillary nerve
Superior lateral cutaneous nerve of arm (C5, 6)

Radial nerve
Inferior lateral cutaneous nerve of arm (C5, 6)

Intercostobrachial nerve (T2) and medial cutaneous nerve of arm (C8, T1, 2)

JOHN A.CRAIG—AD

CRANIAL NERVES
Spinal Accessory (CN 11): Runs on levator scapulae
Sensory: None *Motor:* Trapezius Sternocleidomastoid

CERVICAL PLEXUS
Supraclavicular (C2-3): 3 parts: anterior, middle, posterior
Sensory: Over trapezius, clavicle, deltoid (superior shoulder) *Motor:* None

BRACHIAL PLEXUS
Roots
Dorsal *Scapular* (C3-5): Pierces middle scalene, is deep to levator scapulae.
Sensory: None *Motor:* Levator scapulae Rhomboid major & minor
Long *Thoracic* (C5-7): Runs on anterior surface of serratus anterior with the lateral *thoracic* artery.
Sensory: None *Motor:* Serratus anterior
Upper Trunk
Suprascapular (C5-6): Under the ligament in suprascapular notch, innervates supraspinatus, then through the spinoglenoid notch (where it can be compressed) to infraspinatus fossa (innervates infraspinatus)
Sensory: Shoulder joint capsule *Motor:* Supraspinatus Infraspinatus
Nerve to Subclavius (C5-6): Descends posterior to clavicle
Sensory: None *Motor:* Subclavius

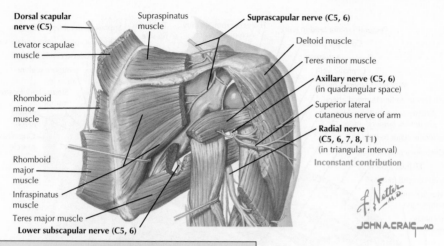

Dorsal scapular nerve (C5)

Levator scapulae muscle

Supraspinatus muscle

Suprascapular nerve (C5, 6)

Deltoid muscle

Teres minor muscle

Axillary nerve (C5, 6) (in quadrangular space)

Superior lateral cutaneous nerve of arm

Rhomboid minor muscle

Radial nerve (C5, 6, 7, 8, T1) (in triangular interval)
Inconstant contribution

Rhomboid major muscle

Infraspinatus muscle

Teres major muscle

Lower subscapular nerve (C5, 6)

JOHN A. CRAIG —AD

BRACHIAL PLEXUS
Lateral Cord
Lateral *Pectoral* (C5-7): Named for the cord, runs medial to the medial *pectoral* nerve with the *pectoral* artery. *Sensory:* None *Motor:*   Pectoralis major (clavicular portion)   Pectoralis minor (via a branch to the medial *pectoral* n.)
Lateral root to median nerve
Medial Cord
Medial *Pectoral* (C5-7): Named for cord, is lateral to the lateral *pectoral* nerve *Sensory:* None *Motor:*   Pectoralis minor   Pectoralis major (sternal portion)
Medial root to median nerve
Posterior Cord
Upper *Subscapular* (C5-6) *Sensory:* None *Motor:*   Upper subscapularis
Thoracodorsal (C7-8): Runs with *thoracodorsal* artery deep to latissimus dorsi muscle *Sensory:* None *Motor:*   Latissimus dorsi
Lower *Subscapular* (C5-6) *Sensory:* None *Motor:*   Lower subscapularis   Teres major
Axillary (C5-6): Directly inferior to joint capsule, it travels posteriorly with post. circumflex humeral art. thru quadrangular space, then bends anteriorly approx. 5cm distal to acromion. It can be injured in glenohumeral dislocations and lateral approaches. *Sensory:* Lateral proximal arm: via **superior lateral cutaneous** n. *Motor:*   Deltoid: via **deep branch**   Teres minor: via **superficial branch**

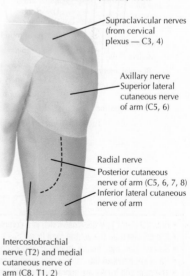

Posterior (dorsal) view

Supraclavicular nerves (from cervical plexus — C3, 4)

Axillary nerve
Superior lateral cutaneous nerve of arm (C5, 6)

Radial nerve
Posterior cutaneous nerve of arm (C5, 6, 7, 8)
Inferior lateral cutaneous nerve of arm

Intercostobrachial nerve (T2) and medial cutaneous nerve of arm (C8, T1, 2)

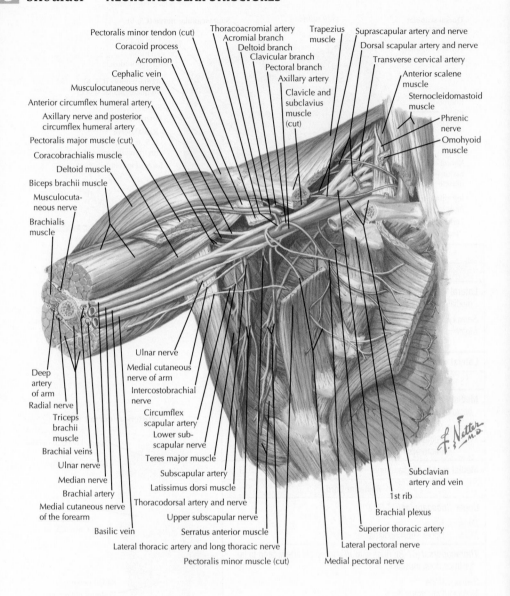

Pectoralis minor tendon (cut)
Coracoid process
Acromion
Cephalic vein
Musculocutaneous nerve
Anterior circumflex humeral artery
Axillary nerve and posterior circumflex humeral artery
Pectoralis major muscle (cut)
Coracobrachialis muscle
Deltoid muscle
Biceps brachii muscle
Musculocutaneous nerve
Brachialis muscle

Thoracoacromial artery
Acromial branch
Deltoid branch
Clavicular branch
Pectoral branch
Axillary artery
Clavicle and subclavius muscle (cut)

Trapezius muscle

Suprascapular artery and nerve
Dorsal scapular artery and nerve
Transverse cervical artery
Anterior scalene muscle
Sternocleidomastoid muscle
Phrenic nerve
Omohyoid muscle

Ulnar nerve
Medial cutaneous nerve of arm
Intercostobrachial nerve
Circumflex scapular artery
Lower subscapular nerve
Teres major muscle
Subscapular artery
Latissimus dorsi muscle
Thoracodorsal artery and nerve
Upper subscapular nerve
Serratus anterior muscle
Lateral thoracic artery and long thoracic nerve
Pectoralis minor muscle (cut)

Deep artery of arm
Radial nerve
Triceps brachii muscle
Brachial veins
Ulnar nerve
Median nerve
Brachial artery
Medial cutaneous nerve of the forearm
Basilic vein

Subclavian artery and vein
1st rib
Brachial plexus
Superior thoracic artery
Lateral pectoral nerve
Medial pectoral nerve

BRACHIAL PLEXUS

- Brachial ("arm") plexus ("network") is a complex of intertwined nerves that innervate the shoulder and upper extremity.
- It is derived from the ventral rami from C5-T1 (variations: C4 [prefixed], T2 [post-fixed]).
- Subdivisions: rami (roots), trunks, divisions, cords, branches (mnemonic: **R**ob **T**aylor **D**rinks **C**old **B**eer)
- Rami exit between the anterior and medial scalene muscles & travel with the subclavian artery in the axillary sheath.
- The rami and trunks are supraclavicular. There are 2 nerves from the rami, and 2 nerves from the trunks (upper)
- The divisions are under (posterior to) the clavicle. Anterior divisions innervate flexors. Posteriors innervate extensors.
- The cords and branches are infraclavicular. The cords are named for their relationship with the axillary artery.
- Terminal branches of the cords are peripheral nerves to the shoulder region and upper extremity.
- Injury to the plexus can be partial or complete. Injuries affect all nerves distal to the injury (e.g., Erb's palsy: C5-6).

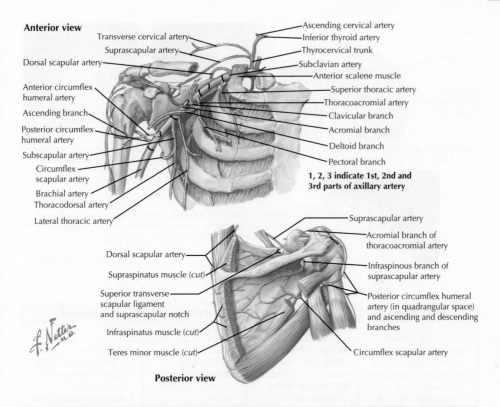

Anterior view

Ascending cervical artery
Transverse cervical artery
Inferior thyroid artery
Suprascapular artery
Thyrocervical trunk
Dorsal scapular artery
Subclavian artery
Anterior scalene muscle
Anterior circumflex humeral artery
Superior thoracic artery
Ascending branch
Thoracoacromial artery
Posterior circumflex humeral artery
Clavicular branch
Acromial branch
Subscapular artery
Deltoid branch
Circumflex scapular artery
Pectoral branch
Brachial artery
Thoracodorsal artery
1, 2, 3 indicate 1st, 2nd and 3rd parts of axillary artery
Lateral thoracic artery

Suprascapular artery
Acromial branch of thoracoacromial artery
Dorsal scapular artery
Supraspinatus muscle (*cut*)
Infraspinous branch of suprascapular artery
Superior transverse scapular ligament and suprascapular notch
Posterior circumflex humeral artery (in quadrangular space) and ascending and descending branches
Infraspinatus muscle (*cut*)
Teres minor muscle (*cut*)
Circumflex scapular artery

Posterior view

COURSE	BRANCHES	COMMENT/SUPPLY
SUBCLAVIAN ARTERY		
Branches off aorta (L) or brachiocephalic trunk (R), b/w anterior & middle scalene muscles with the brachial plexus	Thyrocervical trunk Suprascapular artery Infraspinatus branch Dorsal scapular	3 other branches into the neck Runs over the transverse scapular ligament to rotator cuff muscles Runs around spinoglenoid notch with suprascapular n. Divides around the levator scapulae muscle
AXILLARY ARTERY		
Continuation of subclavian after the 1st rib. Runs through the axilla into the arm, becoming the brachial artery at the lower border of the teres major muscle	I. Superior thoracic II. Thoracoacromial Clavicular branch Acromial branch Deltoid branch *Pectoral* branch Lateral *thoracic* III. Subscapular Circumflex scapular *Thoracodorsal* Anterior circumflex humeral Ascending branch Arcuate artery Posterior circumflex humeral	To serratus anterior and pectoralis muscles Has 4 branches Can be injured in clavicle fractures or surgery With CA ligament, at risk in subacromial decompression With cephalic vein, at risk in deltopectoral approach Runs with lateral *pectoral* nerve Runs with long thoracic nerve to serratus anterior Has 2 main branches Seen posteriorly in triangular space Runs w/*thoracodorsal* nerve. Used for free flap Primary supply of humeral head (via ascending br.) Injury (e.g., anatomic neck fx) leads to osteonecrosis Supplies most of humeral head, also tuberosities Seen in quadrangular space with axillary nerve

The axillary artery is divided into 3 parts by the borders of the pectoralis minor muscle (1st prox., 2nd behind, 3rd distal). The first part (I) has 1 branch, 2nd part (II) has 2 branches, 3rd part (III) has 3 branches.

Adhesive capsulitis

Adhesions of peripheral capsule to distal articular cartilage

Adhesions obliterating axillary fold of capsule

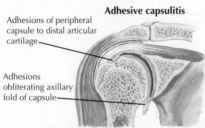

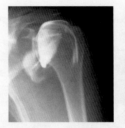

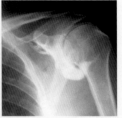

Coronal section of shoulder shows adhesions between capsule and periphery of humeral head

Anteroposterior arthrogram of normal shoulder (left). Axillary fold and biceps brachii sheath visualized. Volume of capsule normal. Anteroposterior arthrogram of frozen shoulder (right). Joint capacity reduced. Axillary fold and biceps brachii sheath not evident.

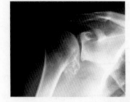

AP radiograph of shoulder demonstrates typical changes of osteoarthritis of the shoulder with narrowing of the joints and prominent osteophyte formation at the inferior aspect of the humeral head.

JOHN A. CRAIG—AD

Glenohumeral arthritis

DESCRIPTION	Hx & PE	WORKUP	TREATMENT
ADHESIVE CAPSULITIS ("FROZEN SHOULDER")			
• Synovial inflammation leads to capsular fibrosis (thickening) & loss of joint space (esp. pouch) • Three stages: pain, stiffness, resolving/"thawing"	**Hx:** Pain, stiffness, +/− PMHx (DM, thyroid dz), trauma, immobilization **PE:** Decreased active AND passive ROM	**XR:** Shoulder series: usually normal **Arthrogram:** shows decreased capsular volume	• Physical therapy (gentle active and passive ROM) and pain management (6+ months) • Arthroscopic lysis of adhesions in refractory cases
ACROMIOCLAVICULAR ARTHROSIS			
• Degeneration of the AC joint • Associated with previous trauma, overuse, rotator cuff disease • Osteolysis in weight-lifters	**Hx:** Pain, +/− grinding **PE:** ACJ TTP, crossbody adduction pain, +/− subtle instability (on palpation)	**XR:** AC narrowing/spurs **MR:** Often not needed; will show edema & degeneration	• Rest, activity modification • Corticosteroid injection • Open vs arthroscopic distal clavicle resection (Mumford)
ARTHRITIS (GLENOHUMERAL)			
• Osteoarthritis #1, also RA • Can be posttraumatic (e.g., fx), 2° to RC tear, or 2° to surgery (e.g., Puddi-Platt)	**Hx:** Usually elderly, pain, stiffness, +/− old trauma **PE:** Decreased ROM, +/− wasting, crepitus	**XR:** Joint narrowing, osteophytes **MR:** For rotator cuff evaluation if indicated	• NSAIDs, physical therapy • Corticosteroid injections • Hemi vs total shoulder arthroplasty
BICEPS TENDINITIS			
• Assoc. w/impingement, RC tear (esp. subscapularis), & tendon subluxation (biceps pulley injury)	**Hx:** Pain, +/− snapping **PE:** Biceps TTP, +Speed & Yergason tests	**XR:** Often normal **MR:** Evaluate for tear	• Physical therapy • Corticosteroid injection • Tenodesis vs tenotomy
BICEPS TENDON RUPTURE (PROXIMAL)			
• Usually in older population • Often degenerative tear • Associated with impingement & RC tears	**Hx:** Pain & deformity **PE:** "Popeye" arm deformity, weak supination	**XR:** Usually normal **MR:** Often not needed, but will show tear	• Physical therapy. Patient often has residual weakness in supination • Consider tenodesis (esp. in younger/active patients)

External impingement

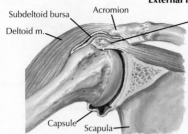

Subdeltoid bursa
Acromion
Deltoid m.
Supraspinatus tendon
Capsule
Scapula

Abduction of arm causes repeated impingement of greater tubercle of humerus on acromion, leading to degeneration and inflammation of supraspinatus tendon, secondary inflammation of bursa, and pain on abduction of arm. Calcific deposit in degenerated tendon produces elevation that further aggravates inflammation and pain.

Rotator cuff tear

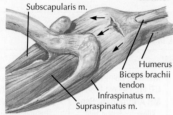

Subscapularis m.

Humerus
Biceps brachii tendon
Infraspinatus m.
Supraspinatus m.

Acute rupture (superior view). Often associated with splitting tear parallel to tendon fibers.

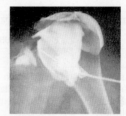

Communication between shoulder joint and subdeltoid bursa is pathognomonic of cuff tear

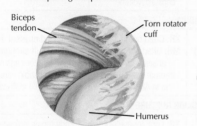

Biceps tendon
Torn rotator cuff

Humerus

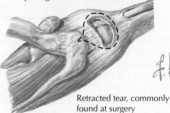

Retracted tear, commonly found at surgery

DESCRIPTION	Hx & PE	WORK-UP	TREATMENT
EXTERNAL (OUTLET) IMPINGEMENT			
• Rotator cuff & bursa trapped b/w acromion & greater tuberosity • Spectrum of disease from bursitis to tendinopathy to partial- to full-thickness RC tear	**Hx:** Pain w/ overhead activities, lifting, etc. **PE:** +Neer sign/test, +Hawkins test. RC: strong +/– painful	**XR:** Outlet view: look for hooked (type 2, 3) acromion or spur **MR:** Best study to evaluate for possible RC tear	• NSAIDs, activity modification • Physical therapy (rotator cuff strengthening) • Subacromial steroid injection • Subacromial decompression
ROTATOR CUFF TEAR			
• Chronic: associated w/impingement (usu. on bursal side) • Acute: in throwers (articular side) or after dislocation (> 40y.o.) • Supraspinatus #1 • Graded by size: <3cm, 3-5cm, >5cm or # of tendons involved	**Hx:** Pain overhead & at night, +/– weakness **PE:** Pain +/– weakness: ∘ SS: FF, + empty can ∘ IS: ER, + hornblower's ∘ Subscap: IR, + lift off, + belly press, incr. ER	**XR:** May show Ca++ of tendon, spurs, or humeral head elevation **MR:** Excellent for cuff tear imaging; contrast shows communication b/w joint & subacromial space	• Activity modification, NSAIDs • PT: ROM, RC strengthening, scapular stabilization • Operative ∘ Partial tear: SA decompression and cuff debridement vs repair ∘ Full tear: RC repair

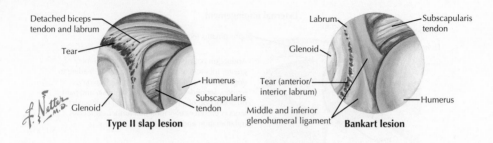

Type II slap lesion

Detached biceps tendon and labrum
Tear
Glenoid
Humerus
Subscapularis tendon

Bankart lesion

Labrum
Glenoid
Tear (anterior-/interior labrum)
Middle and inferior glenohumeral ligament
Subscapularis tendon
Humerus

DESCRIPTION	Hx & PE	WORK-UP	TREATMENT
GLENOHUMERAL INSTABILITY			
"TUBS"			
• Result of a dislocation (**T**rauma) • Most often **U**nilateral • Labral tear (**B**ankart lesion) results from the dislocation • **S**urgery is most often indicated (due to 90% recurrence rate)	**Hx:** Dislocation, pain, & recurrent instability **PE:** + apprehension & relocation, + load & shift (one direction), + jerk (posterior lesion)	**XR:** West point view **CT:** For glenoid lesions **MR Arthrogram:** Sensitive for labral tear; may show increased capsular volume	• Physical therapy (rotator cuff strengthening) & ROM • Bankart (labral) repair with capsular imbrication (open or arthroscopically)
"AMBRI"			
• **A**traumatic (no dislocation) • **M**ultidirectional (ant, inf, post) • **B**ilateral (1 side often worse) • Responds to **R**ehabilitation • **I**nferior capsular shift may help	**Hx:** Pain (from increased joint mobility) **PE:** + load & shift (usu. both ant. & post.), + sulcus sign	**XR:** Often normal **MR:** Often not needed in absence of trauma; labrum normal in AMBRI	• Extended physical therapy (rotator cuff strengthening) • Open inferior capsular shift vs arthroscopic capsular (up to 270°) imbrication
PECTORALIS MAJOR RUPTURE			
• Rare injury, usu. young patients • Most common in weight-lifters • Maximal eccentric contraction	**Hx:** Acute pain **PE:** Axilla deformity, accentuated with adduction	**XR:** Look for avulsion **MR:** Can evaluate for tendon retraction	• Early repair indicated • Late repair controversial • Nonoperative treatment yields adequate results
SCAPULAR WINGING			

• Medial: serratus anterior weakness 2° long thoracic nerve palsy
• Lateral: trapezius weakness 2° spinal accessory (CN11) palsy
	Hx: Weakness
	PE: Winging of scapula observed from back
		XR: Usually normal
		EMG/NCS: Confirm nerve palsy
			• Observation (1-2 years)
			• Refractory cases:
			  Medial: pect. major transfer
			  Lateral: levator scapulae transfer

SUPERIOR LABRAL TEAR (SLAP LESION)			
• Tear of superior labrum (biceps anchor) from ant. to post. • Chronic (with RCT) or acute (load on outstretched arm) • 7 types based on extent of tear	**Hx:** Pain +/− popping, weakness, etc **PE:** + O'Brien's test, + crank test, +/− painful arc of motion	**XR:** Usually normal **MR Arthrogram:** Most sensitive for labral tears	• Rest, activity modification, physical therapy • Superior labral debridement, repair, or biceps tenodesis based on type of lesion (I-VII)
THORACIC OUTLET SYNDROME			
• Compression of neurovascular structure (artery, vein, brachial plexus) in the neck by 1st rib & scalene muscles • Also assoc. w/cervical ribs	**Hx:** Vague sx: pain & numbness/coolness **PE:** + Adson's test, + Wright test, decr. pulses	**XR:** Shoulder: normal C-spine: look for cervical rib **CXR:** r/o lung mass **EMG:** Brachial plexus	• Activity modification • PT & posture training • Rib (esp. cervical rib) or transverse process resection rarely indicated

Sprengel's Deformity

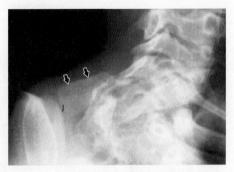

Radiograph shows omovertebral bone (arrows) connecting scapula to spinous processes of cervical vertebrae via osteochondral joint (J)

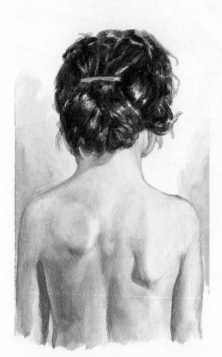

Child with congenital elevation of left scapula. Note shortness of neck on that side and tendency to torticollis

DESCRIPTION	EVALUATION	TREATMENT
SPRENGEL'S DEFORMITY		
• Small (hypoplastic), undescended scapula. Omovertebral bone connects C-spine (spinous process) to scapula • Associated with Klippel-Feil syndrome, scoliosis, kidney disease	**Hx:** Parents notice abnormal neck/scapula **PE:** Neck appears short/full; often decreased ROM (esp. abduction) **XR:** Look for omovertebral bone	• Mild: observation • Symptomatic: omovertebral bone resection, scapula distalization with muscle transfer, +/− clavicle osteotomy to protect brachial plexus

Deltopectoral Approach to Shoulder Joint

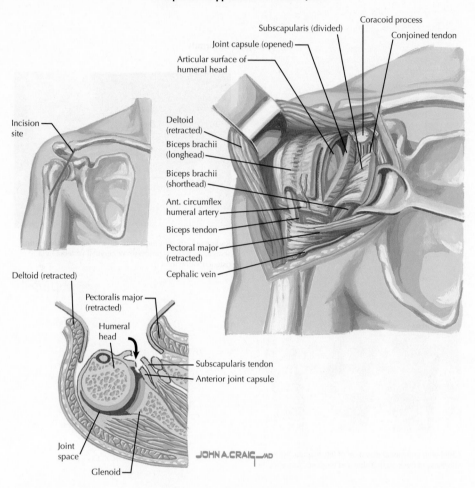

Coracoid process
Conjoined tendon
Subscapularis (divided)
Joint capsule (opened)
Articular surface of humeral head

Incision site

Deltoid (retracted)
Biceps brachii (longhead)
Biceps brachii (shorthead)
Ant. circumflex humeral artery
Biceps tendon
Pectoral major (retracted)
Cephalic vein

Deltoid (retracted)
Pectoralis major (retracted)
Humeral head
Subscapularis tendon
Anterior joint capsule
Joint space
Glenoid

JOHN A. CRAIG—AD

USES	INTERNERVOUS PLANE	DANGERS	COMMENT
ANTERIOR (DELTOPECTORAL) APPROACH			
• Open rotator cuff (esp. subscapularis) or labral repairs • Arthroplasty (hemi vs total) • Proximal humerus fxs	• Deltoid [axillary] • Pectoralis major [lateral & medial pectoral nerves]	• Musculocutaneous n. (with vigorous retraction of conjoined tendon) • Cephalic vein • Axillary nerve	• Subscapularis must be opened and repaired in approach • 3 vessels run along inf. border of subscap.; may need ligation • Adduct/ER protects axillary n.
COMPLICATIONS: Subscapularis rupture; neurapraxia (musculocutaneous or axillary nerve)			

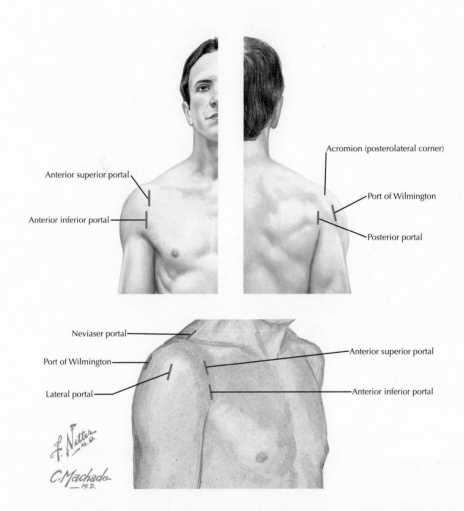

PORTAL	PLACEMENT	DANGERS	COMMENT
ARTHROSCOPY PORTALS			
Posterior	2cm down, 1cm medial to posterolateral corner of acromion (in "soft spot")	Posterior capsule/labrum	Primary viewing portal
Anterior superior	Both anterior portals are b/w the AC joint & lateral coracoid	Coracoacromial ligament and/or artery	Often used for instruments
Anterior inferior	In the rotator interval	Musculocutaneous nerve	Enters just above subscapularis tendon
Lateral	2cm distal to acromial edge	Axillary nerve (5cm distal)	Visualize RC and acromion
Wilmington	1cm ant, 1cm distal to posterolateral acromion corner	Safe portal	Useful in repairs of RC and labrum
Neviaser (supraspinatus)	Posterior to AC joint in sulcus	Rotator cuff	Anterior glenoid view

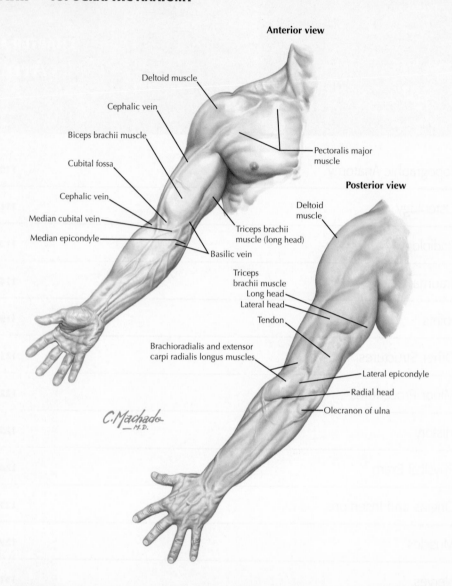

Anterior view

Deltoid muscle

Cephalic vein

Biceps brachii muscle

Cubital fossa

Cephalic vein

Median cubital vein

Median epicondyle

Pectoralis major muscle

Posterior view

Deltoid muscle

Triceps brachii muscle (long head)

Basilic vein

Triceps brachii muscle
Long head
Lateral head

Tendon

Brachioradialis and extensor carpi radialis longus muscles

Lateral epicondyle

Radial head

Olecranon of ulna

C.Machado
—M.D.

STRUCTURE	CLINICAL APPLICATION
Triceps	Can be palpated on the posterior aspect of the arm. A tendon avulsion/rupture can be palpated immediately proximal to the olecranon.
Biceps	Can be palpated on the anterior aspect of the arm.
Cubital fossa	Biceps tendon can be palpated here. If ruptured, the tendon cannot be palpated.
Lateral epicondyle	Site of common extensor origin. Tender in lateral epicondylitis ("tennis elbow")
Medial epicondyle	Site of common flexor origin. Tender in medial epicondylitis ("golfer's elbow")
Olecranon	Proximal tip of ulna. Tenderness can indicate fracture.
Radial head	Proximal end of radius. Tenderness can indicate fracture.

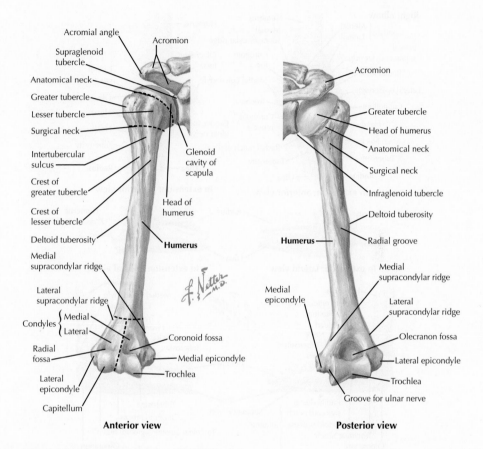

Anterior view   Posterior view

CHARACTERISTICS	OSSIFY		FUSE	COMMENTS
		HUMERUS		
• Cylindrical long bone	**Primary**			• Limited remodeling potential in distal fxs
• Deltoid tuberosity	Shaft	6-7wk (fetal)	Birth	• Deltoid is a deforming force in shaft fractures
• Spiral groove: radial nerve runs in groove	**Secondary**			• Radial nerve can be entrapped in distal ⅓
	Proximal (3):		14-18yr	humeral shaft fractures (Holstein-Lewis fx)
• Lateral condyle	Head	Birth		• Fx of lateral condyle common in pediatrics
∘ Capitellum (articular)	Tuberosities	1-4yr		• Capitellum aligns with radial head on x-ray
∘ Lateral epicondyle	**Distal (4):**		12-17yr	• Lat. epicondyle: origin of extensor mass & LCL
• Medial condyle	Capitellum	1yr		• Supracondylar process present 5%: ligament
∘ Trochlea (articular)	Medial	5yr		of Struthers may entrap median nerve
∘ Medial epicondyle	epicondyle			• Med. epicondyle: origin of flexor mass & MCL
∘ Cubital tunnel	Trochlea	7yr		• Ulnar nerve runs post. to medial epicondyle
• Olecranon and coronoid fossae	Lateral epicondyle	11yr		• Fossae filled with fat; can be displaced in fx, resulting in "fat pad" on x-ray

Elbow ossification order mnemonic: **C**aptain [capitellum] **R**oy [radial head] **M**akes [medial epicondyle] **T**rouble [trochlea] **O**n [olecranon] **L**eave [lateral epicondyle]; can be used to determine approximate age of patient.

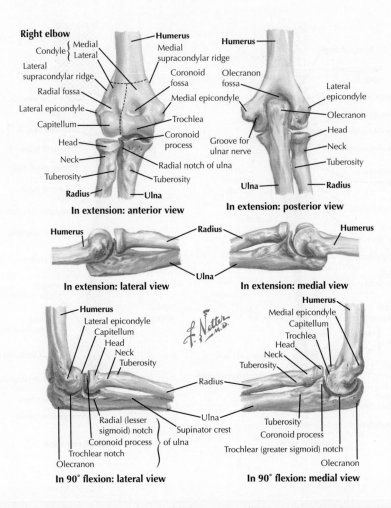

Right elbow

In extension: anterior view

In extension: posterior view

In extension: lateral view

In extension: medial view

In 90° flexion: lateral view

In 90° flexion: medial view

CHARACTERISTICS	OSSIFY		FUSE	COMMENTS
PROXIMAL RADIUS				
• Radial head & physis are intraarticular	**Secondary** Head	2-3yr	16-18yr	• Anterolateral portion of radial head has less subchondral bone & is most susceptible to fracture
• Radial neck: 10-15° angulated				• Radial head should always align with the capitellum
• Tuberosity: biceps insertion				• Tuberosity points ulnarly in supination
PROXIMAL ULNA				
• Olecranon	**Secondary** Olecranon	9yr	16-20yr	• Articulates with trochlea, part of greater notch
• Coronoid process				• Coronoid provides anterior stability & MCL insertion
• Supinator crest				• Lateral ulnar collateral ligament (LUCL) inserts on supinator crest
• Ulnar tuberosity				• Brachialis inserts on ulnar tuberosity
• Greater sigmoid notch				• Greater sigmoid notch: olecranon & coronoid
• Lesser sigmoid notch				• Lesser sigmoid (radial) notch: articulates with RH

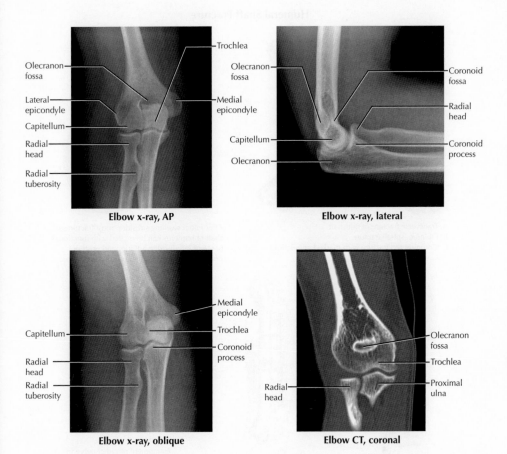

Elbow x-ray, AP

Olecranon fossa
Lateral epicondyle
Capitellum
Radial head
Radial tuberosity
Trochlea

Elbow x-ray, lateral

Olecranon fossa
Medial epicondyle
Capitellum
Olecranon
Coronoid fossa
Radial head
Coronoid process

Elbow x-ray, oblique

Capitellum
Radial head
Radial tuberosity
Medial epicondyle
Trochlea
Coronoid process

Elbow CT, coronal

Radial head
Olecranon fossa
Trochlea
Proximal ulna

RADIOGRAPH	TECHNIQUE	FINDINGS	CLINICAL APPLICATION
Anteroposterior	Elbow extended, beam perpendicular to plate	Elbow joint, distal humerus, proximal radius and ulna	Fractures, dislocations, arthritis/DJD, supracondylar process
Lateral	Elbow flexed 90°, beam from lateral to radial head	Elbow joint, fat pads (fat is displaced by fracture hematoma)	Fractures (esp. peds: fat pads, anterior humeral line), DJD (osteophytes)
Oblique	Elbow extended, rotated 30°	Alignment & position of bones	Subtle fx (radial head, occult fx)
Radiocapitellar	Lateral, beam 45° to elbow	Isolates capitellum/radial head	Fx: radial head, capitellum, coronoid
OTHER STUDIES			
CT	Axial, coronal, and sagittal	Articular congruity, bone healing, bone alignment	Fractures (esp. coronoid, comminuted intraarticular fx)
MR	Sequence protocols vary	Soft tissues (ligaments, tendons, cartilage), bones	Ligament (e.g., MCL) & tendon (e.g., biceps) rupture, OCD
Bone scan		All bones evaluated	Infection, stress fractures, tumors

Humeral Shaft Fracture

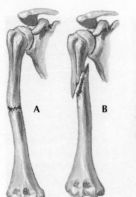
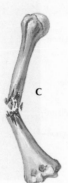
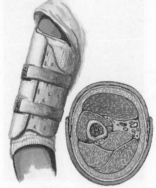

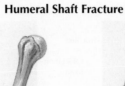

A. Transverse fracture of midshaft
B. Oblique (spiral) fracture
C. Comminuted fracture with marked angulation

After initial swelling subsides, most fractures of shaft of humerus can be treated with functional brace of interlocking anterior and posterior components held together with Velcro straps.

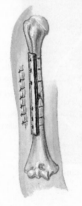
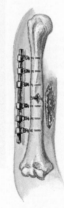
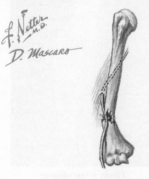

Open reduction and fixation with compression plate indicated under special conditions.

Fracture aligned and held with external fixator. Most useful for wounds requiring frequent changes of dressing.

Entrapment of radial nerve in fracture of shaft of distal humerus may occur at time of fracture; must also be avoided during reduction.

DESCRIPTION	EVALUATION	CLASSIFICATION	TREATMENT
HUMERUS SHAFT FRACTURE			
• Common long bone fracture • Mechanism: fall or direct blow • Displacement based on fracture location and muscle insertion sites. Pectoralis and deltoid are primary deforming forces. • High union rates • Site of pathologic fractures	**Hx:** Trauma/fall, pain and swelling **PE:** Swelling +/− deformity, humerus is TTP. Good neuro. exam (esp. radial n.) **XR:** AP & lateral of arm (also shoulder & elbow series) **CT:** Not usually needed	Descriptive: • Location: site of fracture • Displaced, angulated, or comminuted • Pattern: transverse, spiral, oblique	• Cast/brace: minimally displaced/acceptable alignment • Acceptable: <3cm shortening <20° A/P angulation <30° varus/valgus angulation • Surgical treatment: open fx, floating elbow, segmental fx, polytrauma, vascular injury • Options: ORIF, external fixation, IM nail
COMPLICATIONS: Radial nerve palsy (esp. distal ⅓ fractures [Holstein-Lewis]): most are neurapraxia and resolve spontaneously; nerve exploration is controversial; nonunion/malunion are uncommon.			

Distal Humerus Fracture

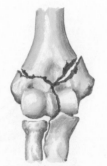

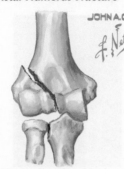

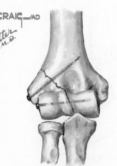

Intercondylar (T or Y) fracture of distal humerus

Fracture of lateral condyle of humerus. Fracture of medial condyle less common

Fractured condyle fixed with one or two compression screws

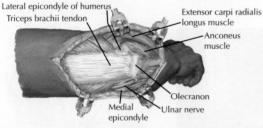

Lateral epicondyle of humerus

Triceps brachii tendon

Extensor carpi radialis longus muscle

Anconeus muscle

Olecranon

Medial epicondyle

Ulnar nerve

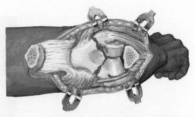

Open (transolecranon) repair. Posterior incision skirts medial margin of olecranon, exposing triceps brachii tendon and olecranon. Ulnar nerve identified on posterior surface of medial epicondyle. Incisions made along each side of olecranon and triceps brachii tendon

Olecranon osteotomized and reflected proximally with triceps brachii tendon

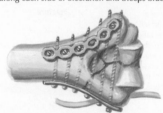

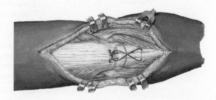

Articular surface of distal humerus reconstructed and fixed with transverse screw and buttress plates with screws. Ulnar nerve may be transposed anteriorly to prevent injury. Lateral column fixed with posterior plate and medial column fixed with plate on the medial ridge.

Olecranon reattached with longitudinal Kirschner wires and tension band wire wrapped around them and through hole drilled in ulna

DESCRIPTION	EVALUATION	CLASSIFICATION	TREATMENT
DISTAL HUMERUS FRACTURE			
• Most often intraarticular (adults); extraarticular (supracondylar) fx uncommon in adults • Mechanism: fall • Unicondylar or bicondylar • Other: epicondyle, capitellum, trochlea fxs all less common	**Hx:** Trauma/fall, pain, esp. w/ elbow ROM (decreased) **PE:** Swelling & tenderness Good neurovascular exam **XR:** Elbow series **CT:** Essential for complete evaluation of fracture/joint	Descriptive: • Uni or bicondylar • T, Y, λ type • Displaced, angulated comminuted (esp. coronal split)	• Nonoperative: rarely indicated • Surgical: ORIF (plates & screws) • Ulnar nerve often needs to be transposed anteriorly • Early ROM is important • Total elbow arthroplasty: if fx is too comminuted for ORIF
COMPLICATIONS: Elbow stiffness, heterotopic ossification (prophylaxis is indicated), ulnar nerve palsy, nonunion			

Supracondylar Fractures

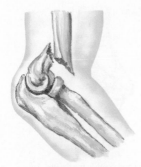

Extension type
Posterior displacement of distal fragment (most common)

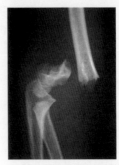

Lateral radiograph

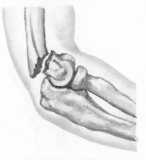

Flexion type
Anterior displacement of distal fragment (uncommon)

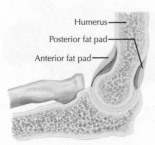

Humerus
Posterior fat pad
Anterior fat pad

Normal

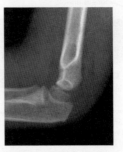

Lateral radiograph of elbow in a 5-year-old sustaining injury to left elbow. Radiograph shows elevation of anterior and posterior fat pads. No apparent fracture on this view, but subsequent radiographs confirmed presence of a nondisplaced supracondylar humerus fracture.

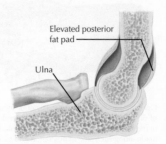

Elevated posterior fat pad
Ulna

Fracture

DESCRIPTION	EVALUATION	CLASSIFICATION	TREATMENT
SUPRACONDYLAR HUMERUS FRACTURE			

• Common pediatric fracture
• Extraphyseal fx at thin portion of bone (1mm) between distal humeral fossae
• Extension type most common
• Malreduction leads to deformity: cubitus varus is most common
• Relatively high incidence of neurovascular injury
	Hx: Fall, pain, will not move arm, +/− deformity
	PE: Swelling +/− deformity. Good neurovascular exam (esp. AIN, radial n., pulses)
	XR: Elbow series. Lateral view: anterior humeral line is anterior to capitellum center in displaced fxs. Posterior fat pad indicates fx.
		• Extension type (Gartland)
		  ∘ I: Nondisplaced
		  ∘ II: Partially displaced (post. cortex intact)
		  ∘ III: Displaced (no cortical continuity)
		• Flexion type (uncommon)
			• Type I: Long arm cast
			• Types II & III: Closed reduction & percutaneous pinning, 2 or 3 pins (crossed or divergent) Medial pins can injure ulnar nerve
			• Open reduction for irreducible fractures (uncommon)
			• Explore pulseless/ unperfused extremity for artery entrapment

COMPLICATIONS: Malunion (cubitus varus #1); neurovascular (median nerve/AIN #1, radial nerve, brachial artery)			

Olecranon fracture

Displaced fracture of olecranon requires open reduction and internal fixation

Open reduction of olecranon fracture. Fracture secured with two Kirschner wires plus tension band wire passed around bent ends of Kirschner wires and through drill

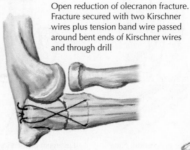

Fracture of head and neck of radius

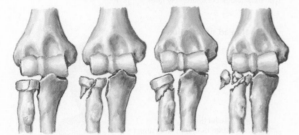

Type I: nondisplaced or minimally displaced.

Type II: displaced single fragment (usually >2 mm) of the head or angulated (usually >30°) of the neck.

Type III: severely comminuted fractures of the radial head and neck.

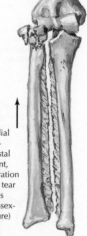

Comminuted fracture of radial head with dislocation of distal radioulnar joint, proximal migration of radius, and tear of interosseous membrane (Essex-Lopresti fracture)

DESCRIPTION	EVALUATION	CLASSIFICATION	TREATMENT
OLECRANON FRACTURE			

• Mechanism: fall directly onto elbow or onto hand
• Intraarticular fracture: congruity important for good results
• Triceps tendon is a deforming force on proximal fragment
	Hx: Trauma (usually fall), pain and swelling
	PE: Tenderness, limited elbow extension. Neuro exam, esp. ulnar nerve
	XR: Elbow series
	CT: Better defines fracture
		Colton:
		• I. Nondisplaced: <2mm
		• II. Displaced
		  ○ Avulsion
		  ○ Transverse/oblique
		  ○ Comminuted
		  ○ Displaced fx-dx
			• Nondisplaced: Long arm cast 3 weeks, then gentle ROM
			• Displaced:
			  ○ Transverse: ORIF tension band or IM screw.
			  ○ Oblique/comminuted: ORIF with contoured plate
			• Excise & reattach tendon

COMPLICATIONS: Painful hardware, elbow stiffness, nonunion, arthritis (posttraumatic), ulnar nerve injury			
RADIAL HEAD FRACTURE			
• Mechanism: fall onto hand • Intraarticular fracture: anterolateral portion is weaker and is most common fracture site • Essex-Lopresti: RH fx w/ disruption of IM membrane & DRUJ • Associated w/ elbow dislocation	**Hx:** Trauma/fall, pain **PE:** Decreased motion (esp. pronosupination) Check DRUJ stability **XR:** Elbow series; radio-capitellar view is helpful, +/− fat pad sign **CT:** Useful in types II-IV	Mason: 4 types • I: Nondisplaced (<2mm) • II: Single displaced fragment • III: Comminuted • IV: Fracture with elbow dislocation	• Type I: Elbow aspiration, sling for 3 days, early ROM • Type II: ORIF (esp. for mechanical block to motion) • Type III: Radial head excision and/or RH arthroplasty • Essex-Lopresti: radial head arthroplasty is required
COMPLICATIONS: Elbow stiffness or instability; Wrist instability (Essex-Lopresti)			

Elbow dislocation

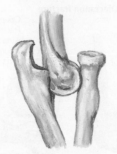

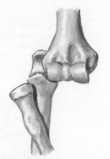

Posterior dislocation. Note prominence of olecranon posteriorly and distal humerus anteriorly.

Divergent dislocation, anterior-posterior type (rare). Medial-lateral type may also occur (extremely rare).

Lateral dislocation (uncommon)

Radial head subluxation

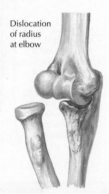

Dislocation of radius at elbow

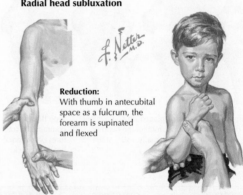

Reduction:
With thumb in antecubital space as a fulcrum, the forearm is supinated and flexed

DESCRIPTION	EVALUATION	CLASSIFICATION	TREATMENT
ELBOW DISLOCATION			

• Mechanism: usually a fall in young patient
 • #3 most common dislocation
 • Associated with fractures: "Terrible triad" = elbow dx with radial head & coronoid fractures
 • Collateral ligaments & anterior capsule are typically all torn
	Hx: Trauma/fall, inability to move elbow
	 PE: Swelling, deformity, limited/no elbow ROM Good neurovasc. exam
	 XR: Elbow series
	 CT: To define associated fractures
		By direction of forearm bones:
		 • Posterior
		   ○ Posterolateral (>80%)
		 • Medial
		 • Lateral (rare)
		 • Anterior (rare)
		 • Divergent (rare)
			• Acute: closed reduction
			   ○ Stable: splint for 7-10d
			   ○ Unstable: splint for 2-3wk
			 • Open reduction for irreducible dxs and/or ORIF fxs
			 • Hinged external fixation for grossly unstable elbows

COMPLICATIONS: Elbow stiffness and instability, neurovascular injury (median and ulnar nerves, brachial artery)			
RADIAL HEAD SUBLUXATION (NURSEMAID'S ELBOW)			
• Mechanism: usually a pull on the hand by an adult • Very common in toddlers • Decreased with increasing age • Annular ligament stretches & radial head subluxates	**Hx:** Child pulled by hand, child will not use arm **PE:** Elbow flexed, pronated. RH tender **XR:** Elbow series; normal, often not needed	None	• Closed reduction: fully extend elbow, fully supinate, then flex with gentle pressure on radial head. Usually a click or pop is felt as it reduces. • Immobilization rarely indicated
COMPLICATIONS: Recurrence			

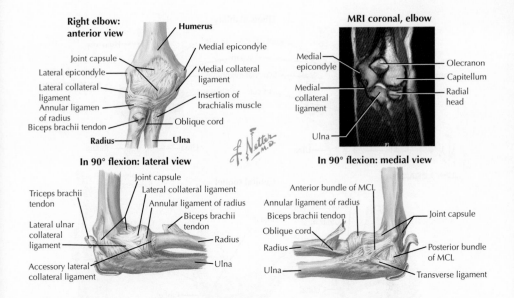

Right elbow: anterior view

MRI coronal, elbow

In 90° flexion: lateral view

In 90° flexion: medial view

LIGAMENTS	ATTACHMENTS	COMMENTS
ELBOW		
• The elbow comprises three articulations: 1. Ulnohumeral (trochlea and greater sigmoid notch): Ginglymus (hinge) joint 2. Radiocapitellar (radial head and capitellum): Trochoid (pivot) joint 3. Proximal radioulnar (radial head and lesser sigmoid notch) • Primary function is as a lever for lifting and placing the hand appropriately in space • Two primary motions: 1. Flexion and extension: 0-150° (functional ROM: 100° [30-130°]); axis is the trochlea 2. Pronosupination: 70° pro. – 80° sup. (functional ROM: 100° [50° pro. – 50° sup.]); axis is RC joint • Stability provided by combination of osseous (articulations) and ligamentous restraints; carrying angle 11-16° valgus		
Medial (Ulnar) Collateral (MCL)		
Anterior bundle	Inf. medial epicondyle to medial coronoid process ("sublime tubercle")	Most important restraint to valgus stress, always taut; usually ruptures off coronoid
Posterior bundle	Medial epicondyle to sigmoid notch	Taut in/resists valgus in flexion (>90º)
Transverse bundle	Med. olecranon to inf. medial coronoid	Stabilizes the greater sigmoid notch
Lateral (Radial) Collateral (LCL)		
Lateral collateral (LCL)	Lat. epicondyle to ant. annular lig.	Varus restraint; stabilizes annular ligament
Lateral ulnar collateral (LUCL)	Lateral epicondyle to supinator crest of the ulna	Buttress to radial head subluxation; injury results in posterolateral rotatory instability
Accessory lateral collateral	Annular ligament to supinator crest	Stabilizes annular ligament during varus stress
Annular ligament	Anterior and posterior portions of sigmoid notch	Allows radial head rotation; stretched or torn in radial head subluxation or dislocation
Other		
Capsule	Surrounds joint	Secondary stabilizer, prone to contracture
Quadrate ligament	Anterolateral ulna to anterior radial neck (under the annular ligament)	Tight in supination, stabilizes the proximal radioulnar joint (PRUJ)
Oblique cord	Proximal lateral ulna to radial neck	Stabilizes joint during pronosupination

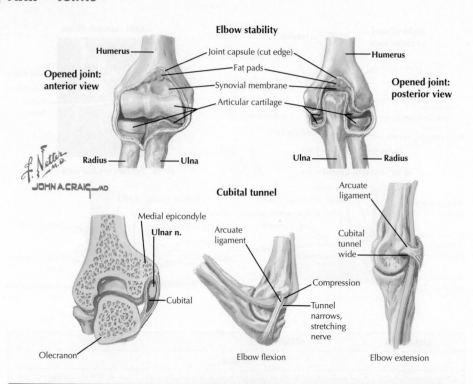

Elbow stability

Opened joint: anterior view

Humerus — Joint capsule (cut edge)
Fat pads
Synovial membrane —
Articular cartilage

Humerus

Opened joint: posterior view

Radius — Ulna — Ulna — Radius

Cubital tunnel

Medial epicondyle
Ulnar n.

Arcuate ligament

Cubital

Olecranon

Elbow flexion

Arcuate ligament

Cubital tunnel wide —

Compression

Tunnel narrows, stretching nerve

Elbow extension

ELBOW STABILITY	
Primary Stabilizers	
Ulnohumeral articulation	Primary restraint to valgus <20° or >120° of flexion
	Primary restraint to varus in extension (2° in flexion)
Medial collateral ligament (MCL) (esp. anterior bundle)	Primary restraint to valgus between 20-120° of flexion
	Anterior bundle is always taut, post. bundle taut >90°
Lateral collateral ligament (LCL) (esp. LUCL)	Primary restraint to varus in flexion (2° in extension)
	LUCL prevents subluxation of radial head (e.g., PLRI)
Secondary Stabilizers	
Radiocapitellar articulation (radial head)	Restraint to valgus from 0-30° of flexion
Anterior and posterior capsule	Restraint to both varus and valgus stress
Common flexor and extensor origins	Dynamic forces act to restrain both varus and valgus stress

STRUCTURE	COMPONENTS	COMMENTS
CUBITAL TUNNEL		
Borders	• Roof: Arcuate (Osborne's) ligament From med. epicondyle to olecranon	• Tightens in flexion, compresses ulnar nerve within cubital tunnel
	• Floor: Medial collateral ligament (MCL)	• Can be injured in decompression surgery
	• Posterior: Medial head of the triceps	• Does not typically compress the nerve
	• Anterior: Medial epicondyle	• Medial epicondylectomy occasionally indicated
	• Lateral: Olecranon	• Does not compress nerve
Contents	• Nerve: Ulnar nerve	• Compressed in cubital tunnel syndrome

• Fractures (malunion) of the medial condyle can cause ulnar nerve entrapment in the cubital tunnel.
• Arcuate ligament is also known as Osborne's ligament/fascia and the cubital tunnel retinaculum.
• See Forearm chapter for radial tunnel.

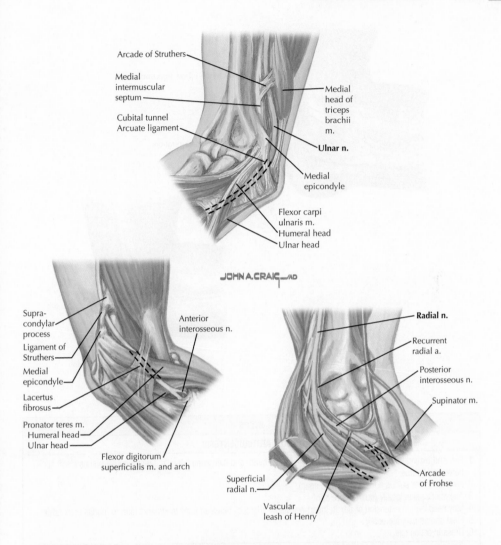

Arcade of Struthers

Medial intermuscular septum

Cubital tunnel
Arcuate ligament

Medial head of triceps brachii m.

Ulnar n.

Medial epicondyle

Flexor carpi ulnaris m.
Humeral head
Ulnar head

JOHN A.CRAIG—AD

Supra-condylar process

Ligament of Struthers

Medial epicondyle

Lacertus fibrosus

Pronator teres m.
Humeral head
Ulnar head

Flexor digitorum superficialis m. and arch

Anterior interosseous n.

Radial n.

Recurrent radial a.

Posterior interosseous n.

Supinator m.

Arcade of Frohse

Superficial radial n.

Vascular leash of Henry

STRUCTURE	DESCRIPTION	COMMENTS
OTHER STRUCTURES		
Fat pads	Located in both the coronoid and olecranon fossae, engaged in full flexion or extension	Can be displaced by fracture hematoma and seen on x-ray as a lucency ("sail sign")
Olecranon bursa	At the tip of the olecranon process	Can become inflamed or infected
Ligament of Struthers	A fibrous band running from an anomalous supracondylar process to medial epicondyle	Can compress the median nerve proximally
Biceps aponeurosis (lacertus fibrosus)	Fascial band from distal biceps and tendon that runs to deep forearm fascia	Covers median nerve and brachial artery and can compress median nerve
Arcade of Struthers	Thickened fascia from IM septum to triceps (medial head), 8cm proximal to epicondyle	Occurs in 70% of population; can compress ulnar nerve proximal to cubital tunnel
Leash of Henry	Branches of recurrent radial artery	Can compress radial nerve/PIN

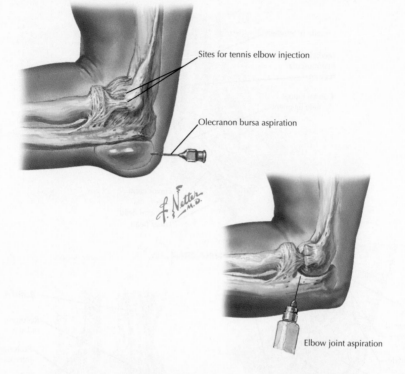

Sites for tennis elbow injection

Olecranon bursa aspiration

Elbow joint aspiration

STEPS
ELBOW ARTHROCENTESIS
1. Flex and extend elbow, palpate lateral condyle, radial head, and olecranon laterally; feel triangular sulcus ("soft spot") between all three
2. Prep skin over sulcus (iodine/antiseptic soap)
3. Anesthetize skin locally (quarter size spot)
4. May keep arm in extension or flex it. Insert needle in "triangle" between bony landmarks (aim to medial epicondyle)
5. Fluid should aspirate easily
6. Dress injection site
OLECRANON BURSA ASPIRATION
1. Prep skin over olecranon (iodine/antiseptic soap)
2. Anesthetize skin locally (quarter size spot)
3. Insert 18-gauge needle into fluctuant portion of the bursa and aspirate fluid
4. If suspicious of infection, send fluid for Gram stain and culture
5. Dress injection site
TENNIS ELBOW INJECTION
1. Ask patient about allergies
2. Flex elbow 90°, palpate ECRB insertion (point of maximal tenderness) on the lateral epicondyle
3. Prep skin over lateral elbow (iodine/antiseptic soap)
4. Anesthetize skin locally (quarter size spot)
5. Insert 22-gauge or smaller needle into ERCB tendon at its insertion on the lateral epicondyle. Aspirate to ensure needle is not in a vessel, then inject 2-3ml of 1:1 local/corticosteroid preparation (fan out injection in broad tendon).
6. Dress insertion site
7. Annotate improvement in symptoms

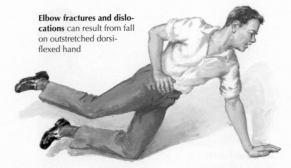

Elbow fractures and dislocations can result from fall on outstretched dorsiflexed hand

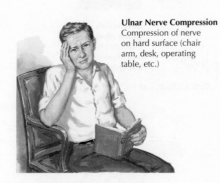

Ulnar Nerve Compression
Compression of nerve on hard surface (chair arm, desk, operating table, etc.)

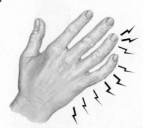

Numbness and tingling in ulnar nerve distribution in hand. Interosseous wasting between thumb and index finger

QUESTION	ANSWER	CLINICAL APPLICATION
1. Age	Young	Dislocation, fracture
	Middle aged, elderly	Tennis elbow (epicondylitis), nerve compression, arthritis
2. Pain		
a. Onset	Acute	Dislocation, fracture, tendon avulsion/rupture, ligament injury
	Chronic	Arthritis, cervical spine pathology
b. Location	Anterior	Biceps tendon rupture, arthritis, elbow contracture
	Posterior	Olecranon bursitis (inflammatory or septic)
	Lateral	Lateral epicondylitis, fracture (especially radial head)
	Medial	Medial epicondylitis, nerve entrapment, fracture, MCL strain
	Night pain/at rest	Infection, tumor
c. Occurrence	With activity	Ligamentous and/or tendinous etiology
3. Stiffness	Without locking	Arthritis, effusions (trauma), contracture
	With locking	Loose body, lateral collateral ligament injury
4. Swelling	Over olecranon	Olecranon bursitis. Other: dislocation, fracture, gout
5. Trauma	Fall on elbow, hand	Dislocation, fracture
6. Activity	Sports, repetitive motion	Epicondylitis, ulnar nerve palsy
	Throwing	MCL strain or rupture
7. Neurologic symptoms	Pain, numbness, tingling	Nerve entrapments (multiple possible sites), cervical spine pathology, thoracic outlet syndrome
8. History of arthritides	Multiple joints involved	Lupus, rheumatoid arthritis, psoriasis, gout

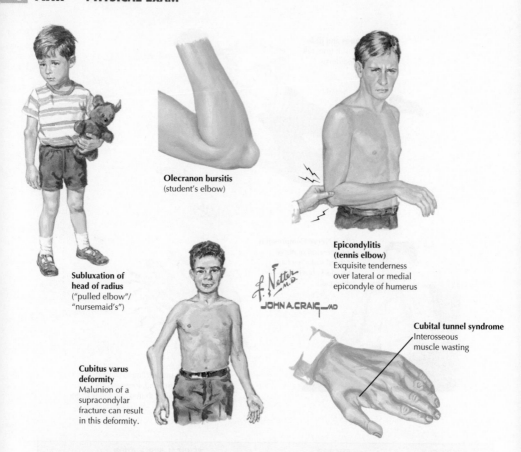

Olecranon bursitis
(student's elbow)

Subluxation of
head of radius
("pulled elbow"/
"nursemaid's")

Cubitus varus
deformity
Malunion of a
supracondylar
fracture can result
in this deformity.

Epicondylitis
(tennis elbow)
Exquisite tenderness
over lateral or medial
epicondyle of humerus

Cubital tunnel syndrome
Interosseous
muscle wasting

EXAM/OBSERVATION	TECHNIQUE	CLINICAL APPLICATION
INSPECTION		
Unwilling to use arm	Observe patient (child)	Fracture, dislocation, radial head subluxation (nursemaid's elbow)
Gross deformity, swelling	Compare both sides	Dislocation, fracture, bursitis
Carrying angle (normal 5-15°)	Negative (<5°) Positive (>15°)	Cubitus varus (e.g., supracondylar fracture) Cubitus valgus (e.g., lateral epicondyle fracture)
Muscle wasting	Inspect hand muscles	Nerve entrapment (e.g., cubital tunnel syndrome)
PALPATION		
Medial	Epicondyle and supracondylar line Ulnar nerve in ulnar groove	Pain: medial epicondylitis (golfer's elbow), fracture, MCL rupture/strain Paresthesias indicate ulnar nerve entrapment
Lateral	Epicondyle and supracondylar line Radial head	Pain: lateral epicondylitis (tennis elbow), fracture Pain: arthritis, fracture, synovitis
Anterior	Biceps tendon in antecubital fossa	Pain: absence of tendon indicates biceps tendon rupture
Posterior	Flex elbow: olecranon, olecranon fossa, triceps tendon	Olecranon bursitis, triceps tendon rupture

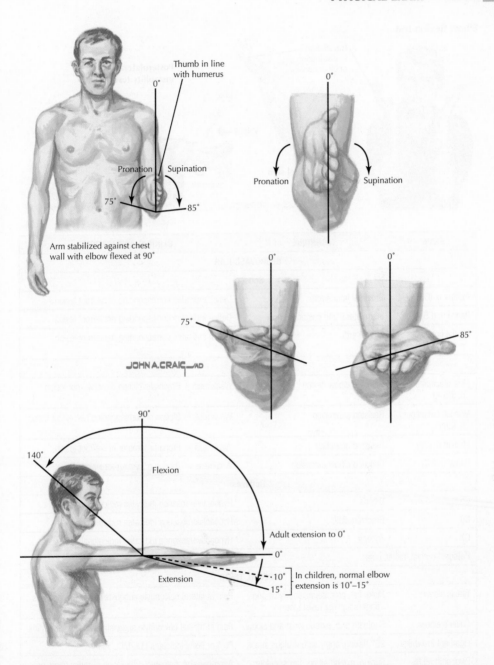

Thumb in line with humerus

0°

Pronation | Supination

75° | 85°

Arm stabilized against chest wall with elbow flexed at 90°

0°

Pronation | Supination

0° | 0°

75° | 85°

JOHN A.CRAIG—MD

90°

140°

Flexion

0°

Adult extension to 0°

Extension

10°
15°

In children, normal elbow extension is 10°–15°

EXAM/OBSERVATION	TECHNIQUE	CLINICAL APPLICATION
RANGE OF MOTION		
Flex and extend	Elbow at side: flex and extend at elbow	Normal: 0° to 140-150°; note if PROM >AROM
Pronate and supinate	Tuck elbows, thumbs up, rotate forearm	Normal: supinate 80-85°, pronate 75-80°

Elbow flexion test

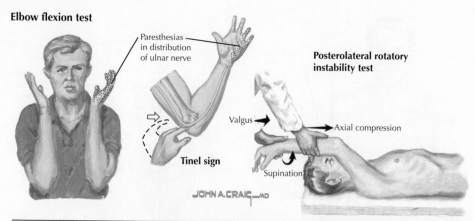

Paresthesias in distribution of ulnar nerve

Tinel sign

Valgus

Posterolateral rotatory instability test

Axial compression

Supination

JOHN A.CRAIG—AD

EXAM	TECHNIQUE	CLINICAL APPLICATION
NEUROVASCULAR		
Sensory		
Axillary n. (C5)	Proximal lateral arm	Deficit indicates corresponding nerve/root lesion
Radial n. (C5)	Inferolateral and posterior arm	Deficit indicates corresponding nerve/root lesion
Medial cutaneous n. of arm (T1)	Medial arm	Deficit indicates corresponding nerve/root lesion
Motor		
Musculocutaneous n. (C5-6)	Resisted elbow flexion	Weakness = Brachialis/biceps or nerve/root lesion
Musculocutaneous n. (C6)	Resisted supination	Weakness = Biceps or corresponding nerve/root lesion
Median n. (C6)	Resisted pronation	Weakness = Pronator teres or nerve/root lesion
Radial n. (C7)	Resisted elbow extension	Weakness = Triceps or nerve/root lesion
Reflexes		
C5	Biceps	Hypoactive/absence indicates radiculopathy
C6	Brachioradialis	Hypoactive/absence indicates radiculopathy
C7	Triceps	Hypoactive/absence indicates radiculopathy
Pulses: brachial, radial, ulnar		
SPECIAL TESTS		
Tennis elbow	Make fist, pronate, extend wrist and fingers against resistance	Pain at lateral epicondyle suggests lateral epicondylitis
Golfer's elbow	Supinate arm, extend wrist and elbow	Pain at medial epicondyle suggests medial epicondylitis
Ligament instability	25° flexion, apply varus/valgus stress	Pain or laxity indicates LCL/MCL injury
Pivot shift (PLRI)	Supine, extend elbow, flex shoulder above head. Supinate, axial load, valgus and flex elbow	Apprehension, palpable subluxation of radial head, or dimpling of skin over radial head positive test for posterolateral rotatory instability (PLRI)
Tinel's sign	Tap on ulnar groove (nerve)	Tingling in ulnar distribution indicates entrapment
Elbow flexion	Maximal elbow flexion for 3 min	Tingling in ulnar distribution indicates entrapment
Pinch grip	Pinch tips of thumb and index finger	Inability (or pinching of pads, not tips): AIN pathology

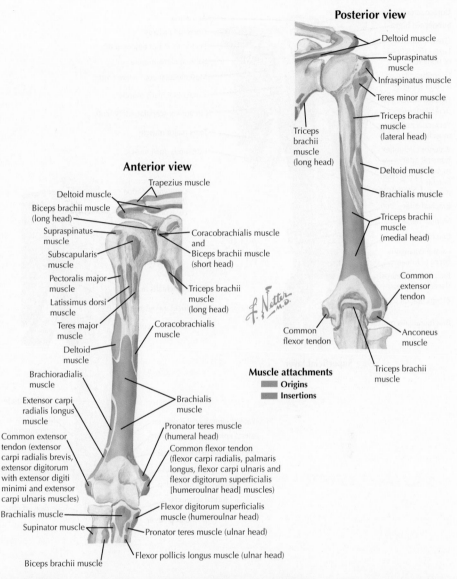

Posterior view

Deltoid muscle

Supraspinatus muscle

Infraspinatus muscle

Teres minor muscle

Triceps brachii muscle (lateral head)

Triceps brachii muscle (long head)

Deltoid muscle

Brachialis muscle

Triceps brachii muscle (medial head)

Common extensor tendon

Common flexor tendon

Anconeus muscle

Triceps brachii muscle

Muscle attachments
- ■ Origins
- ■ Insertions

Anterior view

Trapezius muscle

Deltoid muscle

Biceps brachii muscle (long head)

Supraspinatus muscle

Subscapularis muscle

Pectoralis major muscle

Latissimus dorsi muscle

Teres major muscle

Deltoid muscle

Brachioradialis muscle

Extensor carpi radialis longus muscle

Common extensor tendon (extensor carpi radialis brevis, extensor digitorum with extensor digiti minimi and extensor carpi ulnaris muscles)

Brachialis muscle

Supinator muscle

Biceps brachii muscle

Coracobrachialis muscle and Biceps brachii muscle (short head)

Triceps brachii muscle (long head)

Coracobrachialis muscle

Brachialis muscle

Pronator teres muscle (humeral head)

Common flexor tendon (flexor carpi radialis, palmaris longus, flexor carpi ulnaris and flexor digitorum superficialis [humeroulnar head] muscles)

Flexor digitorum superficialis muscle (humeroulnar head)

Pronator teres muscle (ulnar head)

Flexor pollicis longus muscle (ulnar head)

CORACOID PROCESS	GREATER TUBEROSITY	ANTERIOR PROXIMAL HUMERUS	MEDIAL EPICONDYLE	LATERAL EPICONDYLE
ORIGINS				
Biceps (SH) Coracobrachialis			Pronator teres Common flex. tendon (FCR, PL, FCU, FDS)	Anconeus Common extensor tendon (ECRB, EDC, EDQ, ECU)
INSERTIONS				
Pectoralis minor	Supraspinatus Infraspinatus Teres minor	Pectoralis major Latissimus dorsi Teres major		

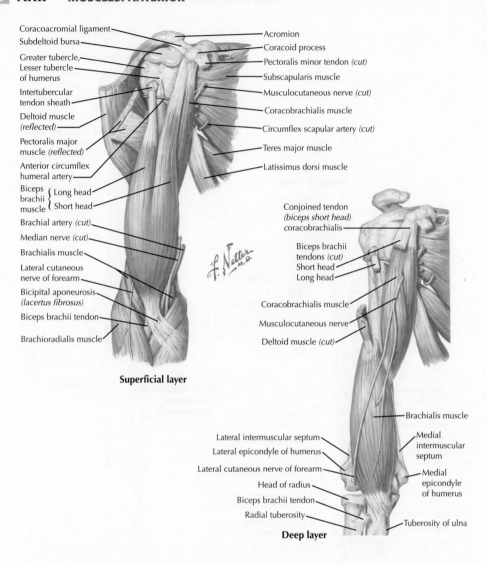

Coracoacromial ligament
Subdeltoid bursa
Greater tubercle,
Lesser tubercle
of humerus
Intertubercular
tendon sheath
Deltoid muscle
(reflected)
Pectoralis major
muscle (reflected)
Anterior circumflex
humeral artery
Biceps { Long head
brachii
muscle { Short head
Brachial artery (cut)
Median nerve (cut)
Brachialis muscle
Lateral cutaneous
nerve of forearm
Bicipital aponeurosis
(lacertus fibrosus)
Biceps brachii tendon
Brachioradialis muscle

Acromion
Coracoid process
Pectoralis minor tendon (cut)
Subscapularis muscle
Musculocutaneous nerve (cut)
Coracobrachialis muscle
Circumflex scapular artery (cut)
Teres major muscle
Latissimus dorsi muscle

Conjoined tendon
(biceps short head)
coracobrachialis

Biceps brachii
tendons (cut)
Short head
Long head

Coracobrachialis muscle

Musculocutaneous nerve

Deltoid muscle (cut)

Superficial layer

Brachialis muscle
Medial
intermuscular
septum
Medial
epicondyle
of humerus

Lateral intermuscular septum
Lateral epicondyle of humerus
Lateral cutaneous nerve of forearm
Head of radius
Biceps brachii tendon
Radial tuberosity

Tuberosity of ulna

Deep layer

MUSCLE	ORIGIN	INSERTION	NERVE	ACTION	COMMENT
Coracobrachialis	Coracoid process	Middle humerus	Musculocutaneous	Flex and adduct arm	Part of "conjoined" tendon
Brachialis	Distal anterior humerus	Ulnar tuberosity (proximal ulna)	Medial: MSC n. Lateral: Radial n.	Flex forearm	Split in anterior surgical approach
Biceps brachii					
Long head	Supraglenoid tubercle	Radial tuberosity (proximal radius)	Musculocutaneous	Supinate and flex forearm	Rupture, results in "Popeye arm"
Short head	Coracoid process	Radial tuberosity (proximal radius)	Musculocutaneous	Supinate and flex forearm	Part of "conjoined" tendon

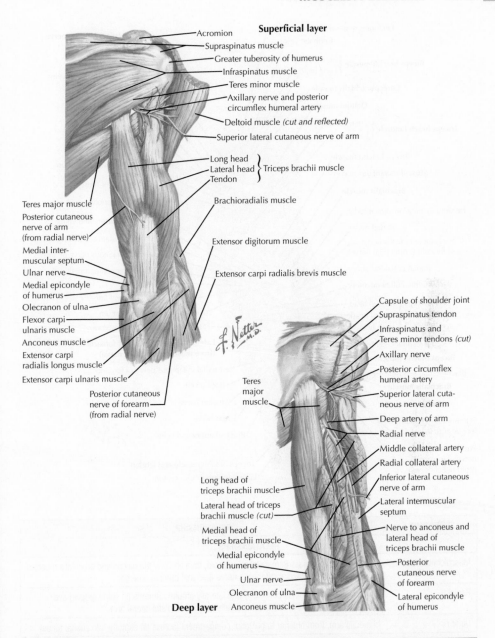

Superficial layer

Acromion
Supraspinatus muscle
Greater tuberosity of humerus
Infraspinatus muscle
Teres minor muscle
Axillary nerve and posterior circumflex humeral artery
Deltoid muscle *(cut and reflected)*
Superior lateral cutaneous nerve of arm

Long head
Lateral head } Triceps brachii muscle
Tendon

Brachioradialis muscle

Teres major muscle
Posterior cutaneous nerve of arm (from radial nerve)
Medial inter-muscular septum
Ulnar nerve
Medial epicondyle of humerus
Olecranon of ulna
Flexor carpi ulnaris muscle
Anconeus muscle
Extensor carpi radialis longus muscle
Extensor carpi ulnaris muscle
Posterior cutaneous nerve of forearm (from radial nerve)

Extensor digitorum muscle

Extensor carpi radialis brevis muscle

Teres major muscle

Capsule of shoulder joint
Supraspinatus tendon
Infraspinatus and Teres minor tendons *(cut)*
Axillary nerve
Posterior circumflex humeral artery
Superior lateral cutaneous nerve of arm
Deep artery of arm
Radial nerve
Middle collateral artery
Radial collateral artery
Inferior lateral cutaneous nerve of arm
Lateral intermuscular septum
Nerve to anconeus and lateral head of triceps brachii muscle
Posterior cutaneous nerve of forearm
Lateral epicondyle of humerus

Long head of triceps brachii muscle
Lateral head of triceps brachii muscle *(cut)*
Medial head of triceps brachii muscle
Medial epicondyle of humerus
Ulnar nerve
Olecranon of ulna
Anconeus muscle

Deep layer

MUSCLE	ORIGIN	INSERTION	NERVE	ACTION	COMMENT
Triceps brachii					
Long head	Infraglenoid tubercle	Olecranon	Radial nerve	Extends elbow	Border of quadrangular & triangular space & interval
Lateral head	Posterior humerus (proximal)	Olecranon	Radial nerve	Extends elbow	Border in lateral approach
Medial head	Posterior humerus (distal)	Olecranon	Radial nerve	Extends elbow	One muscular plane in posterior approach

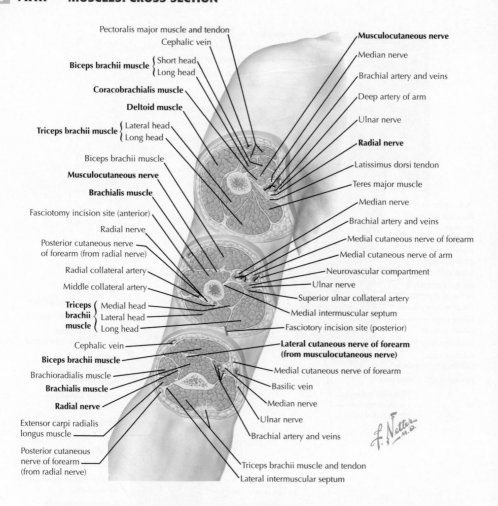

Pectoralis major muscle and tendon
Cephalic vein
Biceps brachii muscle { Short head
Long head
Coracobrachialis muscle
Deltoid muscle
Triceps brachii muscle { Lateral head
Long head
Biceps brachii muscle
Musculocutaneous nerve
Brachialis muscle
Fasciotomy incision site (anterior)
Radial nerve
Posterior cutaneous nerve of forearm (from radial nerve)
Radial collateral artery
Middle collateral artery
Triceps brachii muscle { Medial head
Lateral head
Long head
Cephalic vein
Biceps brachii muscle
Brachioradialis muscle
Brachialis muscle
Radial nerve
Extensor carpi radialis longus muscle
Posterior cutaneous nerve of forearm (from radial nerve)

Musculocutaneous nerve
Median nerve
Brachial artery and veins
Deep artery of arm
Ulnar nerve
Radial nerve
Latissimus dorsi tendon
Teres major muscle
Median nerve
Brachial artery and veins
Medial cutaneous nerve of forearm
Medial cutaneous nerve of arm
Neurovascular compartment
Ulnar nerve
Superior ulnar collateral artery
Medial intermuscular septum
Fasciotory incision site (posterior)
Lateral cutaneous nerve of forearm (from musculocutaneous nerve)
Medial cutaneous nerve of forearm
Basilic vein
Median nerve
Ulnar nerve
Brachial artery and veins
Triceps brachii muscle and tendon
Lateral intermuscular septum

STRUCTURE	RELATIONSHIP
RELATIONSHIPS	
Musculocutaneous n.	Pierces coracobrachialis 8cm distal to coracoid, then lies b/w the biceps and brachialis muscles where lateral antebrachial cutaneous nerve (terminal branch) emerges
Radial n.	Starts medial, then spirals posteriorly and laterally around humerus (in spiral groove) and emerges b/w brachialis and brachioradialis muscles in distal lateral arm
Ulnar n.	In medial arm, from anterior to posterior compartment (across IM septum) into cubital tunnel
Median n.	In anteromedial arm, initially lateral to brachial artery, but crosses over it to become medial
Brachial artery	Runs with median nerve, then crosses under it to become more midline in distal arm/elbow
COMPARTMENTS	
Anterior	Muscles: brachialis, biceps brachii, coracobrachialis Neurovascular: musculocutaneous nerve, median nerve, brachial artery, radial nerve (distally)
Posterior	Muscles: triceps brachii Neurovascular: radial nerve (mid arm), ulnar nerve (distal arm), radial recurrent arteries

Cutaneous Innervation

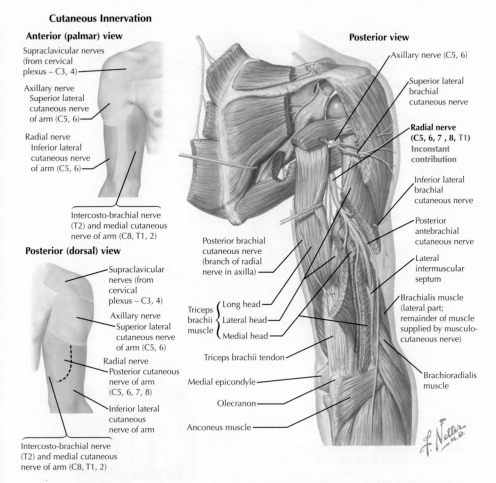

Anterior (palmar) view

Supraclavicular nerves
(from cervical
plexus – C3, 4)

Axillary nerve
Superior lateral
cutaneous nerve
of arm (C5, 6)

Radial nerve
Inferior lateral
cutaneous nerve
of arm (C5, 6)

Intercosto-brachial nerve
(T2) and medial cutaneous
nerve of arm (C8, T1, 2)

Posterior (dorsal) view

Supraclavicular
nerves (from
cervical
plexus – C3, 4)

Axillary nerve
Superior lateral
cutaneous nerve
of arm (C5, 6)

Radial nerve
Posterior cutaneous
nerve of arm
(C5, 6, 7, 8)

Inferior lateral
cutaneous
nerve of arm

Intercosto-brachial nerve
(T2) and medial cutaneous
nerve of arm (C8, T1, 2)

Posterior view

Axillary nerve (C5, 6)

Superior lateral
brachial
cutaneous nerve

**Radial nerve
(C5, 6, 7 , 8, T1)**
Inconstant
contribution

Inferior lateral
brachial
cutaneous nerve

Posterior
antebrachial
cutaneous nerve

Lateral
intermuscular
septum

Brachialis muscle
(lateral part;
remainder of muscle
supplied by musculo-
cutaneous nerve)

Brachioradialis
muscle

Posterior brachial
cutaneous nerve
(branch of radial
nerve in axilla)

Triceps
brachii
muscle
{ Long head
Lateral head
Medial head

Triceps brachii tendon

Medial epicondyle

Olecranon

Anconeus muscle

BRACHIAL PLEXUS		
Lateral and Medial Cord		
Median (C[5]6-T1): runs in medial arm (anterior compartment), medial to biceps and brachialis (lateral to brachial artery), then crosses over (medial) to artery and enters forearm under biceps aponeurosis (lacertus fibrosus)		
Sensory: None (in arm, see Hand chapter) *Motor:* None (in arm, see Forearm & Hand chapters)		
Posterior Cord		
Radial (C5-T1): starts medial to humerus, crosses posterior into spiral groove (where it can be entrapped in a humerus fracture, esp. distal ⅓ fractures) with deep artery of the arm, then exits between the brachioradialis & brachialis, then divides into deep (motor–PIN) and superficial (sensory) branches		
Sensory: Posterior arm: via **posterior cutaneous n. of arm** (posterior brachial cutaneous) Lateral arm: via **inferior lateral cutaneous n. of arm** *Motor:* • Posterior compartment ○ Triceps brachii • Anterior compartment ○ Brachialis (lateral portion)		

Anterior view

Note: Only muscles innervated by musculocutaneous nerve shown

Musculocutaneous nerve (C5, 6, 7)

Coracobrachialis muscle

Biceps brachii muscle *(retracted)*

Brachialis muscle

Articular branch

Lateral cutaneous nerve of forearm

Anterior branch

Posterior branch

Lateral ⎫
Posterior ⎬ Cords of brachial plexus
Medial ⎭

Median nerve

Ulnar nerve

Medial cutaneous nerve of arm

Medial cutaneous nerve of forearm

Radial nerve

Axillary nerve

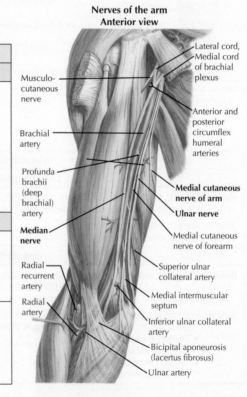

Nerves of the arm
Anterior view

Lateral cord, Medial cord of brachial plexus

Musculo-cutaneous nerve

Brachial artery

Profunda brachii (deep brachial) artery

Median nerve

Radial recurrent artery

Radial artery

Anterior and posterior circumflex humeral arteries

Medial cutaneous nerve of arm

Ulnar nerve

Medial cutaneous nerve of forearm

Superior ulnar collateral artery

Medial intermuscular septum

Inferior ulnar collateral artery

Bicipital aponeurosis (lacertus fibrosus)

Ulnar artery

BRACHIAL PLEXUS
Lateral Cord
Musculocutaneous (C5-7): pierces coracobrachialis (6-8cm below coracoid, where it is at risk from retraction of the conjoined tendon), then runs between the biceps & brachialis, innervating both. Sensory terminal branch exits between the biceps & brachialis at elbow.

Sensory: None (in arm, see Forearm chapter)
Motor: • Anterior compartment
    ◦ Coracobrachialis
    ◦ Biceps brachii
    ◦ Brachialis (medial portion)

Medial Cord
Medial cutaneous n. of arm (brachial cutaneous [C8-T1]): branches from the cord, joins intercostobrachial nerve, and runs subcutaneously in the medial arm.
Sensory: Medial arm *Motor:* None
Ulnar (C[7]8-T1): runs from anterior to posterior compartment in medial arm over the IM septum, then under the arcade of Struthers onto the triceps (medial head), then into cubital tunnel posterior to the medial epicondyle
Sensory: None (in arm, see Forearm & Hand) *Motor:* None (in arm, see Forearm & Hand)

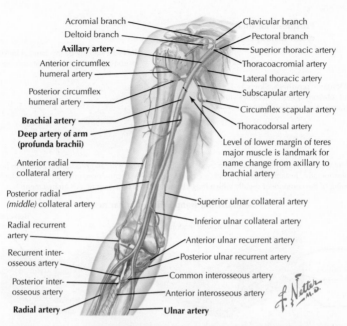

Acromial branch
Deltoid branch
Axillary artery
Anterior circumflex
humeral artery
Posterior circumflex
humeral artery
Brachial artery
**Deep artery of arm
(profunda brachii)**
Anterior radial
collateral artery
Posterior radial
(middle) collateral artery
Radial recurrent
artery
Recurrent inter-
osseous artery
Posterior inter-
osseous artery
Radial artery

Clavicular branch
Pectoral branch
Superior thoracic artery
Thoracoacromial artery
Lateral thoracic artery
Subscapular artery
Circumflex scapular artery
Thoracodorsal artery
Level of lower margin of teres
major muscle is landmark for
name change from axillary to
brachial artery
Superior ulnar collateral artery
Inferior ulnar collateral artery
Anterior ulnar recurrent artery
Posterior ulnar recurrent artery
Common interosseous artery
Anterior interosseous artery
Ulnar artery

BRANCHES	COURSE	COMMENT/SUPPLY
BRACHIAL ARTERY		
The continuation of the axillary artery. It runs with the median n., then crosses under the nerve to be midline.		
Deep artery (profunda brachii)	In the spiral groove	Runs with the radial nerve, can be injured there
Nutrient humeral artery	Enters the nutrient canal	Supplies the humerus
Superior ulnar collateral	With ulnar n. in medial arm	Anastomosis with posterior ulnar recurrent artery
Inferior ulnar collateral	Branches in distal arm	Anastomosis with anterior ulnar recurrent artery
Muscular branches	Usually branch laterally	Supply musculature of the arm
Radial	Terminal branch	One of 2 terminal branches
Ulnar	Terminal branch	One of 2 terminal branches
DEEP ARTERY		
Anterior radial collateral	In anterolateral arm	Anastomosis with radial recurrent artery
Posterior (middle) radial collateral	Posterior to humerus	Anastomosis with recurrent interosseous artery Used as pedicle in lateral arm flap
RADIAL ARTERY		
Radial recurrent	Runs in anterolateral portion of the arm	Anastomosis with anterior radial collateral artery Branches (leash of Henry) can compress radial n.
ULNAR ARTERY		
Anterior ulnar recurrent	In anteromedial arm	Anastomosis with inferior ulnar collateral artery
Posterior ulnar recurrent	In posteromedial arm	Anastomosis with superior ulnar collateral artery
Common interosseous	Midline branch	Is a trunk with multiple branches
Recurrent interosseous	Posterior to elbow	Anastomosis w/ post. radial (middle) collateral artery
Anterior & posterior interosseous	Along intermuscular septum	Supplies forearm musculature

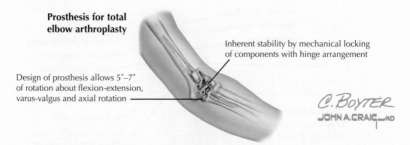

Prosthesis for total elbow arthroplasty

Inherent stability by mechanical locking of components with hinge arrangement

Design of prosthesis allows 5°–7° of rotation about flexion-extension, varus-valgus and axial rotation

C. BOYTER
JOHN A. CRAIG _AD

Three types of total elbow arthroplasty have been used. Results were better with an unrestrained prosthesis but with 5%–20% incidence of postoperative instability, most patients are now treated with a semi-constrained prosthesis, which has inherent stability by linking of the component usually with a hinge (shown above) or a snap-fit axis arrangement.

Submuscular tranposition of ulnar nerve

Medial intermuscular septum

Divided tendon of origin

Repaired flexor-pronator over transposed nerve

Anterior transposition of ulnar nerve

Triceps brachii muscle

DESCRIPTION	Hx & PE	WORKUP/FINDINGS	TREATMENT
ARTHRITIS			
• Less common condition • Osteoarthritis seen in athletes/laborers • Site for arthritides (RA, gout, etc)	**Hx:** Chronic pain, stiffness, +/– previous trauma **PE:** Decreased ROM & tenderness (especially in extension)	• **XR:** OA vs inflammatory • **Blood:** RF, ESR, ANA • **Joint fluid:** crystals, cells, culture	1. Conservative (rest, NSAID) 2. Debridement (osteophytes, loose bodies) 3. Ulnohumeral arthroplasty 4. Total elbow arthroplasty
CUBITAL TUNNEL SYNDROME			

• Entrapment of ulnar nerve at elbow
• Sites:
  ○ IM septum
  ○ Arcade of Struthers
  ○ Cubital tunnel
  ○ FCU fascia
	Hx: Numbness/tingling in ulnar distribution, +/– elbow pain
	PE: +/– decreased grip strength, intrinsic atrophy, + Tinel's and/or elbow flexion text
		XR: Look for abnormal medial epicondyle
		EMG: Confirms diagnosis
			1. Rest, ice, NSAIDs, activity modification
			2. Splints (day and/or night)
			3. Ulnar nerve transposition (submuscular vs subcutaneous)

LATERAL EPICONDYLITIS (TENNIS ELBOW)			
• Degenerative of common extensor tendons (esp. ECRB) • Due to overuse (e.g., tennis) and/or injury (microtrauma) to tendon	**Hx:** Age 30-60, pain at lateral elbow, worse w/wrist extension **PE:** Lateral epicondyle TTP; pain with resisted wrist extension	**XR:** Rule out fracture & OA. Calcification of tendons can occur (esp. ECRB)	1. Activity modification, NSAIDs 2. Use of brace/strap 3. Stretching/strengthening 4. Corticosteroid injection 5. Surgical debridement of tendon (ECRB #1)
OLECRANON BURSITIS			
• Inflammation of bursa (infection/trauma/other)	**Hx:** Swelling, acute or chronic pain **PE:** Palpable/fluctuant mass at olecranon	**LAB:** Aspirate bursa, send fluid for culture, cell count, Gram stain and crystals	1. Compressive dressing 2. Activity modification 3. Corticosteroid injection 4. Surgical debridement

Osteochondral lesion of the capitellum

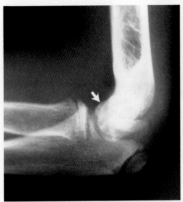

Bone resorption seen as radiolucent areas and irregular surface of capitellum of humerus

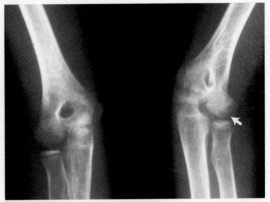

Characteristic changes in capitellum of left humerus (arrow) compared with normal right elbow

DESCRIPTION	Hx & PE	WORKUP/FINDINGS	TREATMENT
DISTAL BICEPS TENDON RUPTURE			
• Mechanism: eccentric overload of partially flexed elbow • Usually male 40-60 y.o. • Early diagnosis important	**Hx:** Acute injury/"pop" **PE:** No palpable tendon, weak and/or painful flexion & supination	**XR:** Usually normal **MR:** Can confirm diagnosis but usually not needed	1. Early: primary repair (1 or 2 incision techniques) 2. Late: no surgery; physical therapy
MEDIAL ELBOW INSTABILITY			
• MCL (anterior bundle) injury from repetitive valgus stress • Acute or chronic, associated with throwers (baseball, javelin)	**Hx:** Pain with throwing or inability to throw **PE:** MCL tenderness, +/− valgus laxity (at >30°)	**XR:** Stress view may show widening (usu. dynamic) postmedial osteophytes. **MR:** Avulsion and tears	1. Rest, activity modification 2. Physical therapy (ROM) 3. Ligament reconstruction & debridement of osteophytes/loose bodies
OSTEOCHONDRITIS DISSECANS OF ELBOW			
• Vascular insufficiency or micro-trauma to capitellum • Adolescent throwers/gymnasts with valgus/compressive loads	**Hx:** Lateral elbow pain, +/− catching, stiffness **PE:** Capitellum TTP, pain w/ valgus stress	**XR:** Lucency, +/− fragmentation of the capitellum **CT:** Helpful to identify loose bodies	1. Rest & physical therapy 2. ORIF of fragments or arthroscopic debridement of loose bodies & chondroplasty
POSTEROLATERAL ROTATORY INSTABILITY			
• Lateral ulnar collateral ligament (LUCL) injury • Allows radial head to subluxate • Mech: traumatic (elbow dx) or iatrogenic (elbow surgery)	**Hx:** Hx of trauma or surgery, pain, +/− clicking **PE:** + lateral pivot shift test (often needs EUA)	**XR:** Often normal **Stress XR:** Shows radial head subluxation **MR:** Identifies LUCL tear	1. Rest, activity modification 2. Physical therapy (ROM) 3. LUCL reconstruction (usually with a palmaris graft)
STIFF ELBOW			
• <30-120° • Intrinsic vs extrinsic etiology • Intrinsic: articular changes/ arthrosis (posttraumatic, etc) • Extrinsic: capsule contracture	**Hx:** Trauma, stiffness, minimal pain **PE:** Limited ROM (esp. in flexion and extension)	**XR:** AP/lateral/oblique Look for osteophytes or other signs of intrinsic joint arthrosis	1. Physical therapy: ROM 2. Operative: Intrinsic: excise osteophytes, LBs Extrinsic: capsular release

Congenital dislocation of radial head

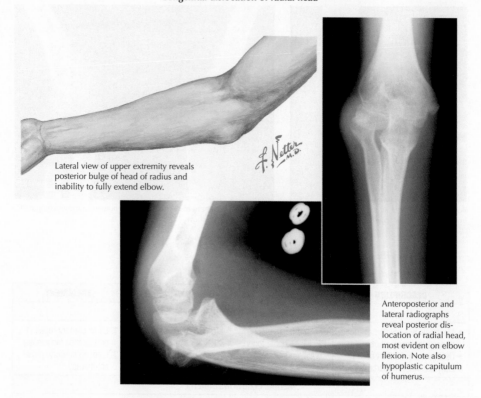

Lateral view of upper extremity reveals posterior bulge of head of radius and inability to fully extend elbow.

Anteroposterior and lateral radiographs reveal posterior dislocation of radial head, most evident on elbow flexion. Note also hypoplastic capitulum of humerus.

DESCRIPTION	EVALUATION	TREATMENT
CONGENITAL RADIAL HEAD DISLOCATION		
• Radial head congenitally dislocated • Usually diagnosed from 2-5y.o. • Patients are typically very functional • Unilateral or bilateral • Associated with other syndromes	**Hx:** Parents notice decreased ROM, +/− pain or deformity (late) **PE:** Decreased ROM, +/− visible radial head and/or tenderness **XR:** Malformed radial head & capitellum	• Asymptomatic: observation • Symptomatic (pain): excision of radial head at skeletal maturity (decreases pain, but does not typically increase ROM)
RADIOULNAR SYNOSTOSIS		
• Failure of separation of radius & ulna • Forearm rotation is absent • Can be assoc. with other syndromes • Bilateral in 60% of cases	**Hx/PE:** Absent pronosupination of the elbow/forearm. Varying degrees of fixed deformity (>60° is severe) **XR:** Radius is thickened, ulna is narrow	• Synostosis resection unsuccessful Mild/unilateral: observation • Osteotomy: dominant hand 20° of pronation, nondominant 30° of supination
OSTEOCHONDROSIS OF CAPITELLUM (PANNER'S DISEASE)		
• Disordered endochondral ossification • Mech: valgus (pitcher's) compression or axial overload (gymnasts) • Usually <10 y.o.; male>female • Favorable long-term prognosis	**Hx:** Insidious onset lateral elbow pain and overuse (baseball, gymnastics) **PE:** Capitellum TTP, decreased ROM **XR:** Irregular borders, +/− fissuring, fragmentation (rarely loose bodies)	1. Rest (no pitching, tumbling, etc) 2. NSAIDs 3. Immobilization (3-4 weeks) Symptoms may persist for months, but most completely resolve

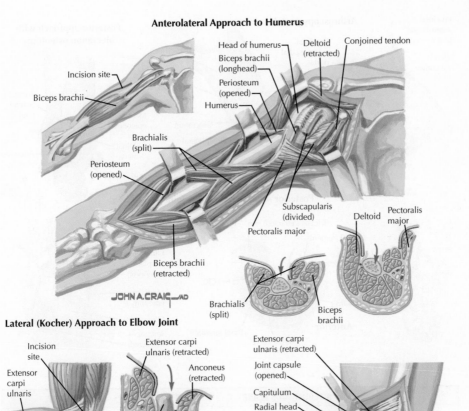

Anterolateral Approach to Humerus

Incision site

Biceps brachii

Head of humerus

Deltoid (retracted)

Conjoined tendon

Biceps brachii (longhead)

Periosteum (opened)

Humerus

Brachialis (split)

Periosteum (opened)

Subscapularis (divided)

Pectoralis major

Deltoid

Pectoralis major

Biceps brachii (retracted)

JOHN A.CRAIG—AD

Brachialis (split)

Biceps brachii

Lateral (Kocher) Approach to Elbow Joint

Incision site

Extensor carpi ulnaris

Extensor carpi ulnaris (retracted)

Anconeus (retracted)

Posterior

Anterior

Anconeus

Capitulum

Olecranon

Ulnar nerve

Radius

Extensor carpi ulnaris (retracted)

Joint capsule (opened)

Capitulum

Radial head

Olecranon

Anconeus (retracted)

Ulna

Supinator

USES	INTERNERVOUS PLANES	DANGERS	COMMENT
HUMERUS: ANTERIOR APPROACH			

• ORIF of fractures
• Bone biopsy/tumor removal
	Proximal
	• Deltoid (axillary)
	• Pectoralis major (pectoral)
	Distal
	• Brachialis splitting
	  ○ Lateral (radial)
	  ○ Medial (MSC)
		Proximal
		• Axillary nerve
		• Humeral circumflex artery
		Distal
		• Radial nerve
		• Musculocutaneous nerve
			• Anterior humeral circumflex artery may need ligation.
			• The brachialis has a split innervation that can be used for an internervous plane.

ELBOW: LATERAL APPROACH (KOCHER)			
Most radial head & lateral condyle procedures	• Anconeus (radial) • ECU (PIN)	• PIN • Radial nerve	• Protect PIN: stay above annular ligament; keep forearm pronated

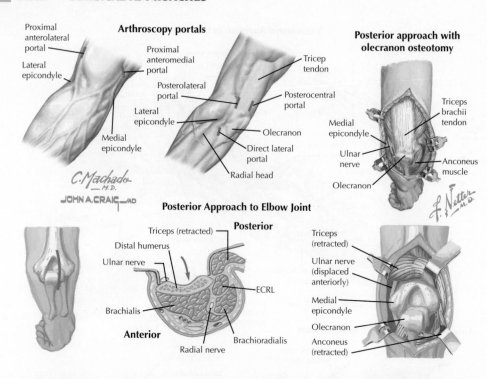

USES	INTERNERVOUS PLANE	DANGERS	COMMENT
POSTERIOR APPROACH			
• Distal humerus fractures • Loose body removal, chondral procedures • Ulnohumeral arthroplasty • Total elbow arthroplasty	• No internervous plane • Olecranon is osteotomized and reflected to expose the distal humerus/joint.	• Ulnar nerve • Nonunion of olecranon osteotomy	• Best exposure of the joint • Olecranon should be drilled and tapped before osteotomy • Chevron osteotomy is best • Olecranon at risk of nonunion
POSTERIOR APPROACH: BRYAN/MORREY			
• Alternative to posterior approach with osteotomy • Same indications as above	• No internervous plane • Triceps is partially detached and reflected laterally	• Ulnar nerve	• Joint visualization is not as good as with osteotomy, no concern for nonunion
ARTHROSCOPY PORTALS			
Uses: Loose body removal/articular injuries, debridements and capsular release, fracture reduction, limited arthroplasty			
Proximal anteromedial	2cm prox. to med. epicondyle anterior to IM septum	Ulnar nerve MAC nerve	Anterior compartment, radial head & capitellum, capsule
Proximal anterolateral	2cm prox. to lat. epicondyle anterior to humerus	Radial nerve	Medial joint, lateral recess, and radiocapitellar joint
Posterocentral	3cm from olecranon tip	Safe (thru tendon)	Posterior compartment, gutters
Posterolateral	3cm from olecranon tip at lat. edge of triceps tendon	Med. & post. antebrachial cutaneous n.	Olecranon tip & fossa, posterior trochlea
Direct lateral ("soft spot")	Between lat. epicondyle, radial head & olecranon	Posterior antebrachial cutaneous nerve	Inferior capitellum and radiocapitellar joint

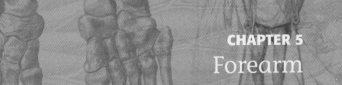

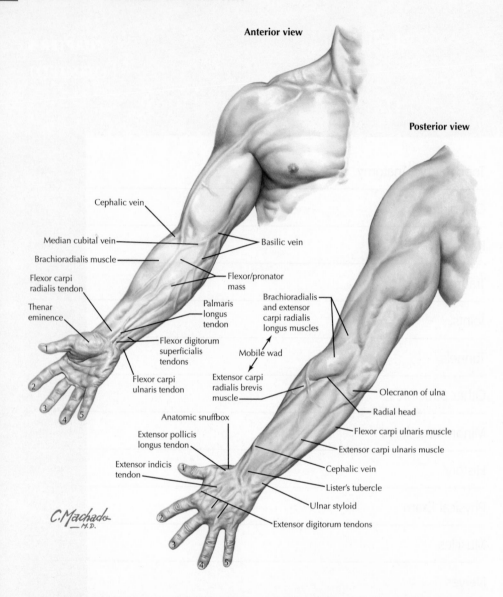

Anterior view

Posterior view

Cephalic vein

Median cubital vein

Brachioradialis muscle

Flexor carpi radialis tendon

Thenar eminence

Basilic vein

Flexor/pronator mass

Palmaris longus tendon

Brachioradialis and extensor carpi radialis longus muscles

Flexor digitorum superficialis tendons

Mobile wad

Flexor carpi ulnaris tendon

Extensor carpi radialis brevis muscle

Anatomic snuffbox

Extensor pollicis longus tendon

Extensor indicis tendon

Olecranon of ulna

Radial head

Flexor carpi ulnaris muscle

Extensor carpi ulnaris muscle

Cephalic vein

Lister's tubercle

Ulnar styloid

Extensor digitorum tendons

C.Machado
—M.D.

STRUCTURE	CLINICAL APPLICATION
Olecranon	Proximal tip of ulna. Tenderness can indicate fracture.
Radial head	Proximal end of radius. Tenderness can indicate fracture.
Flexor radialis tendon	Landmark for volar approach to wrist. Radial pulse is just radial to tendon.
Lister's tubercle	Tubercle on dorsal radius. "Lighthouse of the wrist." EPL tendon runs around it.
Ulnar styloid	Prominent distal end of ulna. Tenderness can indicate fracture.
Palmaris longus tendon	Not present in all people. Can be used for tendon grafts.
Anatomic snuffbox	Site of scaphoid. Tenderness can indicate a scaphoid fracture.

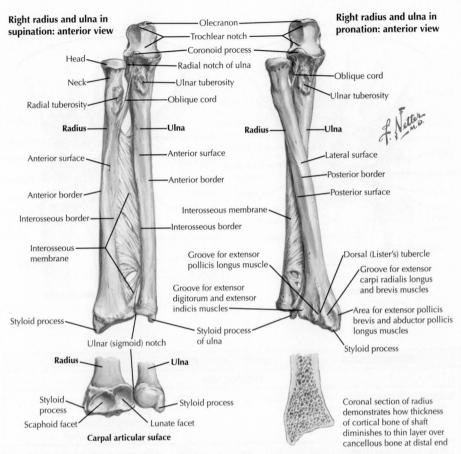

Right radius and ulna in supination: anterior view

Olecranon
Trochlear notch
Coronoid process
Head
Radial notch of ulna
Neck
Ulnar tuberosity
Radial tuberosity
Oblique cord
Radius
Ulna
Anterior surface
Anterior surface
Anterior border
Anterior border
Interosseous border
Interosseous membrane
Interosseous border
Interosseous membrane
Groove for extensor pollicis longus muscle
Groove for extensor digitorum and extensor indicis muscles
Styloid process
Styloid process of ulna
Ulnar (sigmoid) notch

Right radius and ulna in pronation: anterior view

Oblique cord
Ulnar tuberosity
Radius
Ulna
Lateral surface
Posterior border
Posterior surface
Dorsal (Lister's) tubercle
Groove for extensor carpi radialis longus and brevis muscles
Area for extensor pollicis brevis and abductor pollicis longus muscles
Styloid process

f. Netter M.D.

Radius
Ulna
Styloid process
Styloid process
Scaphoid facet
Lunate facet
Carpal articular suface

Coronal section of radius demonstrates how thickness of cortical bone of shaft diminishes to thin layer over cancellous bone at distal end

CHARACTERISTICS	OSSIFY		FUSE	COMMENTS
RADIUS				
• Cylindrical long bone • Head is intraarticular • Tuberosity: biceps inserts • Shaft has a bow • Distal end widens, is made of cancellous bone, has scaphoid & lunate facets, & radial styloid • Ulnar (sigmoid) notch: DRUJ	**Primary** Shaft **Secondary** Head Distal epiphysis	8-9wk 2-3yr 4yr	14yr 16-18yr 16-18yr	• Anterolateral portion of RH has less sub-chondral bone (susceptible to fracture) • Tuberosity points ulnarly in supination • Bow allows rotation around ulna • Cancellous distal radius common fracture site (esp. in peds & older pts) • Distal radius x-ray measurements: 11° volar tilt, 22° radial inclination, 11-12mm radial height
ULNA				
• Long bone: straight bone • Triangular cross-section • Tuberosity: brachialis insertion • Proximal: olecranon, coro-noid process, radial (sigmoid) notch • Distal: ulnar styloid	**Primary** Shaft **Secondary** Olecranon Distal epiphysis	8-9wk 9yr 5-6yr	16-18yr 16-20yr 16-20yr	• The radius rotates around the stationary ulna through proximal & distal notches during pronation/supination • 75% of growth from distal epiphysis • Olecranon & coronoid provide primary bony stability to elbow joint • Coronoid fx can result in instability • Common site of fx (often w/DR fx)

Anterior (palmar) view

Metacarpal bones
4 3 2 1 5

Capitate
Hook of hamate
Hamate
Pisiform
Triquetrum
Lunate
Ulnar styloid process
Ulna

Trapezoid
Tubercle of trapezium
Trapezium
Tubercle of scaphoid
Scaphoid
Radial styloid process
Radius
Ulnar (sigmoid) notch

Posterior (dorsal) view

Metacarpal bones
2 3 4 1 5

Trapezoid
Trapezium
Radial styloid process
Scaphoid
Dorsal tubercle (Lister's) of the radius
Radius

Capitate
Hamate
Triquetrum
Pisiform
Lunate
Ulnar styloid process
Ulna

CHARACTERISTICS	OSSIFY	FUSE	COMMENTS
PROXIMAL ROW			
Scaphoid: boat shape, 80% covered with articular cartilage (not waist)	5th	5yr	14-16yr	• Blood supply enters dorsal waist, bridges both rows • #1 carpal fx. Proximal fractures are at risk of nonunion/AVN
Lunate: moon shape. Four articulations: 1. radius (lunate facet), 2. scaphoid, 3. triquetrum, 4. capitate	4th	4yr	14-16yr	• Dislocations: rare but often missed • Will rotate (carpal instability) if ligamentous attachments to adjacent bones are disrupted
Triquetrum: pyramid shape. Lies under the pisiform and ulnar styloid	3rd	3yr	14-16yr	• 3rd most common carpal fracture • Articulates with TFCC
Pisiform: large sesamoid bone. In FCU tendon, anterolateral to triquetrum	8th	9-10yr	14-16yr	• Multiple attachments: FCU, transverse carpal ligament (TCL), abductor digiti minimi, multiple ligaments
DISTAL ROW			
Trapezium: saddle shape	6th	5-6yr	14-16yr	• Has groove for FCR tendon
Trapezoid: trapezoidal/wedge shape	7th	6-7yr	14-16yr	• Articulates with second metacarpal
Capitate: largest carpal bone, 1st carpal bone to ossify	1st	1yr	14-16yr	• Keystone to carpal arch, floor of CT • Retrograde blood supply
Hamate: has volar-oriented hook that is distal and radial to pisiform	2nd	2yr	14-16yr	• Hook can fx, ulnar a. can be injured • TCL attaches border of Guyon's canal

• Ossification: each from a single center in a counter-clockwise direction (anatomic position) starting with the capitate.
• Each bone has multiple (4-7) tight articulations with adjacent bones.
• Proximal row is considered the "intercalated segment" between the distal radius/TFCC and distal carpal row.
• Scaphoid-lunate angle (measured on lateral x-ray): avg. 47° (range 30-60°; <30=VISI, >60=DISI).

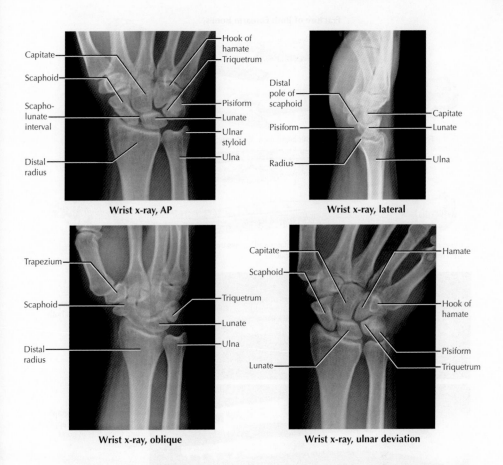

Wrist x-ray, AP

Capitate
Scaphoid
Scapho-
lunate
interval
Distal
radius

Hook of
hamate
Triquetrum
Pisiform
Lunate
Ulnar
styloid
Ulna

Wrist x-ray, lateral

Distal
pole of
scaphoid
Pisiform
Radius

Capitate
Lunate
Ulna

Wrist x-ray, oblique

Trapezium
Scaphoid
Distal
radius

Triquetrum
Lunate
Ulna

Wrist x-ray, ulnar deviation

Capitate
Scaphoid
Lunate

Hamate
Hook of
hamate
Pisiform
Triquetrum

RADIOGRAPH	TECHNIQUE	FINDINGS	CLINICAL APPLICATION
AP (anteroposterior)	Palm down on plate, beam perpendicular to plate	Carpal bones, radiocarpal joint	Distal radius, ulnar, carpal fractures or dislocation
Lateral	Ulnar border of wrist & hand on plate	Alignment of bones, joints	Same as above, carpal (lunate) instability
Oblique	Lateral with 40° rotation	Alignment & position of bones	Same as above
AP-ulnar deviation	AP, deviate wrist ulnarly	Isolates scaphoid	Scaphoid fractures
Carpal tunnel view	Maximal wrist extension, beam at 15°	Hamate, pisiform, trapezium	Fractures (esp. hook of the hamate)
OTHER STUDIES			
CT	Axial, coronal, & sagittal	Articular congruity, bone healing, bone alignment	Fractures (scaphoid, hook of hamate), nonunions
MRI	Sequence protocols vary	Soft tissues (ligaments, tendons, cartilage), bones	Occult fractures (e.g., scaphoid), tears (e.g., TFCC, S-L ligament)
Bone scan		All bones evaluated	Infection, stress fxs, tumors

Fracture of Both Forearm Bones

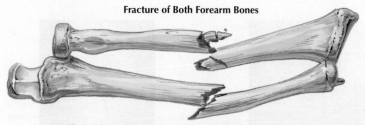

Fracture of both radius and ulna with angulation, shortening, and comminution of radius

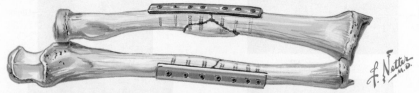

Open reduction and fixation with compression plates and screws through both cortices. Good alignment, with restoration of radial bow and interosseous space.

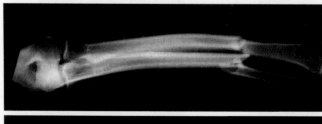

Preoperative radiograph.
Fractures of shafts of both forearm bones

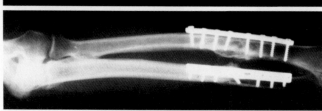

Postoperative radiograph.
Compression plates applied and fragments in good alignment

DESCRIPTION	EVALUATION	CLASSIFICATION	TREATMENT
RADIUS AND ULNA FRACTURES			
Both-Bone Fracture			
• Mech: fall or high energy • Both bones usually fracture as energy passes thru both bones • Fractures can be at different levels	**Hx:** Trauma, pain and swelling, +/− deformity **PE:** Swelling, tenderness, +/− clinical deformity **XR:** AP & lateral forearm	Descriptive: • Proximal, middle, distal ⅓ • Displaced/angulated • Comminuted • Open or closed	• Peds (<10-12y.o.): closed reduction and casting • Adults: ORIF (plates & screws) through separate incisions
COMPLICATIONS: Malunion (loss of radial bow leads to decreased pronosupination), decreased range of motion			
Single-Bone Fracture			
• Mechanism: direct blow; aka "nightstick" fracture • Ulna most common	**Hx:** Direct blow to forearm **PE:** Swelling, tenderness **XR:** AP & lateral forearm	Descriptive: • Displaced, shortened, angulated, comminuted	• Nondisplaced: cast • Displaced: ORIF
COMPLICATIONS: Nonunion, malunion			

Monteggia Fracture

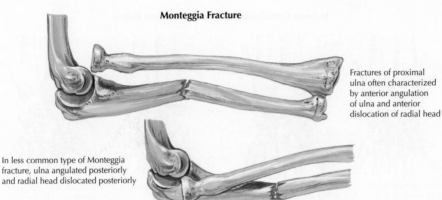

Fractures of proximal ulna often characterized by anterior angulation of ulna and anterior dislocation of radial head

In less common type of Monteggia fracture, ulna angulated posteriorly and radial head dislocated posteriorly

Galeazzi Fracture

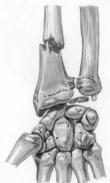

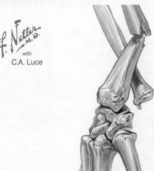

Anteroposterior view of fracture of radius plus dislocation of distal radioulnar joint

Dislocation of distal radioulnar joint better demonstrated in lateral view

DESCRIPTION	EVALUATION	CLASSIFICATION	TREATMENT
MONTEGGIA FRACTURE			
• Proximal ulna fracture, shortening forces result in radial head dislocation • Mechanism: direct blow or fall on outstretched hand	**Hx:** Fall, pain and swelling **PE:** Tenderness, deformity. Check compartments and do neurovascular exam **XR:** AP/lateral: forearm; also, wrist and elbow	Bado (based on RH location): • I: Anterior (common) • II: Posterior • III: Lateral • IV: Anterior with associated both-bone fracture	• Ulna: ORIF (plate/screws) • Radial head: closed reduction (open if irreducible or unstable) • Peds: closed reduction and cast
COMPLICATIONS: Radial nerve/PIN injury (most resolve), decreased ROM, compartment syndrome, nonunion			
GALEAZZI FRACTURE			
• Mechanism: fall on outstretched hand • Distal ⅓ radial shaft fracture, shortening forces result in distal radioulnar dislocation	**Hx:** Fall, pain and swelling **PE:** Tenderness, deformity. Check compartments and do neurovascular exam **XR:** AP/lateral forearm: ulna usually dorsal. Also, wrist and elbow series	By mechanism: • Pronation: Galeazzi • Supination: Reverse Galeazzi (ulna shaft fx with DRUJ dislocation)	• Radius: ORIF • DRUJ: closed reduction, +/– percutaneous pins in supination if unstable (open if unstable) • Cast for 4-6wk • Peds: reduce & cast
COMPLICATIONS: Nerve injury, decreased ROM, nonunion, DRUJ arthrosis			

Frykman Classification of Fractures of Distal Radius

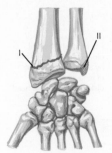
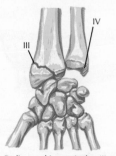
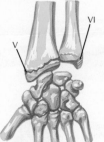
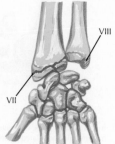

Extraarticular radius: I
Ulnar styloid: II

Radiocarpal intraarticular: III
Ulnar styloid: IV

Intraarticular distal
radioulnar: V
Ulnar styloid: VI

Intraarticular radiocarpal
and distal radioulnar: VII
Ulnar styloid: VIII

Reduction of a Colles Fracture

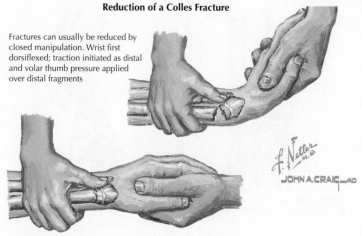

Fractures can usually be reduced by
closed manipulation. Wrist first
dorsiflexed; traction initiated as distal
and volar thumb pressure applied
over distal fragments

With pressure and traction maintained, wrist gently straightened

DESCRIPTION	EVALUATION	CLASSIFICATION	TREATMENT
DISTAL RADIUS FRACTURE			

• Mechanism: fall on out-stretched hand
• Very common (Colles #1)
• Cancellous bone susceptible to fx (incl. osteoporotic fx)
• Colles (#1): dorsal displace-ment (apex volar angulation)
• Smith fx: volar displacement
• Barton fx: articular rim fx
• Radial styloid ("chauffeur fx")
	Hx: Trauma (usually fall), pain and swelling
	PE: Swelling, tenderness, +/– deformity. Do thor-ough neurovascular exam.
	XR: Wrist series (3 views)
	Normal measurements
	  ○ 11° volar tilt
	  ○ 11-12mm radial height
	  ○ 23° radial inclination
	CT: For intraarticular fxs
		Frykman (for Colles):
		• Type I, II: extraarticular
		• Type III, IV: RC joint
		• Type V, VI: RC joint
		• Type VII, VIII: both radio-ulnar & radiocarpal (RC) joints involved
		• Even # fxs have associ-ated ulnar styloid fx
		Other fxs, descriptive: displaced, angulated
			• Nondisplaced: cast
			• Displaced:
			  ○ Stable: closed reduction, well-molded cast, 4-6wk
			  ○ Unstable: closed reduction, percuta-neous pinning +/– ext. fix. or ORIF
			• Intraarticular: ORIF (e.g., volar plate)
			• Elderly: cast, early ROM

COMPLICATIONS: Malunion, posttraumatic osteoarthritis, stiffness/loss of range of motion			

Scaphoid Fracture

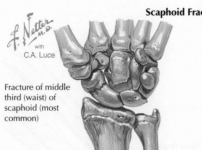

Fracture of middle third (waist) of scaphoid (most common)

Less common fractures

Tubercle   Distal pole

Vertical shear   Proximal pole

Perilunate Dislocation

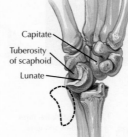

Palmar view shows (A) lunate rotated and displaced volarly, (B) scapholunate space widened, (C) capitate displaced proximally and dorsally

Capitate
Tuberosity of scaphoid
Lunate

Lateral view shows lunate displaced volarly and rotated. Broken line indicates further dislocation to volar aspect of distal radius

DESCRIPTION	EVALUATION	CLASSIFICATION	TREATMENT
SCAPHOID FRACTURE			
• Mechanism: fall on outstretched hand • Most common carpal fx • Retrograde blood suppy to proximal pole is injured in waist fxs, can lead to nonunion or AVN • Distal pole usually heals • High index of suspicion will decrease missed fxs	**Hx:** Trauma (usually fall), pain and swelling **PE:** "Snuffbox" tenderness, decreased ROM **XR:** Wrist & ulnar deviation views **CT:** For most fxs; shows displacement/pattern **MR:** Occult fx, AVN	Location: • Proximal pole • Middle/"waist" (#1) • Distal pole Position: • Displaced • Angulated/shortened	• Nondisplaced: 1. Casting (LAC & SAC) average 10-12wk; 2. Percutaneous screw • Displaced: ORIF +/− bone graft • Nonunion: ORIF with tricortical bone graft or vascularized bone graft
COMPLICATIONS: Nonunion, wrist arthrosis (SLAC wrist from chronic nonunion), osteonecrosis (esp. proximal pole)			
PERILUNATE INSTABILITY/DISLOCATION			
• Mech: fall; axial compression & hyperextension • Instability progresses through 4 stages (Mayfield) as various ligaments are disrupted • Dislocation (stage 4) occurs through weak spot (space of Poirier) • Transscaphoid dislocation is #1 injury pattern	**Hx:** Trauma/fall, pain **PE:** Characteristic volar "fullness", decr. ROM **XR:** S-L gap >3mm S-L angle: >60° or <30° **CT:** Evaluate carpal fxs **MR:** Shows ligament injury in subtle early stages	Instability (Mayfield (4)) • I: Scapholunate disruption • II: Lunocapitate disruption • III: Lunotriquetral disruption • IV: Lunate (peri) dislocation Dislocation (Stage 4 instability) • Lesser arc: ligaments only • Greater arc: assoc. carpal fx	• Instability: closed vs open reduction, percutaneous pinning & primary ligament repair • Dislocation: open reduction of lunate, percutaneous pinning +/− ORIF of carpal fx • Late/wrist arthrosis: proximal row carpectomy or STT fusion
COMPLICATIONS: Wrist arthrosis (e.g., SLAC from instability), nonunion of fracture, chronic pain and/or instability			

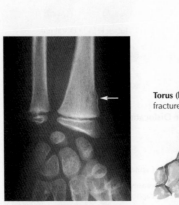

Torus (buckle)
fracture of radius

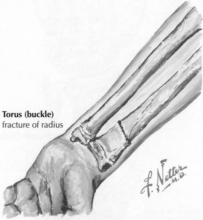

Greenstick fractures
of radius and ulna

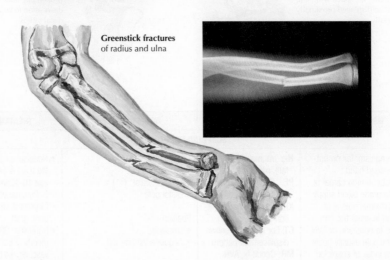

DESCRIPTION	EVALUATION	CLASSIFICATION	TREATMENT
INCOMPLETE FRACTURE: TORUS AND GREENSTICK FRACTURE			
• Common in children (usually 3-12y.o.) • Mechanism: fall on out-stretched hand most common • Distal radius most common • Increased elasticity of pediatric bone allows for plastic deformity and/or unicortical fx	**Hx:** Trauma, pain, inability/unwilling to use hand/extremity **PE:** +/– deformity. Point tenderness & swelling **XR:** AP and lateral. Torus: cortical "buckle." Greenstick: unicortical fracture	• Torus (buckle): concave cortex compresses (buckles), convex/tension side: intact • Greenstick: concave, cortex intact or buckled, convex/ tension side fracture or plastic deformity	• Torus: reduction rarely needed, cast 2-4wk • Greenstick: nondis-placed—SAC 2-4wk. Reduce if >10° of angulation—well-molded LAC 3-4wk
COMPLICATIONS: Deformity, malunion, neurovascular injury (rare)			

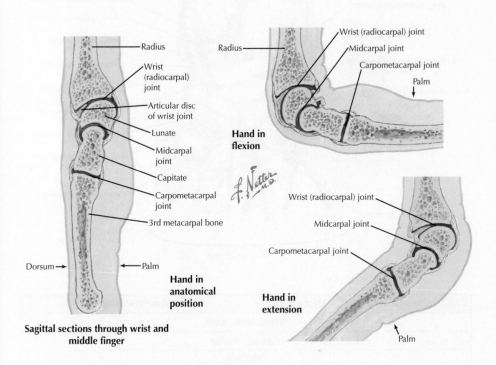

Radius

Wrist (radiocarpal) joint

Articular disc of wrist joint

Lunate

Midcarpal joint

Capitate

Carpometacarpal joint

3rd metacarpal bone

Dorsum → ← Palm

Hand in anatomical position

Sagittal sections through wrist and middle finger

Radius

Hand in flexion

Wrist (radiocarpal) joint

Midcarpal joint

Carpometacarpal joint

Palm

Wrist (radiocarpal) joint

Midcarpal joint

Carpometacarpal joint

Hand in extension

Palm

WRIST
GENERAL

- The wrist is a complex joint comprising 3 main articulations: 1. Radiocarpal (distal radius/TFCC to proximal row), 2. Distal radioulnar joint (DRUJ), 3. Midcarpal (between carpal rows)
- Other articulations: pisotriquetral and multiple intercarpal (between 2 adjacent bones in the same row)
- Proximal row has no muscular attachments, considered the "intercalated segment," & responds to transmitted forces. Distal row bones are tightly connected and act as a single unit in a normal wrist.
- Range of motion:
  - Flexion 65-80° (40% from radiocarpal, 60% midcarpal); extension 55-75° (65% radiocarpal, 35% midcarpal)
  - Radial deviation: 15-25°; ulnar deviation: 30-45° (55% midcarpal, 45% radiocarpal)
- Types of ligaments
  - **Extrinsic:** connect the distal forearm (radius & ulna) to the carpus
  - **Intrinsic:** connect carpal bones to each other (i.e., origin and insertion of ligament both within the carpus)
    - Interosseous: ligaments connecting carpal bones within the same row (proximal or distal)
    - Midcarpal/Intercarpal: ligaments connecting carpal bones between the proximal and distal rows.
- Palmar (volar) ligaments are stronger and more developed; most are intracapsular.

Flexor retinaculum removed: palmar view

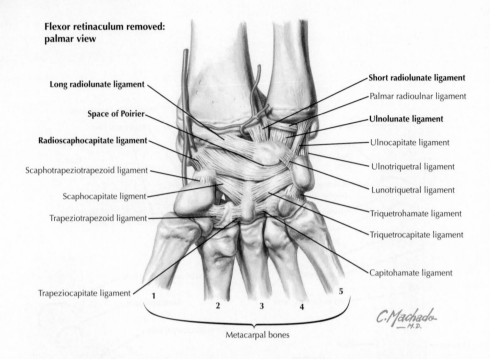

Long radiolunate ligament

Space of Poirier

Radioscaphocapitate ligament

Scaphotrapeziotrapezoid ligament

Scaphocapitate ligment

Trapeziotrapezoid ligament

Trapeziocapitate ligament

Short radiolunate ligament

Palmar radioulnar ligament

Ulnolunate ligament

Ulnocapitate ligament

Ulnotriquetral ligament

Lunotriquetral ligament

Triquetrohamate ligament

Triquetrocapitate ligament

Capitohamate ligament

1 2 3 4 5

Metacarpal bones

C. Machado
—M.D.

LIGAMENTS	ATTACHMENTS	FUNCTION/COMMENT
RADIOCARPAL JOINT		
Extrinsic—Palmar		
Superficial		
Radioscaphocapitate	Radius to carpus	Blends with UC to form distal border of space of Poirier
○ Radioscaphoid (RS)	Radial styloid to scaphoid	Aka "radial collateral" lig. Stabilizes proximal pole
○ Radiocapitate (RC)	Radius to capitate body	Forms a fulcrum around which the scaphoid rotates
Long radiolunate (lRL)	Volar radius to lunate	Blends with palmar LT interosseous ligament
Ulnocapitate (UC)	Ulna/TFC to capitate	Blends with RSC laterally. Distal border of space of Poirier
Deep		
Short radiolunate (sRL)	Distal radius to lunate	**Stout & vertical. Prevents dx in hyperextension**
Ulnolunate (UL)	TFC to lunate	UL & UT blend with UC to help stabilize the DRUJ
Ulnotriquetral (UT)	TFC to triquetrum	UL & UT considered by some to be part of the TFCC
Radioscapholunate	Radius to SL joint	"Ligament of Testut," a neurovascular bundle to SL jt.
Extrinsic—Dorsal		
Dorsal radiocarpal (DRC)	Radius to lunate/triquetrum	Aka radiolunotriquetral (RLT); main dorsal stabilizer
○ Superficial bundle	Radius to triquetrum	The two bundles are typically indistinguishable
○ Deep bundle	Radius to LT joint	Fibers attach to lunate and/or lunotriquetral ligament

- Space of Poirier: weak spot volarly where perilunate dislocations occur (between the proximal edge of RSC & UC ligaments distally and distal edge of lRL ligament proximally).
- No true ulnar collateral ligament exists in the wrist. The ECU & sheath provide some ulnar collateral support.
- Deep volar extrinsic ligaments can be seen easily during wrist arthroscopy; the superficial ones are difficult to visualize.
- The UC, UL, and UT form the ulnocarpal ligamentous complex.

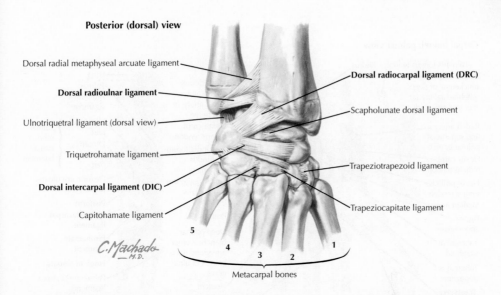

Posterior (dorsal) view

Dorsal radial metaphyseal arcuate ligament

Dorsal radioulnar ligament

Ulnotriquetral ligament (dorsal view)

Triquetrohamate ligament

Dorsal intercarpal ligament (DIC)

Capitohamate ligament

Dorsal radiocarpal ligament (DRC)

Scapholunate dorsal ligament

Trapeziotrapezoid ligament

Trapeziocapitate ligament

5 4 3 2 1

C. Machado
_M.D._

Metacarpal bones

LIGAMENTS	ATTACHMENTS	FUNCTION / COMMENT
INTRINSIC LIGAMENTS		
Midcarpal Joint		
Palmar		
Triquetrohamocapitate (THC) ○ Triquetrohamate (TH) ○ Triquetrocapitate (TC)	Triquetrum to: Hamate Capitate	Medial/ulnar portion of arcuate ligament Short, stout ligament Often confluent with the ulnocapitate part (UC) ligament
Scaphocapitate (SC)	Scaphoid to capitate	Stabilizes distal scaphoid. Radial part of arcuate lig.
Dorsal		
Dorsal intercarpal (DIC)	Triq. to tpzm./tpzd.	A primary dorsal support
Scaphotrapeziotrapezoid (STT)	Scaph. to tpzm./tpzd.	Lateral (radial) and scaphotrapezial joint support
Interosseous Joints		
PROXIMAL ROW: 2 joints. Ligaments are "C" shaped with dorsal and palmar limbs and a membranous portion between. The membrane prevents communication b/w the radiocarpal and midcarpal joints. It does not add stability. 1. Scapholunate (SL) joint: Scaphoid gives a flexion force to the lunate. Arch of motion during ROM: scaphoid>lunate. 2. Lunotriquetral (LT) joint: Triquetrum provides an extension force to the lunate, which is resisted by the LT.		
Scapholunate (SL or SLIL)	Scaphoid to lunate	Dorsal fibers strongest. Disruption: instability, (DISI) Palmar fibers are looser & allow scaphoid rotation
Lunotriquetral (LT)	Lunate to triquetrum	Palmar fibers strongest. Disruption (with DRC ligament injury) leads to carpal instability (VISI)
DISTAL ROW: 3 joints as below. Strong interosseous ligaments keep distal row moving as a single unit.		
Trapeziotrapezium Trapeziocapitate Capitohamate	Trapezoid to trapezium Capitate to trapezoid Capitate to hamate	Each ligament has 3 parts (palmar, dorsal, deep/ interosseous). Distal row ligaments are stronger than in proximal row. CH lig. is strongest distal row ligament.
Pisotriquetral Articulation		
Pisohamate	Pisiform to hamate	Inserts on hook of hamate; part of Guyon's canal
Pisometacarpal	Pisiform to 5th MC base	Assists in FCU flexion

Carpal tunnel: palmar view

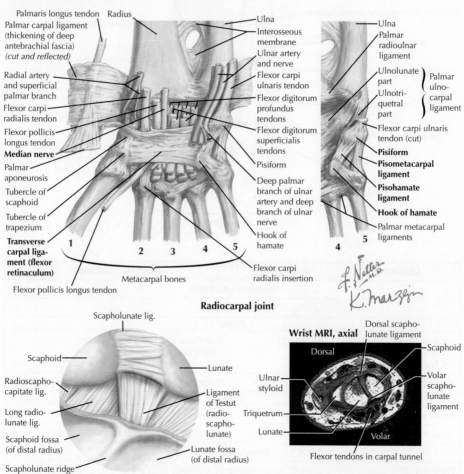

Palmaris longus tendon — Radius — Ulna
Palmar carpal ligament (thickening of deep antebrachial fascia) *(cut and reflected)*
Radial artery and superficial palmar branch
Flexor carpi radialis tendon
Flexor pollicis longus tendon
Median nerve
Palmar aponeurosis
Tubercle of scaphoid
Tubercle of trapezium
Transverse carpal ligament (flexor retinaculum)
Flexor pollicis longus tendon

Interosseous membrane
Ulnar artery and nerve
Flexor carpi ulnaris tendon
Flexor digitorum profundus tendons
Flexor digitorum superficialis tendons
Pisiform
Deep palmar branch of ulnar artery and deep branch of ulnar nerve
Hook of hamate
Flexor carpi radialis insertion
Metacarpal bones
1 2 3 4 5

Ulna
Palmar radioulnar ligament
Ulnolunate part
Ulnotriquetral part
} Palmar ulnocarpal ligament
Flexor carpi ulnaris tendon (cut)
Pisiform
Pisometacarpal ligament
Pisohamate ligament
Hook of hamate
Palmar metacarpal ligaments
4 5

Radiocarpal joint

Scapholunate lig.
Scaphoid
Radioscaphocapitate lig.
Long radiolunate lig.
Scaphoid fossa (of distal radius)
Scapholunate ridge
Lunate
Ligament of Testut (radioscapholunate)
Lunate fossa (of distal radius)

Wrist MRI, axial
Dorsal scapholunate ligament
Dorsal
Scaphoid
Ulnar styloid
Volar scapholunate ligament
Triquetrum
Lunate
Volar
Flexor tendons in carpal tunnel

Triangular fibrocartilage complex

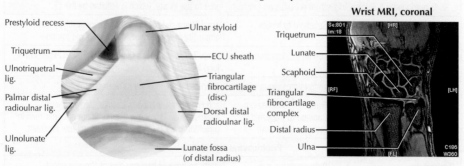

Prestyloid recess
Triquetrum
Ulnotriquetral lig.
Palmar distal radioulnar lig.
Ulnolunate lig.
Ulnar styloid
ECU sheath
Triangular fibrocartilage (disc)
Dorsal distal radioulnar lig.
Lunate fossa (of distal radius)

Wrist MRI, coronal
Triquetrum
Lunate
Scaphoid
Triangular fibrocartilage complex
Distal radius
Ulna

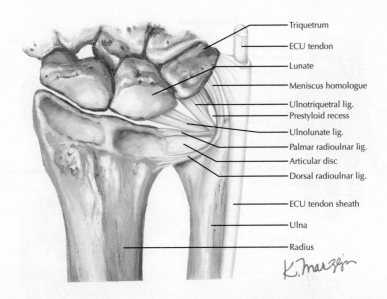

Triquetrum
ECU tendon
Lunate
Meniscus homologue
Ulnotriquetral lig.
Prestyloid recess
Ulnolunate lig.
Palmar radioulnar lig.
Articular disc
Dorsal radioulnar lig.
ECU tendon sheath
Ulna
Radius

LIGAMENTS	ATTACHMENTS	FUNCTION / COMMENT
DISTAL RADIOULNAR JOINT		
• This joint (DRUJ) is stabilized by a combination of structures that form the triangular fibrocartilage complex (TFCC). • Primary motion is pronation (60-80°) & supination (60-85°); the radius rotates around the stationary ulna. • 20% of an axial load is transmitted to ulna in an ulnar neutral wrist. The ulna takes more load when it is ulna positive.		
Triangular Fibrocartilage Complex		
• TFCC is interposed between the distal ulna and the ulnar proximal carpal row (triquetrum). It originates at the articular margin of the sigmoid notch (radius) and inserts at the base of the ulnar styloid. • Vascular supply to TFCC (from ulnar artery & anterior interosseous artery) penetrate the peripheral 10%-25%.		
Triangular fibrocartilage	Radius to ulna fovea (deep fibers) & styloid (superficial fibers)	TFC has 3 portions: central disc and 2 peripheral (radioulnar) ligaments
◦ Central (articular) disc	Blends w/ radial articular cartilage	Resists compression and tension; avascular and aneural
◦ Dorsal radioulnar	Dorsal radius to ulnar fovea (ligamentum subcruentum)	Blends with TFC, tight in pronation, loose in supination
◦ Palmar radioulnar	Volar radius to ulnar fovea (ligamentum subcruentum)	Blends with TFC, tight in supination, loose in pronation
Meniscal homologue	Dorsal radius to volar triquetrum	Highly vascular synovial fold
ECU tendon sheath	Ulna styloid, triquetrum, hamate	Considered an "ulnar collateral ligament"
Other		
• UL, UT, and prestyloid recess are considered by some to be a part of the TFCC.		
Ulnolunate (UL) Ulnotriquetral (UT)	TFC to lunate TFC to triquetrum	UL & UT blend with ulnocapitate lig. to contribute to fxn of TFCC and stabilize the DRUJ.
Prestyloid recess	None	Between palmar radioulnar ligament & meniscus homologue
• Other structures contributing to DRUJ stability: ECU, pronator quadratus, interosseous membrane. • TFCC can be torn (degenerative or traumatic). Peripheral tears can be repaired, central tears need debridement.		

Carpal tunnel

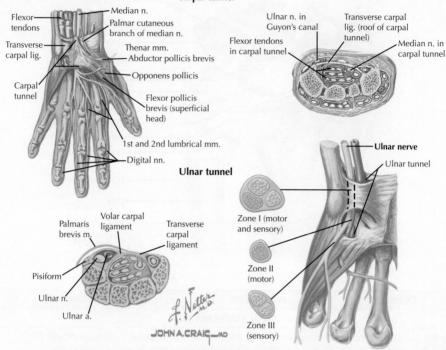

Carpal tunnel labels:
- Flexor tendons
- Transverse carpal lig.
- Carpal tunnel
- Median n.
- Palmar cutaneous branch of median n.
- Thenar mm.
- Abductor pollicis brevis
- Opponens pollicis
- Flexor pollicis brevis (superficial head)
- 1st and 2nd lumbrical mm.
- Digital nn.
- Ulnar n. in Guyon's canal
- Transverse carpal lig. (roof of carpal tunnel)
- Flexor tendons in carpal tunnel
- Median n. in carpal tunnel

Ulnar tunnel

Ulnar tunnel labels:
- Palmaris brevis m.
- Volar carpal ligament
- Transverse carpal ligament
- Pisiform
- Ulnar n.
- Ulnar a.
- Ulnar nerve
- Ulnar tunnel
- Zone I (motor and sensory)
- Zone II (motor)
- Zone III (sensory)

JOHN A. CRAIG—AD

STRUCTURE	COMPONENTS	COMMENTS
CARPAL TUNNEL		
Transverse carpal ligament (TCL, flexor retinaculum)	Attachments: Medial: pisiform and hamate Lateral: scaphoid and trapezium	• Roof of carpal tunnel, can compress median nerve. TCL is incised in a carpal tunnel release. • Tunnel is narrowest at hook of hamate
Borders	Roof: transverse carpal ligament Floor: central carpal bones Medial wall: pisiform and hamate Lateral wall: trapezium and scaphoid	• See above • Especially capitate and trapezoid • Hook of hamate gives medial wall • Trapezium is primary wall structure
Contents	Tendons: FDS (4), FDP (4), FPL Nerve: median	• 9 tendons within the carpal tunnel • Compressed in carpal tunnel syndrome
• Thenar motor branch of median nerve can exit under, through, or distal to the transverse carpal ligament. • A persistent median artery or aberrant muscle can occur in the tunnel and may cause carpal tunnel syndrome.		
ULNAR TUNNEL / GUYON'S CANAL		
Borders	Floor: transverse carpal ligament Roof: volar carpal ligament Medial wall: pisiform Lateral wall: hook of hamate	• Can be released simultaneously with CTR • Continuous with deep antebrachial fascia • Neurovascular bundle is under pisohamate ligament • Fracture can cause nerve compression.
Contents	Ulnar nerve Ulnar artery	• Divides in canal to deep & superficial branches • Terminates as superficial arch around hamate
• Fractures (malunion) or masses (e.g., ganglion cysts #1) can compress the ulnar nerve or artery within the canal.		

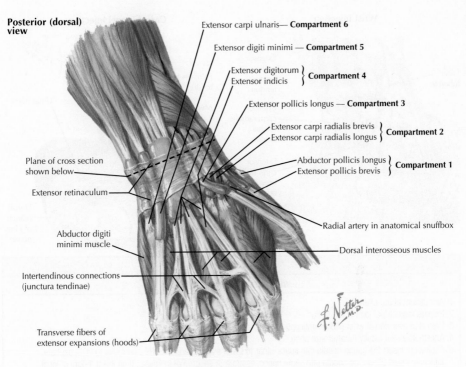

Posterior (dorsal) view

Extensor carpi ulnaris— **Compartment 6**

Extensor digiti minimi — **Compartment 5**

Extensor digitorum
Extensor indicis } **Compartment 4**

Extensor pollicis longus — **Compartment 3**

Extensor carpi radialis brevis
Extensor carpi radialis longus } **Compartment 2**

Abductor pollicis longus
Extensor pollicis brevis } **Compartment 1**

Plane of cross section shown below

Extensor retinaculum

Radial artery in anatomical snuffbox

Abductor digiti minimi muscle

Dorsal interosseous muscles

Intertendinous connections (junctura tendinae)

Transverse fibers of extensor expansions (hoods)

Cross section of most distal portion of forearm

Extensor retinaculum

Extensor pollicis longus — **Compartment 3**

Compartment 4 { Extensor digitorum and extensor indicis

Extensor carpi radialis brevis
Extensor carpi radialis longus } **Compartment 2**

Compartment 5 { Extensor digiti minimi

Compartment 6 { Extensor carpi ulnaris

Extensor pollicis brevis
Abductor pollicis longus } **Compartment 1**

Ulna

Radius

STRUCTURE	FUNCTION		COMMENTS
EXTENSOR COMPARTMENTS			
Extensor retinaculum	Covers the wrist dorsally		Forms six fibro-osseous compartments through which the extensor tendons pass
	Number	**Tendon**	**Clinical Condition**
Dorsal compartments	I	EPB, APL	de Quervain's tenosynovitis can develop here
	II	ECRL, ECRB	Tendinitis can occur here
	III	EPL	Travels around Lister's tubercle, can rupture
	IV	EDC, EIP	This compartment split in dorsal wrist approach
	V	EDQ (EDM)	Rupture (Jackson-Vaughn syndrome) in RA
	VI	ECU	Tendon can snap over ulnar styloid causing pain

• EIP and EDQ tendons are ulnar to EDC tendons to the index and small fingers, respectively.
• 1st compartment may have multiple slips that all need to be released in de Quervain's disease for a full release.

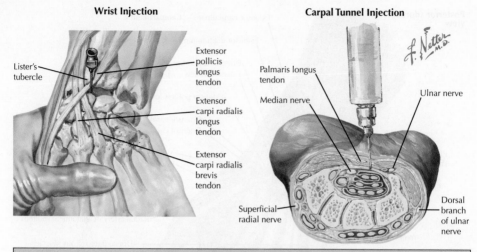

Wrist Injection

Carpal Tunnel Injection

Lister's tubercle

Extensor pollicis longus tendon

Extensor carpi radialis longus tendon

Extensor carpi radialis brevis tendon

Palmaris longus tendon

Median nerve

Ulnar nerve

Superficial radial nerve

Dorsal branch of ulnar nerve

STEPS
WRIST ASPIRATION/INJECTION

1. Ask patient about allergies
2. Palpate radiocarpal joint dorsally, find Lister's tubercle and the space ulnar to it
3. Prep skin over dorsal wrist (iodine/antiseptic soap)
4. Anesthetize skin locally (quarter size spot)
5. Aspiration: insert 20-gauge needle into space ulnar to Lister's tubercle/EPL/ECRB and radial to EDC, aspirate.
   Injection: insert 22-gauge needle into same space, aspirate to ensure not in vessel, then inject 1-2ml of local
   or local/steroid preparation into RC joint.
6. Dress injection site
7. If suspicious for infection, send fluid for Gram stain and culture

CARPAL TUNNEL INJECTION/MEDIAN NERVE BLOCK

1. Ask patient about allergies
2. Ask patient to pinch thumb and small finger tips; palmaris longus (PL) tendon will protrude (10% -20% do not have
   one). Median nerve is beneath PL, just ulnar to FCR within the carpal tunnel.
3. Prep skin over volar wrist (iodine/antiseptic soap)
4. Anesthetize skin locally (quarter size spot)
5. Insert 22-gauge or smaller needle into wrist ulnar to PL at flexion crease at 45° angle. Aspirate to ensure needle is
   not in a vessel. Inject 1-2ml of local or local/steroid preparation.
6. Dress injection site

WRIST BLOCK

Four separate nerves are blocked. Based on the necessary anesthesia, a complete or partial block can be performed:
1. Ask patient about allergies
2. Prep skin over each landmark (iodine/antiseptic soap)
3. **Ulnar nerve:** palpate the FCU tendon just proximal to volar wrist crease. Insert needle under the FCU tendon.
   Aspirate to ensure needle is not in ulnar artery (nerve is ulnar to the artery). Inject 3-4ml of local anesthetic into
   the space dorsal to the FCU tendon.
4. **Dorsal cutaneous branch** of ulnar nerve: palpate the distal ulna/styloid. Inject a large subcutaneous wheal on the
   dorsal and ulnar aspect of the wrist, just proximal to the ulnar styloid.
5. **Superficial radial nerve:** block at radial styloid with a large subcutaneous wheal on the dorsoradial aspect of
   the wrist.
6. **Median nerve:** block in carpal tunnel as described above
7. **Palmar cutaneous branch** of median nerve: raise a wheal over the central volar wrist.

• Median and superficial radial nerve blocks are effective for thumb, index finger, and most middle finger injuries.
• Ulnar and dorsal cutaneous branch blocks are used for small finger injuries. Most ring finger injuries require complete
  wrist block.

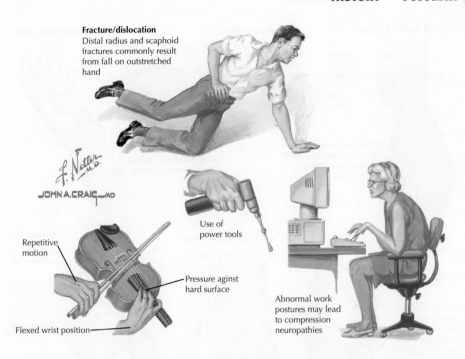

Fracture/dislocation
Distal radius and scaphoid fractures commonly result from fall on outstretched hand

F. Netter M.D.

JOHN A. CRAIG MD

Repetitive motion

Flexed wrist position

Use of power tools

Pressure aginst hard surface

Abnormal work postures may lead to compression neuropathies

QUESTION	ANSWER	CLINICAL APPLICATION
1. Age	Young	Trauma: fractures and dislocations, ganglions
	Middle aged, elderly	Arthritis, nerve entrapments, overuse
2. Pain		
a. Onset	Acute	Trauma
	Chronic	Arthritis
b. Location	Dorsal	Kienböck's disease, ganglion
	Volar	Carpal tunnel syndrome (CTS), ganglion (esp. radiovolar)
	Radial	Scaphoid fracture, de Quervain's tenosynovitis, arthritis
	Ulnar	Triangular fibrocartilage complex (TFCC) tear, tendinitis (e.g., ECU)
3. Stiffness	With dorsal pain	Kienböck's disease
	With volar pain (at night)	Carpal tunnel syndrome
4. Swelling	Joint: after trauma	Fracture or sprain
	Joint: no trauma	Arthritides, infection, gout
	Along tendons	Flexor or extensor tendinitis (calcific), de Quervain's disease
5. Instability	Popping, snapping	Carpal instability (e.g., scapholunate dislocation)
6. Mass	Along wrist joint	Ganglion
7. Trauma	Fall on hand	Fractures: distal radius, scaphoid; dislocation: lunate; TFCC tear
8. Activity	Repetitive motion (e.g., typing)	CTS, de Quervain's tenosynovitis
9. Neurologic symptoms	Numbness, tingling	Nerve entrapment (e.g., CTS), thoracic outlet syndrome, radiculopathy (cervical spine)
	Weakness	Nerve entrapment (median, ulnar, radial)
10. History of arthritides	Multiple joints involved	Arthritides

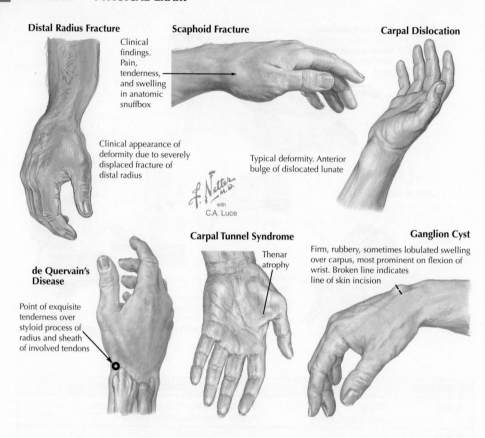

Distal Radius Fracture

Scaphoid Fracture

Clinical findings. Pain, tenderness, and swelling in anatomic snuffbox

Carpal Dislocation

Clinical appearance of deformity due to severely displaced fracture of distal radius

Typical deformity. Anterior bulge of dislocated lunate

F. Netter M.D.
with
C.A. Luce

de Quervain's Disease

Point of exquisite tenderness over styloid process of radius and sheath of involved tendons

Carpal Tunnel Syndrome

Thenar atrophy

Ganglion Cyst

Firm, rubbery, sometimes lobulated swelling over carpus, most prominent on flexion of wrist. Broken line indicates line of skin incision

EXAMINATION	TECHNIQUE	CLINICAL APPLICATION
INSPECTION		
Gross deformity	Bones and soft tissues	Fractures, dislocations: forearm and wrist
Swelling	Especially dorsal or radial Diffuse	Ganglion cyst Trauma (fracture/dislocation), infection
Wasting	Loss of muscle	Peripheral nerve compression (e.g., CTS)
PALPATION		
Skin changes	Warm, red Cool, dry	Infection, gout Neurovascular compromise
Radial and ulnar styloids	Palpate each separately	Tenderness may indicate fracture

Carpal bones	Both proximal and distal row
	
	Proximal row
	Pisiform
		Snuffbox tenderness: scaphoid fracture; lunate
		  tenderness: Kienböck's disease
		Scapholunate dissociation
		Tenderness: pisotriquetral arthritis or FCU
		  tendinitis

Soft tissues	6 dorsal extensor compartments TFCC: distal to ulnar styloid Compartments	Tenderness over 1st compartment: de Quervain's disease Tenderness indicates TFCC injury Firm/tense compartments = compartment synd.

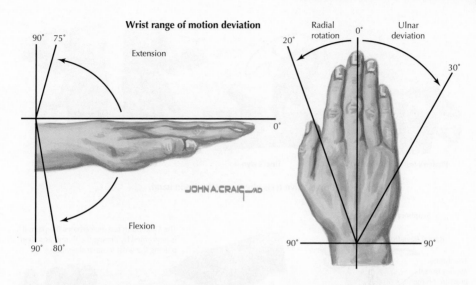

Wrist range of motion deviation

Extension

Flexion

90° 75°

90° 80°

0°

Radial
rotation

Ulnar
deviation

20°

0°

30°

90°

90°

JOHN A.CRAIG—MD

EXAMINATION	TECHNIQUE	CLINICAL APPLICATION
RANGE OF MOTION		
Flex and extend	Flex (toward palm), extend opposite	Normal: flexion 80°, extension 75°
Radial/ulnar deviation	In same plane as the palm	Normal: radial 15-25°, ulnar 30-45°
Pronate and supinate	Flex elbow 90°, rotate wrist	Normal: supinate 90°, pronate 80-90° (only 10-15° in wrist; most motion is in elbow)
NEUROVASCULAR		
Sensory		
Lateral cutaneous nerve of forearm (C6)	Lateral forearm	Deficit indicates corresponding nerve/root lesion
Medial cutaneous nerve of forearm (T1)	Medial forearm	Deficit indicates corresponding nerve/root lesion
Posterior cutaneous nerve of forearm	Posterior forearm	Deficit indicates corresponding nerve/root lesion
Motor		
Radial nerve (C6-7)	Resisted wrist extension	Weakness = ECRL/B or corresponding nerve/root lesion
PIN (C6-7)	Resisted ulnar deviation	Weakness = ECU or corresponding nerve/root lesion
Ulnar nerve (C8)	Resisted wrist flexion	Weakness = FCU or corresponding nerve/root lesion
Median nerve (C7)	Resisted wrist flexion	Weakness = FCR or corresponding nerve/root lesion
Median nerve (C6)	Resisted pronation	Weakness = pronator teres or corresponding nerve/root lesion
Musculocutaneous (C6)	Resisted supination	Weakness = biceps or corresponding nerve/root lesion
Reflex		
C6	Brachioradialis	Hypoactive/absence indicates corresponding radiculopathy
Pulses		
	Radial, ulnar	Diminished/absent = vascular injury or compromise (perform Allen test)

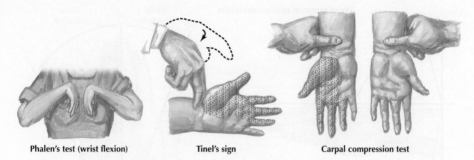

Phalen's test (wrist flexion)   Tinel's sign   Carpal compression test

Provocative tests elicit paresthesias in hand.

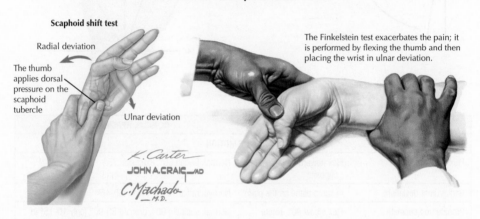

Scaphoid shift test

Radial deviation

The thumb applies dorsal pressure on the scaphoid tubercle

Ulnar deviation

The Finkelstein test exacerbates the pain; it is performed by flexing the thumb and then placing the wrist in ulnar deviation.

EXAMINATION	TECHNIQUE	CLINICAL APPLICATION / DDX
SPECIAL TESTS		
Durkan carpal compression	Manual pressure on median nerve at carpal tunnel	Reproduction of symptoms (e.g., tingling, numbness): median nerve compression (most sensitive test for carpal tunnel syndrome [CTS])
Phalen test	Flex both wrists for 1 minute	Reproduction of symptoms (e.g., tingling): median n. compression (CTS)
Tinel	Tap volar wrist (CT/TCL)	Reproduction of symptoms (e.g., tingling): median n. compression (CTS)
Finkelstein	Flex thumb into palm, ulnarly deviate the wrist	Pain in 1st dorsal compartment (APL/EPB tendons) suggests de Quervain's tenosynovitis
"Piano key"	Stabilize ulnar and translate radius dorsal and volar	Laxity or subluxation (click) indicates instability of DRUJ
Watson (scaphoid shift)	Push dorsally on distal pole of scaphoid, bring wrist from ulnar to radial deviation	A click or clunk (scaphoid subluxating dorsally over rim of distal radius) is positive for carpal instability (scapholunate dissociation)
Allen test	Occlude both radial and ulnar arteries manually, pump fist, then release one artery only	Delay or absence of "pinking up" of the palm and fingers suggests arterial compromise of the artery released

Anterior (volar)

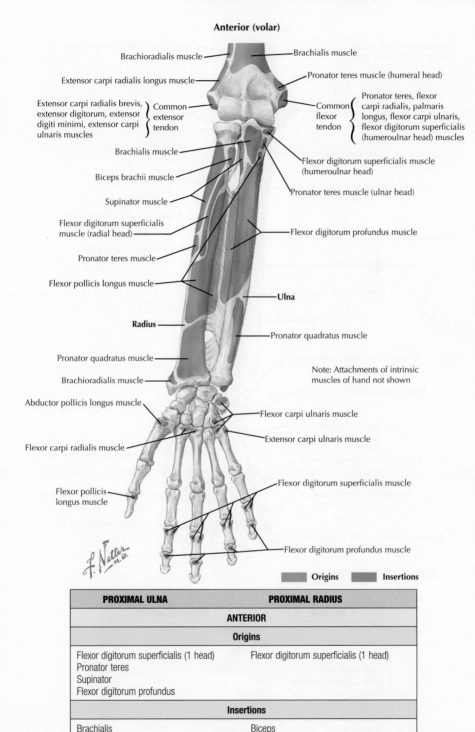

Brachioradialis muscle

Brachialis muscle

Extensor carpi radialis longus muscle

Pronator teres muscle (humeral head)

Extensor carpi radialis brevis, extensor digitorum, extensor digiti minimi, extensor carpi ulnaris muscles } Common extensor tendon

Common flexor tendon { Pronator teres, flexor carpi radialis, palmaris longus, flexor carpi ulnaris, flexor digitorum superficialis (humeroulnar head) muscles

Brachialis muscle

Biceps brachii muscle

Flexor digitorum superficialis muscle (humeroulnar head)

Supinator muscle

Pronator teres muscle (ulnar head)

Flexor digitorum superficialis muscle (radial head)

Flexor digitorum profundus muscle

Pronator teres muscle

Flexor pollicis longus muscle

Ulna

Radius

Pronator quadratus muscle

Pronator quadratus muscle

Brachioradialis muscle

Note: Attachments of intrinsic muscles of hand not shown

Abductor pollicis longus muscle

Flexor carpi ulnaris muscle

Extensor carpi ulnaris muscle

Flexor carpi radialis muscle

Flexor digitorum superficialis muscle

Flexor pollicis longus muscle

Flexor digitorum profundus muscle

Origins Insertions

PROXIMAL ULNA	PROXIMAL RADIUS
ANTERIOR	
Origins	
Flexor digitorum superficialis (1 head) Pronator teres Supinator Flexor digitorum profundus	Flexor digitorum superficialis (1 head)
Insertions	
Brachialis	Biceps Supinator

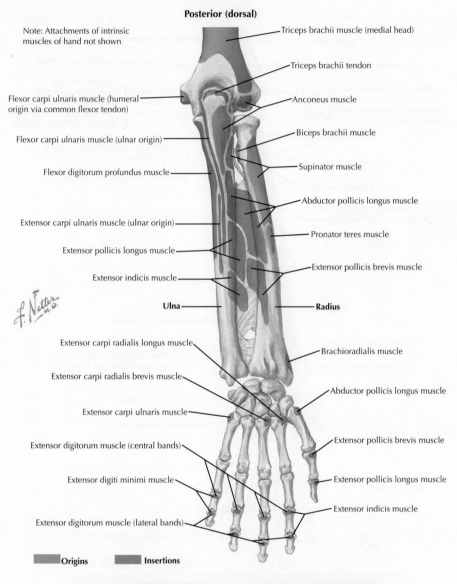

Posterior (dorsal)

Note: Attachments of intrinsic muscles of hand not shown

Triceps brachii muscle (medial head)

Flexor carpi ulnaris muscle (humeral origin via common flexor tendon)

Triceps brachii tendon

Anconeus muscle

Flexor carpi ulnaris muscle (ulnar origin)

Biceps brachii muscle

Flexor digitorum profundus muscle

Supinator muscle

Abductor pollicis longus muscle

Extensor carpi ulnaris muscle (ulnar origin)

Pronator teres muscle

Extensor pollicis longus muscle

Extensor pollicis brevis muscle

Extensor indicis muscle

Ulna

Radius

Extensor carpi radialis longus muscle

Brachioradialis muscle

Extensor carpi radialis brevis muscle

Abductor pollicis longus muscle

Extensor carpi ulnaris muscle

Extensor pollicis brevis muscle

Extensor digitorum muscle (central bands)

Extensor digiti minimi muscle

Extensor pollicis longus muscle

Extensor indicis muscle

Extensor digitorum muscle (lateral bands)

Origins   Insertions

PROXIMAL ULNA	PROXIMAL RADIUS
POSTERIOR	
Origins	
Flexor carpi ulnaris Flexor digitorum profundus Supinator	none
Insertions	
Triceps Anconeus	Biceps Supinator

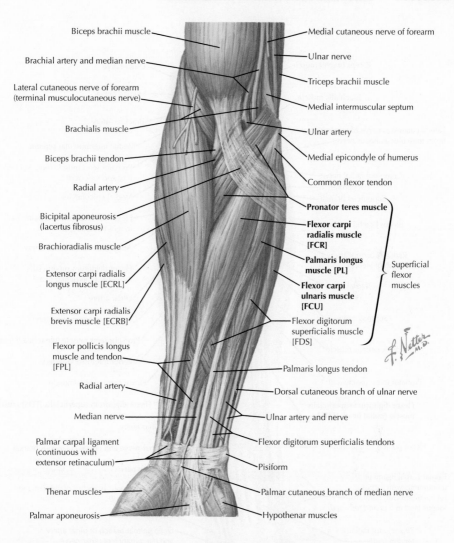

Biceps brachii muscle

Brachial artery and median nerve

Lateral cutaneous nerve of forearm
(terminal musculocutaneous nerve)

Brachialis muscle

Biceps brachii tendon

Radial artery

Bicipital aponeurosis
(lacertus fibrosus)

Brachioradialis muscle

Extensor carpi radialis
longus muscle [ECRL]

Extensor carpi radialis
brevis muscle [ECRB]

Flexor pollicis longus
muscle and tendon
[FPL]

Radial artery

Median nerve

Palmar carpal ligament
(continuous with
extensor retinaculum)

Thenar muscles

Palmar aponeurosis

Medial cutaneous nerve of forearm

Ulnar nerve

Triceps brachii muscle

Medial intermuscular septum

Ulnar artery

Medial epicondyle of humerus

Common flexor tendon

Pronator teres muscle

**Flexor carpi
radialis muscle
[FCR]**

**Palmaris longus
muscle [PL]**

**Flexor carpi
ulnaris muscle
[FCU]**

Flexor digitorum
superficialis muscle
[FDS]

Superficial
flexor
muscles

Palmaris longus tendon

Dorsal cutaneous branch of ulnar nerve

Ulnar artery and nerve

Flexor digitorum superficialis tendons

Pisiform

Palmar cutaneous branch of median nerve

Hypothenar muscles

MUSCLE	ORIGIN	INSERTION	NERVE	ACTION	COMMENT
SUPERFICIAL FLEXORS					
Pronator teres (PT) Humeral head Ulnar (deep) head	Medial epicondyle Proximal ulna	Lateral radius middle ⅓	Median	Pronate and flex forearm	Can compress me- dian nerve (prona- tor syndrome)
Flexor carpi radialis (FCR)	Medial epicondyle	Base of 2nd (and 3rd) metacarpal	Median	Flex wrist, ra- dial deviation	Radial artery is im- mediately lateral
Palmaris longus (PL)	Medial epicondyle	Flexor retinaculum/ palmar aponeurosis	Median	Flex wrist	Used for tendon transfers, 10% congenitally absent
Flexor carpi ulnaris (FCU)	1. Medial epicondyle 2. Posterior ulna	Pisiform, hook of hamate, 5th MC	Ulnar	Flex wrist, ulnar deviation	Most powerful wrist flexor. May com- press ulnar nerve

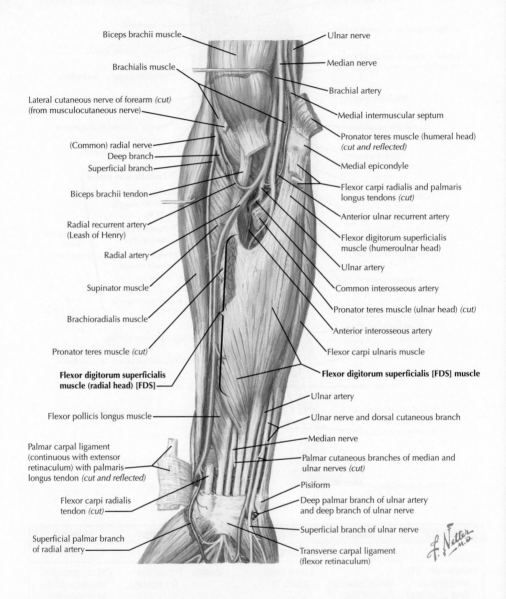

Biceps brachii muscle

Brachialis muscle

Lateral cutaneous nerve of forearm *(cut)*
(from musculocutaneous nerve)

(Common) radial nerve
Deep branch
Superficial branch

Biceps brachii tendon

Radial recurrent artery
(Leash of Henry)

Radial artery

Supinator muscle

Brachioradialis muscle

Pronator teres muscle *(cut)*

**Flexor digitorum superficialis
muscle (radial head) [FDS]**

Flexor pollicis longus muscle

Palmar carpal ligament
(continuous with extensor
retinaculum) with palmaris
longus tendon *(cut and reflected)*

Flexor carpi radialis
tendon *(cut)*

Superficial palmar branch
of radial artery

Ulnar nerve

Median nerve

Brachial artery

Medial intermuscular septum

Pronator teres muscle (humeral head)
(cut and reflected)

Medial epicondyle

Flexor carpi radialis and palmaris
longus tendons *(cut)*

Anterior ulnar recurrent artery

Flexor digitorum superficialis
muscle (humeroulnar head)

Ulnar artery

Common interosseous artery

Pronator teres muscle (ulnar head) *(cut)*

Anterior interosseous artery

Flexor carpi ulnaris muscle

Flexor digitorum superficialis [FDS] muscle

Ulnar artery

Ulnar nerve and dorsal cutaneous branch

Median nerve

Palmar cutaneous branches of median and
ulnar nerves *(cut)*

Pisiform

Deep palmar branch of ulnar artery
and deep branch of ulnar nerve

Superficial branch of ulnar nerve

Transverse carpal ligament
(flexor retinaculum)

MUSCLE	ORIGIN	INSERTION	NERVE	ACTION	COMMENT
		SUPERFICIAL FLEXORS			
Flexor digito-rum superficialis (FDS)	1. Medial epicondyle proximal ulna 2. Anteroproximal radius	Middle phalan-ges of digits (not thumb)	Median	Flex PIPJ (also flex digit and wrist)	Sublimus test will isolate and test function
FDS is often considered a "middle flexor" because of its position between muscles.					

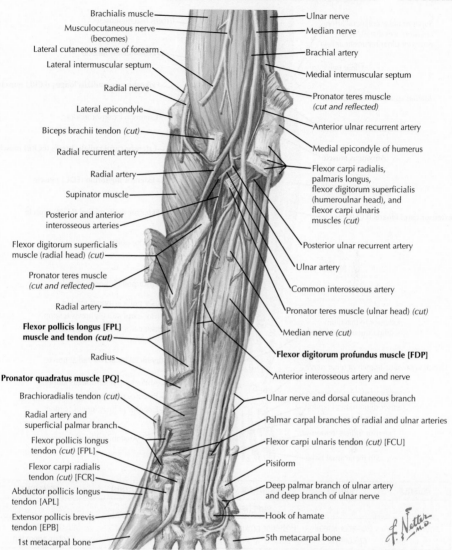

MUSCLE	ORIGIN	INSERTION	NERVE	ACTION	COMMENT
DEEP FLEXORS					
Flexor digitorum profundus (FDP)	Anterior ulna & interosseous membrane	Distal phalanx (IF, +/− MF) Distal phalanx (RF, SF, +/− MF)	Median/AIN Ulnar	Flex DIPJ (also flex digit and wrist)	Avulsion: Jersey finger Profundus test will isolate and test function
Flexor pollicis longus (FPL)	Anterior radius & proximal ulna	Distal phalanx of thumb	Median/AIN	Flex thumb IP	FDP and FPL are most susceptible to Volkmann's contracture
Pronator quadratus (PQ)	Medial distal ulna	Anterior distal radius	Median/AIN	Pronate forearm	Primary pronator (initiates pronation)
• AIN innervates all three deep flexors. It is tested by making "OK" signs.					

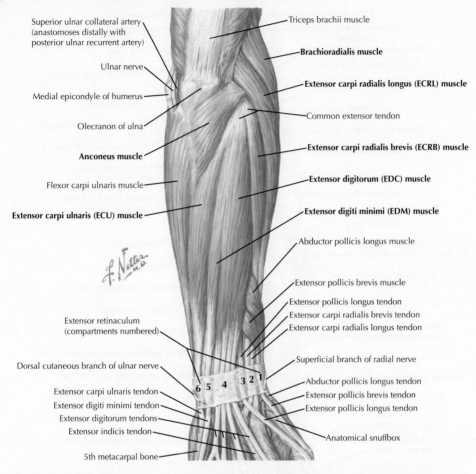

Superior ulnar collateral artery (anastomoses distally with posterior ulnar recurrent artery)

Ulnar nerve

Medial epicondyle of humerus

Olecranon of ulna

Anconeus muscle

Flexor carpi ulnaris muscle

Extensor carpi ulnaris (ECU) muscle

Extensor retinaculum (compartments numbered)

Dorsal cutaneous branch of ulnar nerve

Extensor carpi ulnaris tendon
Extensor digiti minimi tendon
Extensor digitorum tendons
Extensor indicis tendon

5th metacarpal bone

Triceps brachii muscle

Brachioradialis muscle

Extensor carpi radialis longus (ECRL) muscle

Common extensor tendon

Extensor carpi radialis brevis (ECRB) muscle

Extensor digitorum (EDC) muscle

Extensor digiti minimi (EDM) muscle

Abductor pollicis longus muscle

Extensor pollicis brevis muscle
Extensor pollicis longus tendon
Extensor carpi radialis brevis tendon
Extensor carpi radialis longus tendon

Superficial branch of radial nerve

Abductor pollicis longus tendon
Extensor pollicis brevis tendon
Extensor pollicis longus tendon

Anatomical snuffbox

MUSCLE	ORIGIN	INSERTION	NERVE	ACTION	COMMENT
SUPERFICIAL EXTENSORS					
Anconeus	Posterior-lateral epicondyle	Posterior-proximal ulna	Radial	Forearm extension	Muscular plane in Kocher approach
Extensor digito-rum commu-nis (EDC)	Lateral epicondyle	MCP: Sag. band P2: Central slip P3: Term. insert	Radial-PIN	Digit extension	Tendon avulsion: P2: boutonniere P3: mallet finger
Extensor digiti minimi (EDM)	Lateral epicondyle	Same as above in small finger	Radial-PIN	SF extension	Aka EDQ: In 5th dorsal compartment
Extensor carpi ulnaris (ECU)	Lateral epicondyle	Base of 5th MC	Radial-PIN	Hand extension and adduction	Can cause painful snapping over ulna
Mobile Wad					
Brachioradialis (BR)	Lateral condyle	Lateral distal radius	Radial	Forearm flexion	Is a deforming force in radius fractures
Extensor carpi radialis longus	Lateral condyle	Base of 2nd MC	Radial	Wrist extension	Aka ECRL
Extensor carpi radialis brevis	Lateral epicondyle	Base of 3rd MC	Radial-PIN	Wrist extension	ECRB degenerates in tennis elbow

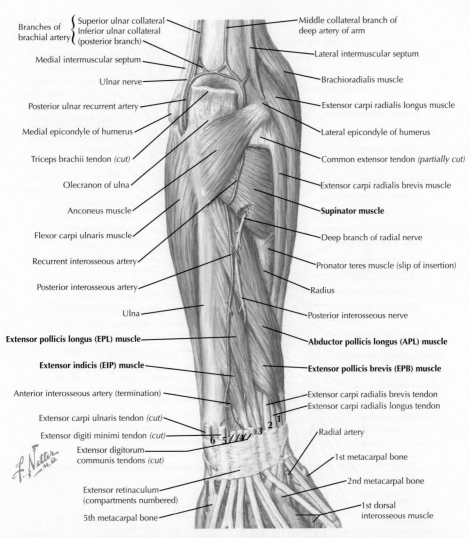

Branches of brachial artery { Superior ulnar collateral / Inferior ulnar collateral (posterior branch)

Medial intermuscular septum

Ulnar nerve

Posterior ulnar recurrent artery

Medial epicondyle of humerus

Triceps brachii tendon *(cut)*

Olecranon of ulna

Anconeus muscle

Flexor carpi ulnaris muscle

Recurrent interosseous artery

Posterior interosseous artery

Ulna

Extensor pollicis longus (EPL) muscle

Extensor indicis (EIP) muscle

Anterior interosseous artery (termination)

Extensor carpi ulnaris tendon *(cut)*

Extensor digiti minimi tendon *(cut)*

Extensor digitorum communis tendons *(cut)*

Extensor retinaculum (compartments numbered)

5th metacarpal bone

Middle collateral branch of deep artery of arm

Lateral intermuscular septum

Brachioradialis muscle

Extensor carpi radialis longus muscle

Lateral epicondyle of humerus

Common extensor tendon *(partially cut)*

Extensor carpi radialis brevis muscle

Supinator muscle

Deep branch of radial nerve

Pronator teres muscle (slip of insertion)

Radius

Posterior interosseous nerve

Abductor pollicis longus (APL) muscle

Extensor pollicis brevis (EPB) muscle

Extensor carpi radialis brevis tendon
Extensor carpi radialis longus tendon

Radial artery

1st metacarpal bone

2nd metacarpal bone

1st dorsal interosseous muscle

MUSCLE	ORIGIN	INSERTION	NERVE	ACTION	COMMENT
DEEP EXTENSORS					
Supinator	Posterior medial ulna	Proximal lateral radius	Radial-PIN	Forearm supination	PIN pierces muscles, can be compressed
Abductor pollicis longus (APL)	Posterior radius/ ulna	Base of 1st thumb meta-carpal	Radial-PIN	Abduct and ex-tend thumb (CMCJ)	de Quervain's dis-ease (may have multiple slips)
Extensor pollicis brevis (EPB)	Posterior radius	Base of thumb prox. phalanx	Radial-PIN	Extend thumb (MCPJ)	Radial border of snuffbox
Extensor pollicis longus (EPL)	Posterior ulna	Base of thumb distal phalanx	Radial-PIN	Extend thumb (IPJ)	Tendon turns 45° on Lister's tubercle
Extensor indicis proprius (EIP)	Posterior ulna	Same as EDC & EDM	Radial-PIN	Index finger extension	Ulnar to EDC tendon; last PIN muscle

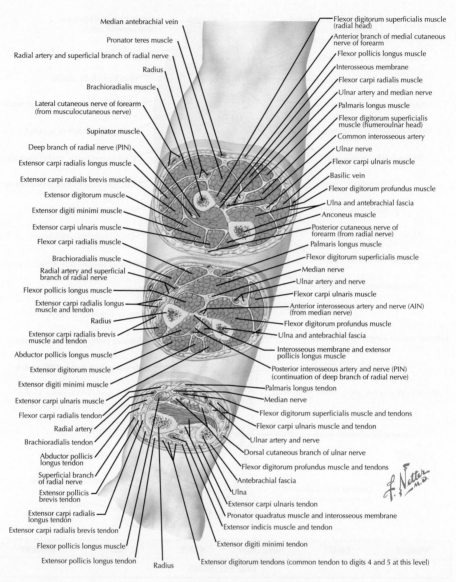

Median antebrachial vein

Pronator teres muscle

Radial artery and superficial branch of radial nerve

Radius

Brachioradialis muscle

Lateral cutaneous nerve of forearm (from musculocutaneous nerve)

Supinator muscle

Deep branch of radial nerve (PIN)

Extensor carpi radialis longus muscle

Extensor carpi radialis brevis muscle

Extensor digitorum muscle

Extensor digiti minimi muscle

Extensor carpi ulnaris muscle

Flexor carpi radialis muscle

Brachioradialis muscle

Radial artery and superficial branch of radial nerve

Flexor pollicis longus muscle

Extensor carpi radialis longus muscle and tendon

Radius

Extensor carpi radialis brevis muscle and tendon

Abductor pollicis longus muscle

Extensor digitorum muscle

Extensor digiti minimi muscle

Extensor carpi ulnaris muscle

Flexor carpi radialis tendon

Radial artery

Brachioradialis tendon

Abductor pollicis longus tendon

Superficial branch of radial nerve

Extensor pollicis brevis tendon

Extensor carpi radialis longus tendon

Extensor carpi radialis brevis tendon

Flexor pollicis longus muscle

Extensor pollicis longus tendon

Radius

Flexor digitorum superficialis muscle (radial head)

Anterior branch of medial cutaneous nerve of forearm

Flexor pollicis longus muscle

Interosseous membrane

Flexor carpi radialis muscle

Ulnar artery and median nerve

Palmaris longus muscle

Flexor digitorum superficialis muscle (humeroulnar head)

Common interosseous artery

Ulnar nerve

Flexor carpi ulnaris muscle

Basilic vein

Flexor digitorum profundus muscle

Ulna and antebrachial fascia

Anconeus muscle

Posterior cutaneous nerve of forearm (from radial nerve)

Palmaris longus muscle

Flexor digitorum superficialis muscle

Median nerve

Ulnar artery and nerve

Flexor carpi ulnaris muscle

Anterior interosseous artery and nerve (AIN) (from median nerve)

Flexor digitorum profundus muscle

Ulna and antebrachial fascia

Interosseous membrane and extensor pollicis longus muscle

Posterior interosseous artery and nerve (PIN) (continuation of deep branch of radial nerve)

Palmaris longus tendon

Median nerve

Flexor digitorum superficialis muscle and tendons

Flexor carpi ulnaris muscle and tendon

Ulnar artery and nerve

Dorsal cutaneous branch of ulnar nerve

Flexor digitorum profundus muscle and tendons

Antebrachial fascia

Ulna

Extensor carpi ulnaris tendon

Pronator quadratus muscle and interosseous membrane

Extensor indicis muscle and tendon

Extensor digiti minimi tendon

Extensor digitorum tendons (common tendon to digits 4 and 5 at this level)

STRUCTURE	RELATIONSHIP
RELATIONSHIPS	
Ulnar nerve/artery	Run under FDS on top of FDP muscles, ulnar to the artery
Superior branch of radial nerve	Runs under the brachioradialis muscle/tendon, radial to the artery
Radial artery	Is radial (lateral) to FCR muscle and tendon
Median nerve	Is radial (lateral) to ulnar nerve, runs between FDP and FPL muscles into the carpal tunnel
Post. interosseous nerve (PIN)	Pierces supinator muscle proximally, runs between APL & EPL along interosseous membrane

Incisions for Compartment Syndrome of Forearm and Hand

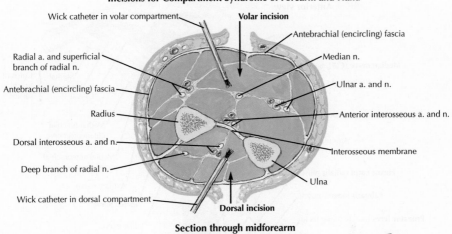

Wick catheter in volar compartment
Volar incision
Antebrachial (encircling) fascia
Radial a. and superficial branch of radial n.
Median n.
Antebrachial (encircling) fascia
Ulnar a. and n.
Radius
Anterior interosseous a. and n.
Dorsal interosseous a. and n.
Interosseous membrane
Deep branch of radial n.
Ulna
Wick catheter in dorsal compartment
Dorsal incision

Section through midforearm

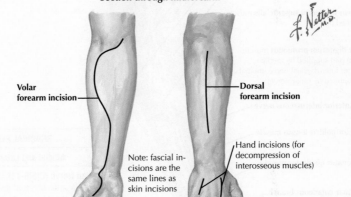

Volar forearm incision
Dorsal forearm incision
Note: fascial incisions are the same lines as skin incisions
Hand incisions (for decompression of interosseous muscles)

STRUCTURE	CONTENTS
COMPARTMENTS	
Anterior	
Superficial	Pronator teres (PT), flexor carpi radialis (FCR), palmaris longus (PL), flexor carpi ulnaris (FCU)
Middle	Flexor digitorum superficialis (FDS)
Deep	Flexor digitorum profundus (FDP), flexor pollicis longus (FPL), pronator quadratus (PQ)
Posterior	
Superficial	Anconeus, ext. digit. communis (EDC), ext. digit. minimi (EDM), ext. carpi ulnaris (ECU)
Deep	Supinator, abd. poll. longus (APL), ext. poll. brevis (EPB), ext. poll. longus (EPL), ext. indicis proprius (EIP)
Mobile Wad	
	Brachioradialis, extensor carpi radialis longus (ECRL), extensor carpi radialis brevis (ECRB)
FASCIOTOMIES	
Palmar incision	Releases the entire anterior compartment
Dorsal incision	Releases the entire posterior compartment and mobile wad

Anterior view

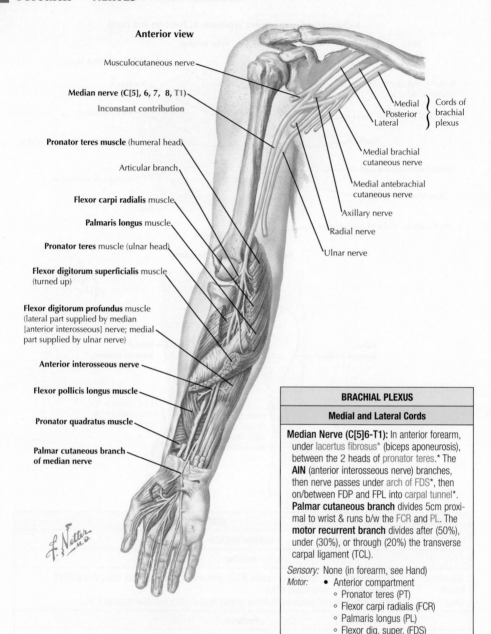

Musculocutaneous nerve

Median nerve (C[5], 6, 7, 8, T1)

Inconstant contribution

Pronator teres muscle (humeral head)

Articular branch

Flexor carpi radialis muscle

Palmaris longus muscle

Pronator teres muscle (ulnar head)

Flexor digitorum superficialis muscle (turned up)

Flexor digitorum profundus muscle (lateral part supplied by median [anterior interosseous] nerve; medial part supplied by ulnar nerve)

Anterior interosseous nerve

Flexor pollicis longus muscle

Pronator quadratus muscle

Palmar cutaneous branch of median nerve

Medial
Posterior } Cords of brachial plexus
Lateral

Medial brachial cutaneous nerve

Medial antebrachial cutaneous nerve

Axillary nerve

Radial nerve

Ulnar nerve

BRACHIAL PLEXUS
Medial and Lateral Cords

Median Nerve (C[5]6-T1): In anterior forearm, under lacertus fibrosus* (biceps aponeurosis), between the 2 heads of pronator teres.* The **AIN** (anterior interosseous nerve) branches, then nerve passes under arch of FDS*, then on/between FDP and FPL into carpal tunnel*. **Palmar cutaneous branch** divides 5cm proximal to wrist & runs b/w the FCR and PL. The **motor recurrent branch** divides after (50%), under (30%), or through (20%) the transverse carpal ligament (TCL).

Sensory: None (in forearm, see Hand)
Motor: • Anterior compartment
      ○ Pronator teres (PT)
      ○ Flexor carpi radialis (FCR)
      ○ Palmaris longus (PL)
      ○ Flexor dig. super. (FDS)

Anterior Interosseous Nerve (AIN): Branches proximally, then runs along the interosseous membrane with anterior interosseous artery, between FPL & FDP

Sensory: Volar wrist capsule
Motor: • Anterior compartment—deep flexors
      ○ Flexor digitorum profundus (FDP) to 2nd (3rd) digits
      ○ Flexor pollicis longus (FPL)
      ○ Pronator quadratus (PQ)

*Potential site of nerve compression.

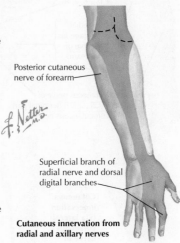

Radial nerve (C5, 6, 7, 8, [T1]) Inconstant contribution
Superficial (terminal) branch
Deep (terminal) branch (PIN) **Posterior view**
Lateral epicondyle
Anconeus muscle
Brachioradialis muscle
Extensor carpi radialis longus muscle
Supinator muscle
Extensor carpi radialis brevis muscle Posterior cutaneous
Extensor carpi ulnaris muscle nerve of forearm
Extensor digitorum muscle and
extensor digiti minimi muscle
Extensor indicis muscle
Extensor pollicis longus muscle
Abductor pollicis longus muscle
Extensor pollicis brevis muscle
Posterior interosseous nerve Superficial branch of
(continuation of deep branch of radial nerve and dorsal
radial nerve distal to supinator muscle) digital branches
Superficial (sensory) branch of radial nerve

**Cutaneous innervation from
radial and axillary nerves**

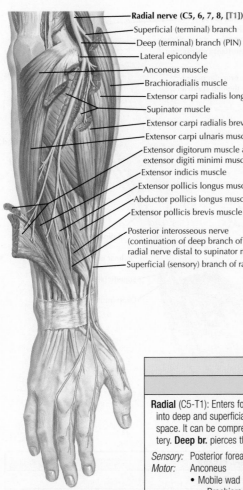

BRACHIAL PLEXUS
Posterior Cord
Radial (C5-T1): Enters forearm b/w brachioradialis (BR) & brachialis, then divides into deep and superficial branches. **Superficial br.** runs under BR to thumb web space. It can be compressed under the BR tendon.* It is lateral to the radial artery. **Deep br.** pierces the supinator, then becomes the **PIN**.

Sensory: Posterior forearm: via **posterior cutaneous nerve of forearm**
 Motor: Anconeus
   • Mobile wad
     ○ Brachioradialis (BR)
     ○ Extensor carpi radialis longus (ECRL)

Posterior Interosseous Nerve (PIN): Runs past vascular Leash of Henry* (recurrent radial artery) and ECRB, through the arcade of Frohse* (proximal supinator), into the supinator, past its distal edge,* then along interosseous membrane under EDC and between APL and EPL.

Sensory: Dorsal wrist capsule (in 4th dorsal compartment)
Motor: • Mobile wad
    ○ Extensor carpi radialis brevis (ECRB)
  • Posterior compartment—superficial extensors
    ○ Supinator
    ○ Extensor digitorum communis (EDC)
    ○ Extensor digiti minimi (EDM or EDQ)
    ○ Extensor carpi ulnaris (ECU)
  • Posterior compartment—deep extensors
    ○ Abductor pollicis longus (APL)
    ○ Extensor pollicis brevis (EPB)
    ○ Extensor pollicis longus (EPL)
    ○ Extensor indicis proprius (EIP)

*Potential site of nerve compression.

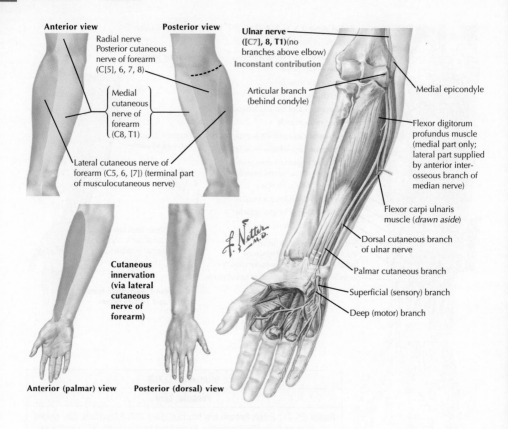

Anterior view

Radial nerve
Posterior cutaneous
nerve of forearm
(C[5], 6, 7, 8)

Medial
cutaneous
nerve of
forearm
(C8, T1)

Lateral cutaneous nerve of
forearm (C5, 6, [7]) (terminal part
of musculocutaneous nerve)

Posterior view

Ulnar nerve
([C7], **8, T1**)(no
branches above elbow)
Inconstant contribution

Articular branch
(behind condyle)

Medial epicondyle

Flexor digitorum
profundus muscle
(medial part only;
lateral part supplied
by anterior inter-
osseous branch of
median nerve)

Flexor carpi ulnaris
muscle (*drawn aside*)

Dorsal cutaneous branch
of ulnar nerve

Palmar cutaneous branch

Superficial (sensory) branch

Deep (motor) branch

Cutaneous
innervation
(via lateral
cutaneous
nerve of
forearm)

F. Netter M.D.

Anterior (palmar) view   **Posterior (dorsal) view**

BRACHIAL PLEXUS
Lateral Cord
Musculocutaneous (C5-7): Exits between biceps & brachialis, purely sensory, runs in subcutaneous tissues above the brachioradialis *Sensory:* Radial forearm: via **lateral cutaneous nerve of forearm** *Motor:* None (in forearm)
MEDIAL CORD
Medial Cutaneous Nerve of Forearm (Antebrachial Cutaneous) (C8-T1): Branches directly from the cord, runs subcutaneously anterior to medial epicondyle into the medial forearm *Sensory:* Medial forearm *Motor:* None

Ulnar (C[7]8-T1): Runs posterior to medial epicondyle in cubital tunnel,* then through FCU heads/aponeurosis,* then runs on FDP (under FDS) to wrist. The **dorsal** and **palmar cutaneous branches** divide 4-5cm proximal to wrist, then the nerve runs into the ulnar tunnel (Guyon's canal*), where it divides into deep/**motor** & superficial/**sensory branches**
Sensory: None (in forearm)
Motor: • Anterior compartment
   ◦ Flexor carpi ulnaris (FCU)
   ◦ Flexor digitorum profundus (FDP) to (3rd), 4th, 5th digits

*Potential site of nerve compression.

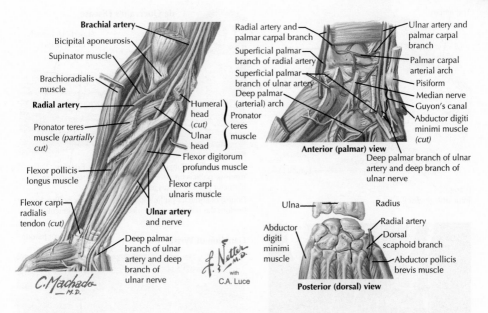

Anterior (palmar) view

Posterior (dorsal) view

COURSE	BRANCHES	
FOREARM		
Radial Artery		
Runs over the pronator teres, on FDS & FPL lateral to the FCR	Radial recurrent (leash of Henry) Muscular branches	
Ulnar Artery		
Runs under the ulnar head of the pronator teres, on the FDP muscle, lateral and adjacent to the ulnar nerve	Anterior ulnar recurrent Posterior ulnar recurrent Common interosseous ○ Anterior interosseous ○ Posterior interosseous ○ Recurrent interosseous Muscular branches	
WRIST		
Radial Artery		
Lateral to FCR tendon, wraps dorsally, under the APL & EPB tendons, between the 2 heads of 1st dorsal interosseous muscles, to the palm ending in deep arch	Palmar carpal branch Dorsal carpal branch **Superficial palmar branch** ○ Palmar scaphoid branch Dorsal scaphoid branch **Deep palmar arch**	Deep to flexor tendons Deep to extensor tendons Anastomoses w/super. palmar arch Supplies 25% of scaphoid (distal) Supplies 75% of scaphoid (proximal) Terminal branch of radial artery in hand
Ulnar Artery		
On transverse carpal ligament (TCL) into Guyon's canal, divides into deep and superficial palmar branches	Palmar carpal branch Dorsal carpal branch **Deep palmar** branch **Superficial palmar arch**	Deep to flexor tendons Deep to extensor tendons Anastomoses with deep palmar arch Terminal branch of the *ulnar* artery
• Allen test: Occlude both radial and ulnar arteries at the wrist. Patient squeezes fist to exsanguinate the hand. Release one artery and check for hand perfusion. Repeat with the other artery. Test confirms patency of arches/vessels.		

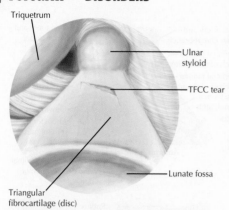

Triquetrum

Ulnar styloid

TFCC tear

Lunate fossa

Triangular fibrocartilage (disc)

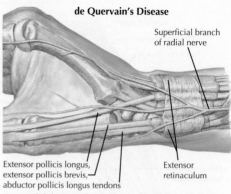

de Quervain's Disease

Superficial branch of radial nerve

Extensor pollicis longus, extensor pollicis brevis, abductor pollicis longus tendons

Extensor retinaculum

Course of abductor pollicis longus and extensor pollicis brevis tendons through 1st compartment of extensor retinaculum

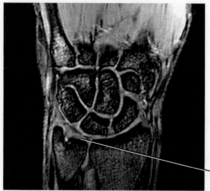

Triangular fibrocartilage tear (TFCC)

TFCC tear

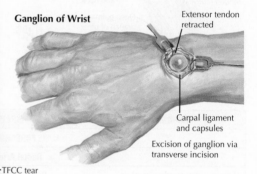

Ganglion of Wrist

Extensor tendon retracted

Carpal ligament and capsules

Excision of ganglion via transverse incision

DESCRIPTION	Hx & PE	WORKUP/FINDINGS	TREATMENT
TRIANGULAR FIBROCARTILAGE COMPLEX (TFCC) TEAR			
• Can be traumatic (class 1) or degenerative (class 2) • Only periphery is vascular (i.e., peripheral tear can be repaired)	**Hx:** Ulnar wrist pain, +/− popping/grinding **PE:** TFC is TTP, + TFCC, grind, +/− piano key	**XR:** Usually normal; tears assoc. w/styloid base fx **MRA:** Study of choice for diagnosis of tears	1. Class 1: repair or debride tear (fix styloid fracture if needed) 2. Class 2: NSAIDs, splint; ulnar shortening procedure
de QUERVAIN'S TENOSYNOVITIS			
• Inflammation of first dorsal compartment (APL/EPB tendons) • Middle age women #1. • Assoc. w/tendon abnormality	**Hx:** Radial pain/swelling **PE:** Tenderness at 1st dorsal compartment, + Finkelstein's test	**XR:** Usually normal **MR:** No indication	1. Splint and NSAIDs 2. Corticosteroid injection into sheath 3. Surgical release
GANGLION CYST			
• Synovial fluid–filled cyst arising from a wrist joint • Most common mass in wrist • Dorsal wrist most common site (usually from SL joint)	**Hx:** Mass, +/− pain **PE:** Palpable, mobile mass, +/− tenderness, + transillumination	**XR:** Wrist series usually normal **MR:** Will show cyst well, needed only if diagnosis is uncertain	1. Observation if asymptomatic 2. Aspiration (recurrence 20%) 3. Excision (including stalk of cyst; recurrence <10%)

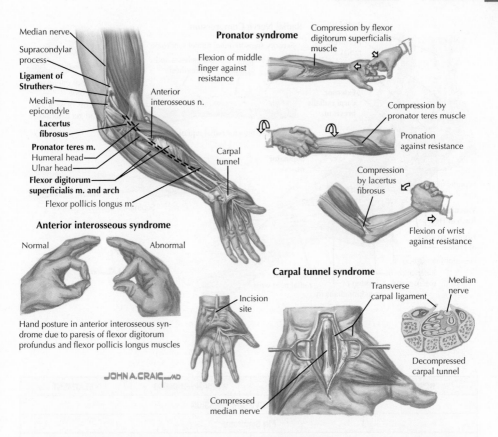

Median nerve
Supracondylar process
Ligament of Struthers
Medial epicondyle
Lacertus fibrosus
Pronator teres m.
Humeral head
Ulnar head
Flexor digitorum superficialis m. and arch
Flexor pollicis longus m.
Anterior interosseous n.
Carpal tunnel

Anterior interosseous syndrome

Normal   Abnormal

Hand posture in anterior interosseous syndrome due to paresis of flexor digitorum profundus and flexor pollicis longus muscles

JOHN A.CRAIG—AD

Pronator syndrome

Flexion of middle finger against resistance

Compression by flexor digitorum superficialis muscle

Compression by pronator teres muscle

Pronation against resistance

Compression by lacertus fibrosus

Flexion of wrist against resistance

Carpal tunnel syndrome

Transverse carpal ligament
Median nerve

Incision site

Compressed median nerve

Decompressed carpal tunnel

DESCRIPTION	Hx & PE	WORKUP/FINDINGS	TREATMENT
MEDIAN NERVE COMPRESSION			
Pronator Syndrome			
• Proximal median nerve compression • Sites: 1. Ligament of Struthers, 2. Pronator teres, 3. Lacertus fibrosis, 4. FDS aponeurosis/arch	**Hx:** Numbness, tingling, +/− weakness **PE:** Decreased palm sensation, + pronator or FDS sign	**XR:** Look for supracondylar process off humerus **EMG/NCS:** Can confirm dx (can also be normal)	1. Activity modification/rest 2. Splinting, NSAIDs 3. Surgical decompression of all proximal compression sites
AIN Syndrome			
• Rare nerve compression • Same sites at pronator syndrome • Motor symptoms only	**Hx:** Weakness, +/− pain **PE:** Weak thumb (FPL) and IF (FDP) pinch	**XR:** Usually normal **EMG/NCS:** Will confirm diagnosis if unclear	1. Activity modification 2. Splinting, NSAIDs 3. Surgical decompression
Carpal Tunnel Syndrome			
• Compression in carpal tunnel • Most common neuropathy • Associated with metabolic diseases (thyroid, diabetes), pregnancy	**Hx:** Numbness, +/− pain **PE:** +/− thenar atrophy, + Durkin's, +/− Phalen's, & Tinel's tests	**XR:** Usually normal **EMG/NCS:** Will confirm diagnosis if unclear (incr. latency, decr. velocity)	1. Activity modification 2. Night splints, NSAIDs 3. Corticosteroid injection 4. Carpal tunnel release

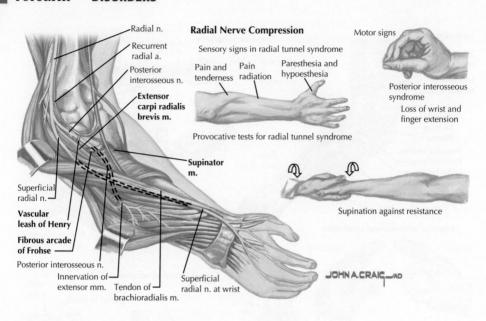

Radial n.
Recurrent radial a.
Posterior interosseous n.
Extensor carpi radialis brevis m.
Superficial radial n.
Vascular leash of Henry
Fibrous arcade of Frohse
Posterior interosseous n.
Innervation of extensor mm.
Tendon of brachioradialis m.
Superficial radial n. at wrist
Supinator m.

Radial Nerve Compression

Sensory signs in radial tunnel syndrome

Pain and tenderness | Pain radiation | Paresthesia and hypoesthesia

Provocative tests for radial tunnel syndrome

Motor signs

Posterior interosseous syndrome
Loss of wrist and finger extension

Supination against resistance

JOHN A.CRAIG—AD

DESCRIPTION	Hx & PE	WORKUP/FINDINGS	TREATMENT
RADIAL NERVE COMPRESSION			
PIN Syndrome			
• Compression in radial tunnel • Sites: 1. Fibrous bands, 2. Leash of Henry, 3. ECRB, 4. Arcade of Frohse (proximal supinator edge), 5. Distal edge of supinator	Hx: Hand & wrist weakness, +/– elbow pain PE: Weak thumb/ finger ext., TTP at radial tunnel	XR: Look for radiocapitellar abnormality MR: Evaluate for masses EMG/NCS: Confirms diagnosis & localizes lesion	1. Activity modification 2. Splint, NSAIDs 3. Surgical decompression (complete release)
Radial Tunnel Syndrome			
• Compression in radial tunnel • Same sites as above • Pain only, no weakness	Hx: Lat. elbow pain PE: Radial tunnel TTP, no weakness	XR: Evaluate RC joint MR: Evaluate for masses EMG/NCS: Not useful	1. Activity modification 2. Splint, NSAIDs 3. Surgical decompression
Wartenberg's Syndrome			
• Compression of superficial radial nerve at wrist (b/w ERCL and BR tendons) • Sensory symptoms only	Hx: Numbness/pain PE: Decr. sensation IF/thumb. + Tinel's, sx w/pronation	XR: Usually normal MR: Usually not helpful EMG/NCS: May confirm diagnosis	1. Activity modification 2. Wrist splint, NSAIDs 3. Surgical decompression
ULNAR NERVE COMPRESSION			
Ulnar Tunnel (Guyon's Canal) Syndrome			
• Compression in Guyon's canal • Etiology: ganglion, hamate malunion, thrombotic a., muscle • Sensory (zone 3), motor (zone 2), or mixed (zone 1) symptoms	Hx: Numbness, weakness in hand PE: Decr. sensation, +/– atrophy, clawing, weakness	XR: Look for fracture CT: Evaluate for fx/malunion MR: Useful for masses US: Evaluate for thrombosis EMG: Confirm diagnosis	1. Activity modification 2. Splint, NSAIDs 3. Surgical decompression (address underlying cause of compression)

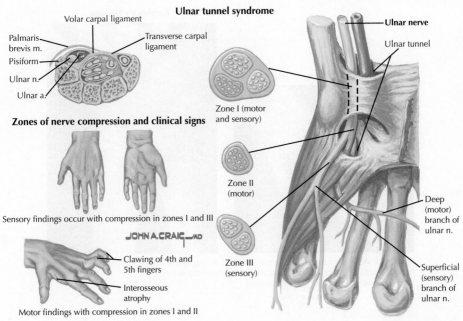

Ulnar tunnel syndrome

Volar carpal ligament

Palmaris brevis m.

Pisiform

Ulnar n.

Ulnar a.

Transverse carpal ligament

Ulnar nerve

Ulnar tunnel

Zone I (motor and sensory)

Zones of nerve compression and clinical signs

Sensory findings occur with compression in zones I and III

JOHN A.CRAIG—AD

Zone II (motor)

Deep (motor) branch of ulnar n.

Clawing of 4th and 5th fingers

Interosseous atrophy

Motor findings with compression in zones I and II

Zone III (sensory)

Superficial (sensory) branch of ulnar n.

DESCRIPTION	EVALUATION	TREATMENT
CARPAL INSTABILITY		
Carpal Instability, Dissociative (CID)		
Instability within a carpal row; two main types: 1. Dorsal intercalated segment instability (**DISI**) ○ Due to scapholunate (SL) ligament disruption or scaphoid fracture/nonunion ○ Deformity: scaphoid flexes, lunate extends ○ May lead to STT arthritis or SLAC wrist 2. Volar intercalated segment instability (**VISI**) ○ Due to lunotriquetral ligament disrupted (also requires dorsal radiocarpal lig. injury)	**Hx:** Trauma, pain +/− popping **PE:** +/− decreased ROM, +/− snuffbox or SL/LT interval tenderness, + Watson test (DISI) or Regan test (VISI) **XR:** Wrist & clenched fist views ○ DISI: SL gap >3mm, SL angle >70°, "ring sign" ○ VISI: disrupted carpal arches **MRA:** Can confirm ligament inj.	**Acute/early treatment:** 1. Fx: ORIF of scaphoid 2. Ligament: SL or LT ligament repair or reconstruction with pin fixation 3. Capsulodesis **Chronic/late treatment:** 1. Limited fusion (e.g., STT fusion for DISI)
Carpal Instability, Nondissociative (CIND)		
• Instability between carpal rows • Midcarpal or radiocarpal variations • Associated with generalized hyperlaxity or trauma to ligaments (e.g., ulnar translation at RCJ) or to bones (e.g., distal radius fracture)	**Hx:** Fall/trauma or ligament hyperlaxity; popping/clunking **PE:** Tenderness, instability **XR:** Evaluate for fxs & static carpal translation **Fluoro:** Dynamic carpal transl.	1. Nonoperative: splint/cast (esp. midcarpal) 2. Arthrodesis (fusion) ○ Midcarpal ○ Radiocarpal
Carpal Instability, Combined (CIC)		
• Instability both within a row & between rows • Perilunate dislocation most common • Greater arc injury = transosseous injury • Lesser arc injury = ligamentous injury	**Hx:** Fall/trauma, pain **PE:** Tenderness, instability **XR:** Disruption of carpal arches, lunate abnormality (angle &/or position)	1. ORIF of bones with primary repair of ligaments 2. Late: arthrodesis

Kienböck's Disease

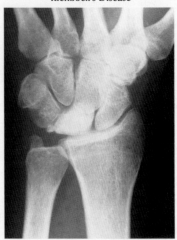

Rheumatoid Arthritis

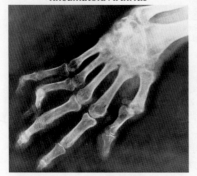

Radiograph shows cartilage thinning at proximal interphalangeal joints, erosion of carpus and wrist joint, osteoporosis, and finger deformities

Radiograph of wrist shows characteristic sclerosis of lunate

DESCRIPTION	Hx & PE	WORKUP/FINDINGS	TREATMENT
DEGENERATIVE/ARTHRITIC CONDITIONS			
• Primary osteoarthritis in the wrist is uncommon. It is usually posttraumatic (distal radius/scaphoid fx or lig. injury).			
Scapholunate Advanced Collapse (SLAC)			

• Wrist arthritis due to posttraumatic scaphoid flexion deformity (SL ligament injury or scaphoid fracture [SNAC])
• Arthritis progresses over four stages (I-IV)
	Hx: Prior trauma/fall (often untreated), pain
	PE: +/− decreased ROM with pain, tenderness to palpation
		XR: 4 stages. DJD at:
		I. Rad. styloid & scaphoid
		II. Radioscaphoid joint
		III. Capitolunate joint
		IV. Capitate migration
		   (radiolunate joint is
		   spared)
			I. Styloidectomy & STT fusion
			II. Proximal row carpectomy or scaphoidectomy & 4 corner (lun., tri., cap., ham.) fusion
			III. 4 corner fusion
			IV. Wrist arthrodesis (fusion)

Rheumatoid Arthritis			
• Inflammatory disorder attacks synovium and destroys joint • Radiocarpal (supination &, ulnar volar translation) & DRUJ (ulna subluxates dorsally) affected	**Hx:** Pain (esp. in AM), stiffness, deformity **PE:** Swelling, deformity (volar, ulnar translation of the carpus)	**XR:** Wrist series. Depends on severity. Mild degeneration to destruction of joint. **LABS:** RF, ANA, ESR	1. Medical management 2. Synovectomy 3. Tendon transfers 4. Wrist fusion or arthroplasty
Kienböck's Disease			
• Osteonecrosis of the lunate • Etiology: traumatic or repetitive microtrauma to lunate • 4 radiographic stages • Associated with ulnar negative variance of wrist	**Hx:** Pain, stiffness, and disability of wrist **PE:** Lunate/proximal row tenderness, decreased ROM, decreased grip strength	**XR:** Stage I: Normal x-ray; II: Lunate sclerosis IIIA: Lunate fragmented IIIB: IIIA + scaphoid flexed IV. DJD of adjacent joints **MR:** Needed to dx stage I	Stage: I: Immobilization I-IIIA: Radial shortening IIIB: STT fusion or proximal row carpectomy (PRC) IV: Wrist fusion or PRC

Madelung's Deformity

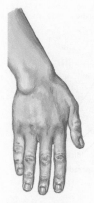

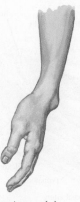

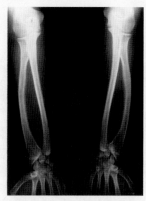

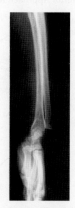

Dorsal view of hand reveals prominence of ulnar heads

Prominence of ulnar head, palmar deviation of hand, and bowing of forearm clearly seen on radial view

Radiograph shows ulnar inclination of articular surfaces of distal radius, wedging of carpal bones into resulting space, and bowing of radius

Lateral radiograph demonstrates dorsal prominence of ulnar head with palmar deviation of carpal bones

Radial Club Hand

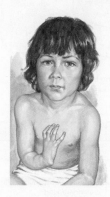

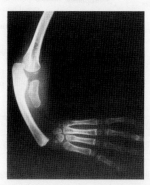

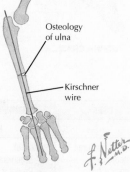

Osteology of ulna

Kirschner wire

Short, bowed forearm with marked radial deviation of hand. Thumb absent. Radiograph shows partial deficit of radial ray (vestige of radius present). Scaphoid, trapezium, and metacarpal and phlanges of thumb absent.

Centralization procedure

DESCRIPTION	EVALUATION	TREATMENT
MADELUNG'S DEFORMITY		
• Deformity of the distal radius • Volar ulnar physis disrupted causes increased volar tilt & radial inclination • Ages 6-12; females>males	**Hx:** Pain in wrists & deformity **PE:** Deformity & prominent ulna head **XR:** Distal radius deformity (incr. tilt & inclination) & dorsal ulna sublux-ation	Asymptomatic: observation and/or activity modification Symptomatic: radial osteotomy +/- ulna recession
RADIAL CLUB HAND (RADIAL HEMIMELIA)		
• Failure of formation (partial or com-plete: stages I-IV) of the radius • Associated with syndromes (TAR, VATER)	**Hx/PE:** Bowing of forearm, radial de-viation of hand **XR:** Radius short or absent, bowed ulna	1. Elbow ROM (no surgery if stiff) 2. Hand centralization (age 1)

Posterior Approach to Forearm

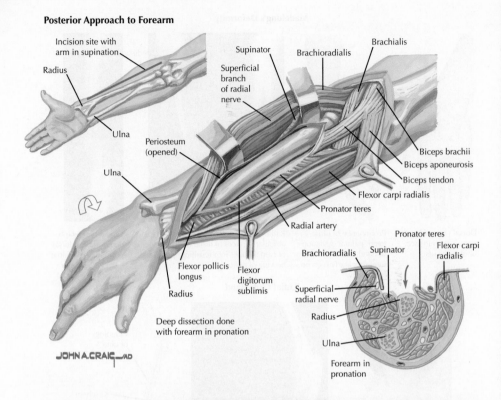

Incision site with arm in supination
Radius
Ulna
Periosteum (opened)
Ulna
Flexor pollicis longus
Radius
Flexor digitorum sublimis
Deep dissection done with forearm in pronation

Supinator
Superficial branch of radial nerve
Brachioradialis
Brachialis
Biceps brachii
Biceps aponeurosis
Biceps tendon
Flexor carpi radialis
Pronator teres
Radial artery

Pronator teres
Flexor carpi radialis
Brachioradialis
Supinator
Superficial radial nerve
Radius
Ulna
Forearm in pronation

JOHN A.CRAIG—AD

USES	INTERNERVOUS PLANE	DANGERS	COMMENT
FOREARM: ANTERIOR APPROACH (HENRY)			

• ORIF of fractures
• Osteotomy
• Biopsy & bone tumors
	Proximal
	  ○ Brachioradialis (radial)
	  ○ Pronator teres (median)
	Distal
	  ○ Brachioradialis (radial)
	  ○ FCR (median)
		• Radial artery
		• Superficial radial nerve
		• Posterior interosseous nerve (PIN)
			• Most commonly only a portion of the incision is needed/used
			• Proximally, must ligate the radial recurrent artery
			• Distally, must detach pronator quadratus to get to distal radius

WRIST: DORSAL APPROACH			
• ORIF of fractures • Wrist fusion or carpectomy • Tendon repair	• No internervous plane (muscles all innervated by radial nerve [PIN]) • 4th dorsal compartment is opened & tendons are retracted	• Superficial radial nerve • Radial artery	• If needed, a compartment other than the 4th can be opened • The capsular sensory branch of the PIN is in the 4th compartment
WRIST: VOLAR APPROACH			

• ORIF (e.g., distal radius, scaphoid)
• Carpal tunnel release
• Tendon repair
	Proximal (same as Henry)
	  ○ Brachioradialis (radial)
	  ○ FCR (median)
	Distal (over wrist & palm)
	  ○ None
		• Median nerve
		  ○ Palmar cutaneous br.
		  ○ Motor recurrent branch
		• Superficial palmar arch
			• Incise transverse carpal ligament to access volar wrist capsule/bones
			• Must detach pronator quadratus to expose distal radius

Dorsal Approach to Wrist Joint

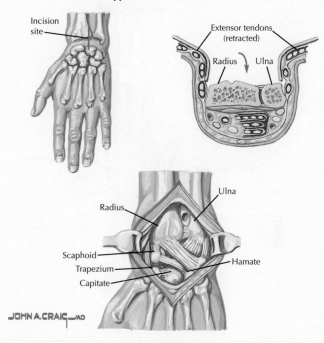

Volar Approach to Wrist Joint

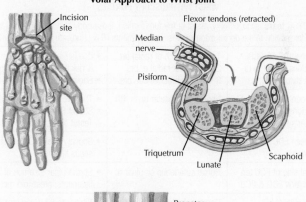

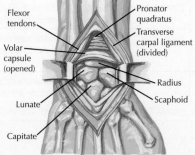

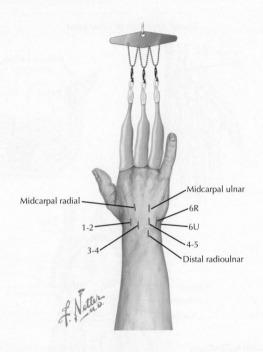

Midcarpal radial

Midcarpal ulnar

6R

1-2

6U

3-4

4-5

Distal radioulnar

PORTAL	LOCATION	DANGERS	COMMENT
WRIST ARTHROSCOPY PORTALS			
• Uses: Diagnostic, TFCC **tears**, synovectomy, assist in fracture fixation, loose body removal, chondral lesions • Portals are named for relation to the dorsal extensor wrist compartments (*R & U* indicate radial or ulnar side of tendon).			
1-2	Between APL & ECRL tendons. Distal to radial styloid	1. Deep branch of radial art. 2. Superficial radial n. brs. 3. Lat. antebrachial cut. brs.	• Use is limited b/c of close proximity to & risk of neurovascular injury • Shows distal scaphoid & radial styloid
3-4	Between EPL & EDC tendons, 1cm distal to Lister's tubercle	None (PIN capsular br. in 4th comp)	• The "workhorse" portal of arthroscopy • Shows SL interosseous lig., ligament of Testut (RSL), distal radius fossae
4-5	Between EDC & EDQ tendons	None	• Shows radial TFCC attachment, LT interosseous ligament
6R	Radial side of ECU tendon (b/w EDQ & ECU)	Dorsal cutaneous br. ulnar n.	• Shows ulnar insertion of TFCC, UT, & UL ligaments, prestyloid recess
6U	Ulnar side of ECU tendon	Dorsal cutaneous br. ulnar n.	• Similar to 6R. Used less due to risk of nerve injury. Can be used for outflow.
Midcarpal radial	1cm distal to 3-4 portal, along radial border of 3rd MC	None	• Distal scaphoid, proximal capitate, SL ligament, STT articulation
Midcarpal ulnar	1cm distal to 4-5 portal, in line with 4th MC	None	• Lunotriquetral joint, LT ligament, triquetrohamate articulation
Other portals: Midcarpal: STT and triquetrohamate. Distal radioulnar: proximal and distal to ulnar head.			
FASCIOTOMIES			
See page 169.			

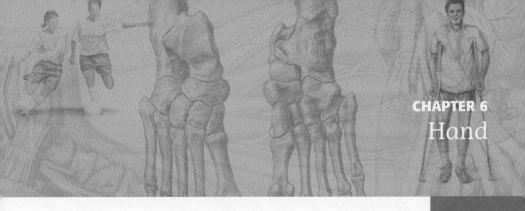

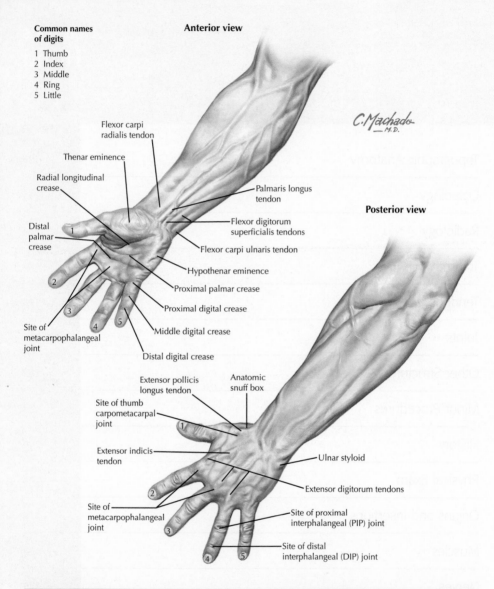

Common names of digits

1 Thumb
2 Index
3 Middle
4 Ring
5 Little

Anterior view

C.Machado
—M.D.

Flexor carpi radialis tendon

Thenar eminence

Radial longitudinal crease

Palmaris longus tendon

Posterior view

Distal palmar crease

Flexor digitorum superficialis tendons

Flexor carpi ulnaris tendon

Hypothenar eminence

Proximal palmar crease

Proximal digital crease

Middle digital crease

Site of metacarpophalangeal joint

Distal digital crease

Extensor pollicis longus tendon

Anatomic snuff box

Site of thumb carpometacarpal joint

Extensor indicis tendon

Ulnar styloid

Site of metacarpophalangeal joint

Extensor digitorum tendons

Site of proximal interphalangeal (PIP) joint

Site of distal interphalangeal (DIP) joint

STRUCTURE	CLINICAL APPLICATION
Palmaris longus tendon	Not present in all people. Can be used for tendon grafts.
Anatomic snuffbox	Site of scaphoid. Tenderness can indicate a scaphoid fracture.
Thumb carpometacarpal joint	Common site of arthritis and source of radial hand pain.
Thenar eminence	Atrophy can indicate median nerve compression (e.g., carpal tunnel syndrome).
Hypothenar eminence	Atrophy can indicate ulnar nerve compression (e.g., ulnar or cubital tunnel syndrome).
Proximal palmar crease	Approximate location of the superficial palmar arch of the palm.
Distal palmar crease	Site of metacarpophalangeal joints on volar side of hand.

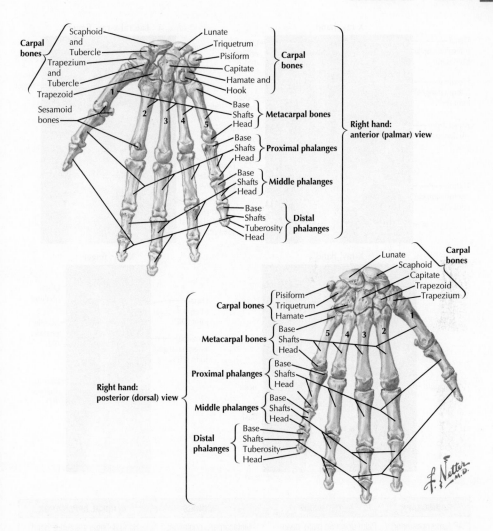

Carpal bones
Scaphoid and Tubercle
Trapezium and Tubercle
Trapezoid
Sesamoid bones

Lunate
Triquetrum
Pisiform
Capitate
Hamate and Hook

Carpal bones

1 2 3 4 5

Base
Shafts
Head — Metacarpal bones

Base
Shafts
Head — Proximal phalanges

Base
Shafts
Head — Middle phalanges

Base
Shafts
Tuberosity
Head — Distal phalanges

Right hand: anterior (palmar) view

Right hand: posterior (dorsal) view

Carpal bones
Pisiform
Triquetrum
Hamate

Metacarpal bones
Base
Shafts
Head

Proximal phalanges
Base
Shafts
Head

Middle phalanges
Base
Shafts
Head

Distal phalanges
Base
Shafts
Tuberosity
Head

Lunate
Scaphoid
Capitate
Trapezoid
Trapezium

Carpal bones

5 4 3 2 1

CHARACTERISTICS	OSSIFY		FUSE	COMMENT
METACARPALS				
• Triangular in cross section: gives 2 volar muscular attachment sites	**Primary:** body	9wk (fetal)	18yr	• Named I-V (thumb to small finger)
• Thumb MC has saddle-shaped base: increases it mobility	**Secondary** epiphysis	2yr	18yr	• Only one physis per bone in the head; base in thumb MC
PHALANGES				
• Volar surface is almost flat	**Primary:** body	8wk (fetal)	14-18yr	• 3 in each digit except thumb (two)
• Tubercles and ridges are sites for attachment	**Secondary** epiphysis	2-3yr	14-18yr	• Only one physis per bone; it is in the base
• Nomenclature for digits: thumb, index finger (IF), middle finger (MF), ring finger (RF), small/little finger (SF or LF), proximal phalanx (P1), middle phalanx (P2), distal phalanx (P3)				

X-ray, hand

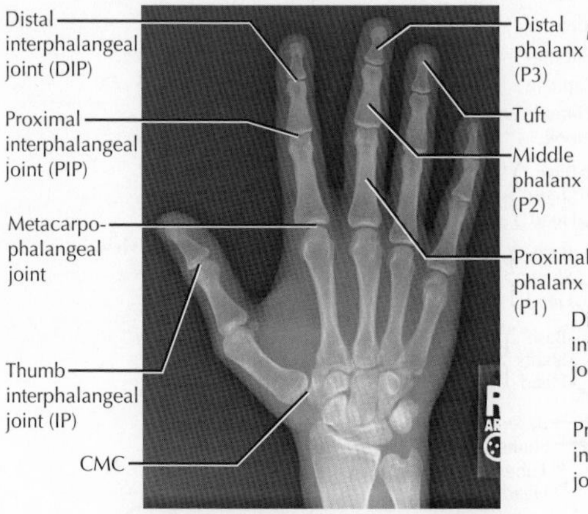

Distal interphalangeal joint (DIP)

Proximal interphalangeal joint (PIP)

Metacarpophalangeal joint

Thumb interphalangeal joint (IP)

CMC

Distal phalanx (P3)

Tuft

Middle phalanx (P2)

Proximal phalanx (P1)

Lateral x-ray, finger

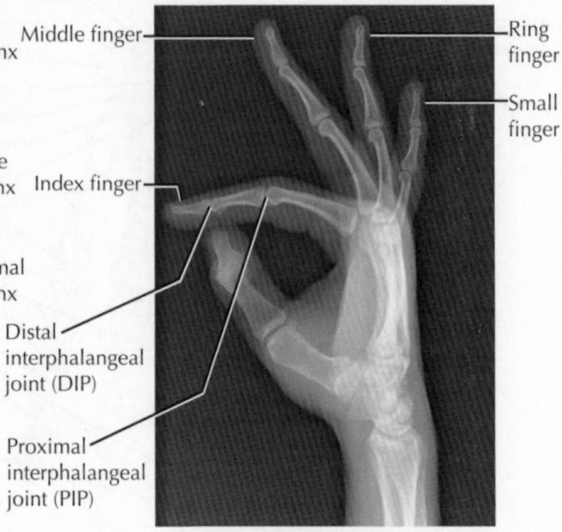

Middle finger

Ring finger

Small finger

Index finger

Distal interphalangeal joint (DIP)

Proximal interphalangeal joint (PIP)

X-ray, hand

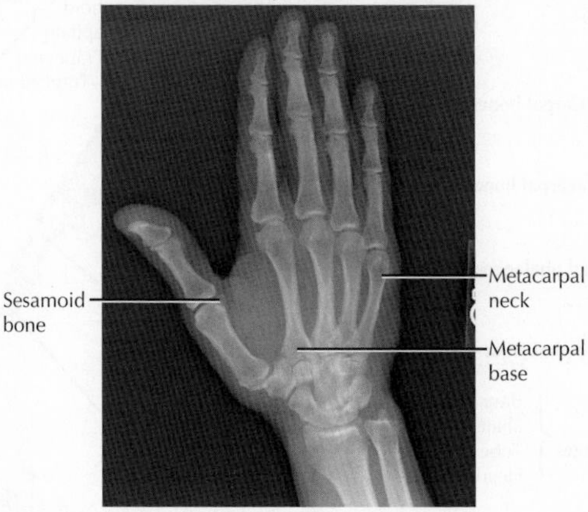

Sesamoid bone

Metacarpal neck

Metacarpal base

X-ray, finger

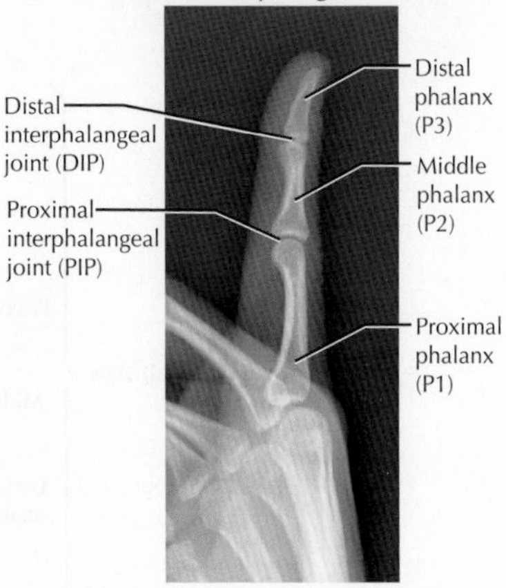

Distal interphalangeal joint (DIP)

Proximal interphalangeal joint (PIP)

Distal phalanx (P3)

Middle phalanx (P2)

Proximal phalanx (P1)

RADIOGRAPH	TECHNIQUE	FINDINGS	CLINICAL APPLICATION
AP (anteroposterior)	Palm down on plate, beam perpendicular to plate	Metacarpals, phalanges, CMC, MCP, and IP joints	Hand & finger fractures, hand joint dislocations and DJD
Lateral	Ulnar wrist and hand on plate, stagger finger flexion	Alignment of bones, joints	Same as above
Oblique	Lateral with 40° rotation	Alignment and position of bones	Same as above
Thumb stress view	Abduct thumb at 0° & 30° of flexion, beam at MCPJ	Thumb MCPJ under stress	Evaluate ulnar collateral ligament integrity (gamekeeper's thumb)
OTHER STUDIES			
CT	Axial, coronal, and sagittal	Articular congruity, bone healing, bone alignment	Fractures (esp. scaphoid, hook of hamate), nonunions
MRI	Sequence protocols vary	Soft tissues (ligaments, tendons), bones	Occult fractures (e.g., scaphoid), ligament/tendon injuries
Bone scan		All bones evaluated	Infection, stress fxs, tumors

Metacarpal Fractures

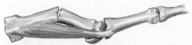

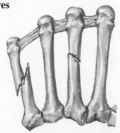

Transverse fractures of metacarpal shaft usually angulated dorsally by pull of interosseous muscles

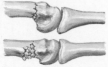

In fractures of metacarpal neck, volar cortex often comminuted, resulting in marked instability after reduction, which often necessitates pinning

Oblique fractures tend to shorten and rotate metacarpal, particularly in index and little fingers because metacarpals of middle and ring fingers are stabilized by deep transverse metacarpal ligaments

Fracture of Base of Metacarpals of Thumb

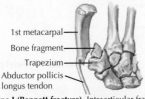

1st metacarpal—
Bone fragment—
Trapezium—
Abductor pollicis longus tendon

Type I (Bennett fracture). Intraarticular fracture with proximal and radial dislocation of 1st metacarpal. Triangular bone fragment sheared off

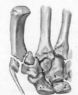

Type II (Rolando fracture). Intraarticular fracture with Y-shaped configuration

Fracture of Proximal Phalanx

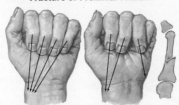

Reduction of fractures of phalanges or metacarpals requires correct rotational as well as longitudinal alignment. In normal hand, tips of flexed fingers point toward tuberosity of scaphoid, as in hand at left.

DESCRIPTION	EVALUATION	CLASSIFICATION	TREATMENT
METACARPAL FRACTURES			

• Common in adults, usually a fall or punching mechanism
• 5th MC most common (boxer fx)
• Thumb MC base fractures: displaced, intraarticular fractures problematic
  ○ Bennett's fx: APL deforms fx
  ○ Rolando's fx: can lead to DJD
• 4th & 5th MCs can tolerate some angulation, 2nd & 3rd cannot
	Hx: Trauma, pain, swelling,+/− deformity
	PE: Swelling, tenderness. Check for rotational deformity. Check neurovascular integrity.
	XR: Hand. Evaluate for angulation & shortening
	CT: Useful to evaluate for nonunion of fracture
		By location:
		• Head
		• Neck (most common)
		• Shaft (transverse, spiral)
		• Base
		  ○ Thumb MC
		    ○ Bennett: volar lip fx
		    ○ Rolando: comminuted
		  ○ Small finger MC: "Baby Bennett"
			• Nondisplaced: cast
			• Displaced: reduce
			  ○ Stable: cast
			  ○ Unstable: CR-PCP vs. ORIF
			  ○ Shortened: ORIF
			• Intraarticular
			  ○ Head: ORIF
			  ○ Thumb base:
			    ○ Bennett: CR-PCP
			    ○ Rolando: ORIF

COMPLICATIONS: Nonunion/malunion, grip strength deficiency, posttraumatic osteoarthritis (esp. Rolando fractures)			

Phalangeal Fractures

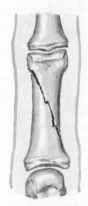

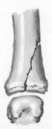

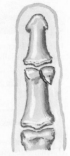

Extraarticular oblique shaft (diaphysis) **fracture.**

Intraarticular phalangeal base **fracture.** Intraarticular fractures of phalanx that are non-displaced and stable may be treated with buddy taping, careful observation, and early active exercise.

Intraarticular condyle fractures.

Fractures of distal phalanx

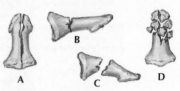

Types of fractures.
A. Longitudinal
B. Nondisplaced transverse
C. Angulated transverse
D. Comminuted

Fracture dislocation of middle phalanx.

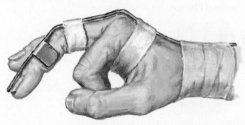

Extension block splint useful for fracture dislocation of proximal

DESCRIPTION	EVALUATION	CLASSIFICATION	TREATMENT
PHALANGEAL FRACTURES			

• Common injury
• Mechanism: jamming, crush, or twisting
• Distal phalanx most common
• Stiffness is common problem; early motion and occupational therapy needed for best results
• Intraarticular fractures can lead to early osteoarthritis
• Nail bed injury common w/ tuft (distal phalanx) fx
	Hx: Trauma, pain, swelling, +/– deformity
	PE: Swelling, tenderness. Check for rotational deformity. Check neurovascular integrity.
	XR: Hand. Evaluate for angulation & shortening
	CT: Useful to evaluate for nonunion of fracture
		Description:
		• Intra- vs extraarticular
		• Displaced/nondisplaced
		• Transverse, spiral, oblique
		Location:
		• Condyle
		• Neck
		• Shaft/diaphysis
		• Base
		• Tuft
			• Extraarticular:
			  ∘ Stable: buddy tape/splint
			  ∘ Unstable: CR-PCP vs ORIF
			• Intraarticular: ORIF
			• Middle phalanx volar base fx:
			  ∘ Stable: extension block splint
			  ∘ Unstable: ORIF
			• Tuft fx: irrigate wound, repair nail bed as needed, splint fx/digit

COMPLICATIONS: Stiffness/loss of range of motion (esp. intraarticular fractures), nonunion/malunion, osteoarthritis			

Gamekeeper's thumb

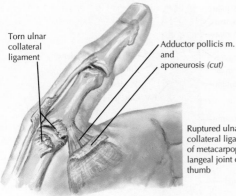

Torn ulnar collateral ligament

Adductor pollicis m. and aponeurosis (cut)

Ruptured ulnar collateral ligament of metacarpophalangeal joint of thumb

Mallet finger

A. Tendon torn from its insertion. B. Bone fragment avulsed with tendon. In A and B there is a 40°- 45° flexion deformity and loss of active extension

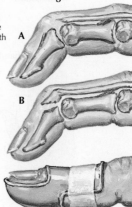

A

B

Splinted Mallet Finger

Jersey finger

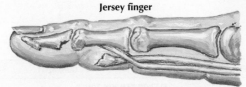

Flexor digitorum profundus tendon may be torn directly from distal phalanx or may avulse small or large bone fragment.

DESCRIPTION	Hx & PE	WORKUP/FINDINGS	TREATMENT
MALLET FINGER—EXTENSOR DIGITORUM AVULSION			
• Rupture of extensor tendon from distal phalanx • Soft tissue or bony form • Mech: jamming finger	**Hx:** "Jammed" finger; pain, DIPJ deformity **PE:** Extensor lag at DIPJ; inability to actively extend DIPJ	**XR:** Hand series. Look for bony avulsion (EDC) fx from dorsal base of P3 in bony form of injury	1. DIPJ extension splint, 6wk for most injuries 2. Bony mallet with DIPJ subluxation: consider PCP vs ORIF
JERSEY FINGER—FLEXOR DIGITORUM PROFUNDUS AVULSION			
• FDP tendon rupture from P3 • Mech: forced extension against a flexed finger • Tendon retracts variably	**Hx:** Forced DIPJ extension; injury; pain **PE:** Inability to flex DIPJ (−profundus test)	**XR:** Hand series. Look for avulsion fracture from volar base of P3. May be retracted to finger/palm.	Leddy classification: Type: • 1: to palm. Early repair • 2: to PIPJ. Repair <6wk • 3: bony to A4: ORIF
GAMEKEEPER'S THUMB			
• Thumb MCP joint proper ulnar collateral ligament injury • Mech: forced radial deviation • Often a ski pole injury	**Hx:** Pain, decreased grip **PE:** Pain & laxity of MCPJ at 30° of flexion, +/− palpable mass (Stener lesion)	**XR:** Hand; r/o avulsion fx **Stress Fluoro:** Can compare side to side asym. **MR:** If diagnosis is unclear	• Incomplete tear (sprain) or no Stener lesion: splint 4-6wk • Complete tear or Stener lesion: primary repair

• **Stener lesion:** when adductor aponeurosis falls under torn ulnar collateral ligament, producing a palpable mass/bump
• Stress testing of the thumb MCP in extension tests the accessory collateral ligament and volar plate integrity

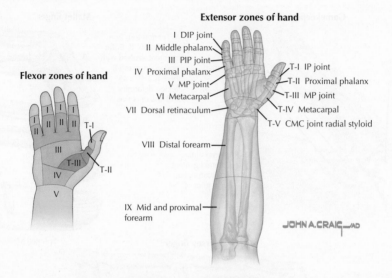

Flexor zones of hand

Extensor zones of hand

I DIP joint
II Middle phalanx
III PIP joint
IV Proximal phalanx
V MP joint
VI Metacarpal
VII Dorsal retinaculum
VIII Distal forearm
IX Mid and proximal forearm

T-I IP joint
T-II Proximal phalanx
T-III MP joint
T-IV Metacarpal
T-V CMC joint radial styloid

JOHN A.CRAIG AD

ZONE	BOUNDARIES	COMMENT
FLEXOR TENDON ZONES		
I	Distal to FDS insertion	Single tendon (FDP) injury. Primary repair. DIPJ contracture results if tendon shortened >1cm. Quadriga effect can also result
II	Finger flexor retinaculum	"No man's land." Both tendons(FDS, FDP) require early repair (within 7 days) and mobilization. Lacerations may be at different locations on each tendon and away from skin laceration. Preserve A2 & A4 pulleys during repair
III	Palm	Primary repair. Arterial arch & median nerve injuries common.
IV	Carpal tunnel	Must release & repair the transverse carpal ligament during tendon repair.
V	Wrist & forearm	Primary repair (+ any neurovascular injury). Results are usually favorable.
Thumb I	Distal to FPL insertion	Primary tendon repair. Rerupture rate is high.
Thumb II	Thumb flexor retinaculum	Primary tendon repair. Preserve either A1 or oblique pulley.
Thumb III	Thenar eminence	Do not operate in this zone. Recurrent motor branch is at risk of injury.
EXTENSOR TENDON ZONES		
I	DIP joint	"Mallet finger." Splint in extension for 6 wk continuously.
II	Middle phalanx	Complete lacerations: primary repair and extension splint.
III	PIP joint	Central slip injury. Splint in extension for 6 wk. If triangular ligament is also disrupted, lateral bands migrate volarly, resulting in "boutonniere finger"
IV	Proximal phalanx	Primary repair of tendon (and lateral bands if needed), then extension splint
V	MCP joint	Often from "fight bite." Repair tendon and sagittal bands as needed.
VI	Metacarpal	Primary repair and early mobilization/dynamic splinting.
VII	Wrist	Retinaculum likely injured. Primary tendon repair, early mobilization.
VIII	Distal forearm	At musculotendinous jxn. Primary repair of tendinous tissue & immobilize
IX	Proximal forearm	Often muscle injury. Neurovascular injury high. Repair muscle & immobilize.

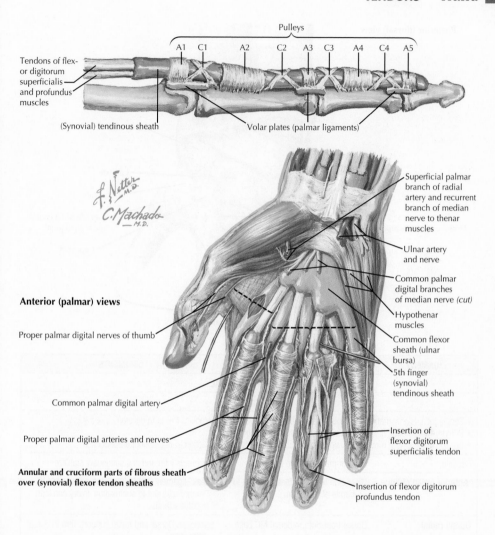

Pulleys

A1 C1   A2   C2   A3   C3   A4   C4   A5

Tendons of flexor digitorum superficialis and profundus muscles

(Synovial) tendinous sheath

Volar plates (palmar ligaments)

Anterior (palmar) views

Superficial palmar branch of radial artery and recurrent branch of median nerve to thenar muscles

Ulnar artery and nerve

Common palmar digital branches of median nerve *(cut)*

Hypothenar muscles

Common flexor sheath (ulnar bursa)

5th finger (synovial) tendinous sheath

Proper palmar digital nerves of thumb

Common palmar digital artery

Proper palmar digital arteries and nerves

Annular and cruciform parts of fibrous sheath over (synovial) flexor tendon sheaths

Insertion of flexor digitorum superficialis tendon

Insertion of flexor digitorum profundus tendon

STRUCTURE	DESCRIPTION	COMMENT
FLEXOR TENDON SHEATH		
Flexor tendon sheath	Fibroosseous tunnel lined with tenosynovium Protects, lubricates, and nourishes the tendon	Site of possible infection; check for Kanavel signs (see Disorders table)
Pulleys	Thickenings of sheath to stabilize tendons 5 annular (A1[MCPJ], A3[PIPJ], A5[DIPJ] over joints; A2, A4 over phalanges) 3 or 4 cruciate pulleys	A2 & A4 (over P1 & P2) most important; must be intact to prevent "bowstringing" of tendons Tight A1 can cause a trigger finger A3 covers PIPJ volar plate: incise to access
Vincula	Within sheath, give vascular supply to tendons: 2 vincula (longa and brevia)	Vincula torn in type 1 FDP rupture (dysvascular), preserved in types 2 & 3 rupture
Volar plate (palmar ligament)	Thickening of volar capsule of interphalangeal joints	FDS & FDP tendons insert here to flex the PIP & DIP joints, respectively. Prevent hyperextension.

Posterior (dorsal) view

Scaphoid

Triquetrum

Capitate

Hamate

Trapezium

Dorsal carpometacarpal ligaments

Capsule of 1st carpo-metacarpal joint

Dorsal metacarpal ligaments

Trapezoid

1

5 4 3 2

Metacarpal bones

LIGAMENT	ATTACHMENTS	COMMENTS
CARPOMETACARPAL		
Thumb		
• Saddle joint. Highly mobile, has both inherent bony and ligamentous stability. Prone to develop osteoarthritis • Primary movements: flexion, extension, adduction, abduction • Complex (combined) movements: opposition, retropulsion, palmar abduction, radial abduction/adduction		
Capsule	Base of metacarpal to trapezium	Surrounds joint and is a secondary stabilizer
Anterior (volar) **oblique**	Ulnar side of 1st metacarpal base to tubercle of trapezium	"Beak" ligament. Holds fragment in Bennett's fx. Primary restraint to subluxation. Injury can lead to osteoarthritis.
Dorsal radial	Dorsal trapezium to dorsal MC base	Strongest. Dorsal and radial support. Torn in dorsal dislocation.
1st intermetacarpal	Ulnar 1st MC base to radial 2nd MC base	Prevents 1st metacarpal from translating radially
Posterior oblique	Trapezium to dorsal ulnar MC base	Secondary stabilizer
Ulnar collateral	Volar ulnar trapezium to ulnar MC base	Limits abduction and extension
Radial lateral	Radially on trapezium and MC base	Under the APL tendon/insertion
Finger		
• Gliding joints. 2nd & 3rd CMC have little motion, so minimal metacarpal fx angulation is acceptable b/c of immobility. 4th & 5th CMC have more anteroposterior motion, so more metacarpal fx angulation is acceptable b/c of mobility.		
Capsule	Base of metacarpal to carpus	Adds stability
CMC ligaments	Base of metacarpal to carpus	Dorsal (strongest), volar, interosseous ligaments
Intermetacarpal	Between adjacent metacarpal bases	Adds ulnar and radial stability to CMC joint

Anterior (palmar) view

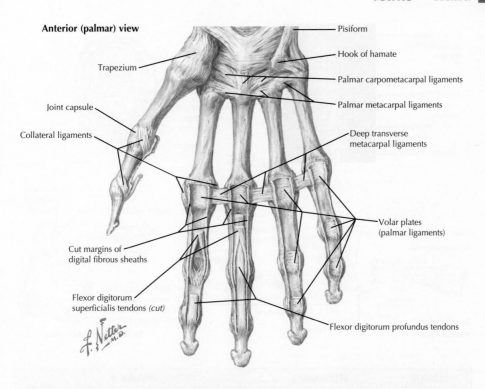

Pisiform

Hook of hamate

Trapezium

Palmar carpometacarpal ligaments

Palmar metacarpal ligaments

Joint capsule

Collateral ligaments

Deep transverse
metacarpal ligaments

Volar plates
(palmar ligaments)

Cut margins of
digital fibrous sheaths

Flexor digitorum
superficialis tendons *(cut)*

Flexor digitorum profundus tendons

LIGAMENT	ATTACHMENTS	COMMENTS
METACARPOPHALANGEAL		
Thumb		
• Diarthrodial joint. Motion: primary = flexion & extension; secondary = rotation, adduction, abduction		
Capsule	Surrounds joint	Secondary stabilizer dorsally. Taut in flexion
Proper collateral	Center of metacarpal head to palmar proximal phalanx	Primary stabilizer. Taut in flexion, test in 30° flexion. Ulnar collateral injured in "gamekeeper's/skier's" thumb
Accessory collateral	Palmar to proper collateral lig.	Taut in extension. Test integrity in extension.
Volar (palmar) **plate**	Palmar metacarpal head to palmar proximal phalanx base	Primary stabilizer in extension. Laxity in extension indicates injury to volar plate (+/− accessory collateral lig.)
Finger		
• Diarthrodial joint. Motion: primary = flexion & extension (ROM 0-90°); secondary = radial & ulnar deviation		
• Asymmetry of metacarpal head & collateral ligament origin result in "cam effect" (tight in flexion, loose in extension)		
Capsule	Surrounds joint	Secondary stabilizer; synovial reflections volar & dorsal
Proper collateral	Dorsal MC head to palmar P1 base	Primary stabilizer; tight in flexion, loose in extension
Accessory collateral	Palmar MC head to volar plate	Palmar to proper collaterals; stabilizes the volar plate
Volar (palmar) **plate**	Palmar MC head to palmar P1 base	Limits extension; volar support
Deep transverse (inter)**metacarpal**	Between adjacent metacarpal bases and MCPJ volar plates	Interconnects the volar plates, MCPJs, and metacarpals. Can prevent shortening of isolated metacarpal fractures.

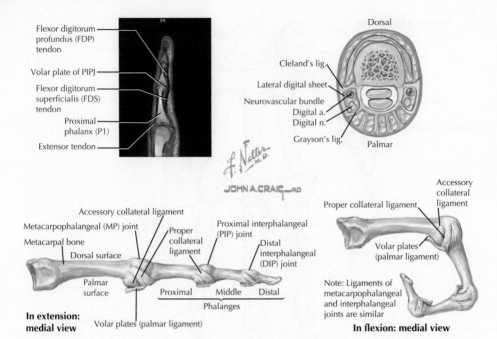

In extension:
medial view

In flexion: medial view

LIGAMENT	ATTACHMENTS	COMMENTS
PROXIMAL INTERPHALANGEAL		
• Hinge joints: Primary motion = flexion & extension (PIPJ: ROM 0-110°, DIPJ: ROM 0-60°). Minimal rotation or deviation motion. No "cam effect" in this joint. PIPJ is prone to stiffness/contracture after injury and/or immobilization.		
Capsule	Surrounds joint	Weak stabilizer esp. dorsally (central slip adds most support)
Proper collateral	Center of P1 head to volar P2	Primary stabilizer to deviation. Constant tension through ROM
Accessory collateral	Volar proximal phalanx head to volar plate (not bone)	Origin volar to axis of rotation: tight in ext., loose in flexion This can result in a contracture (do not immobilize in flexion)
Volar (palmar) **plate**	Volar middle phalanx to volar proximal phalanx (via check-rein ligaments)	Primary restraint to hyperextension. Firm distal attachment, looser proximal attachment (more prone to injury). Checkrein ligaments often contract after injury: contracture
OTHER INTERPHALANGEAL		
• Thumb interphalangeal (IPJ) and finger distal interphalangeal joints (DIPJ) • Hinge joints: Primary motion = flexion & extension (IPJ: ROM 0-90°; DIPJ: ROM 0-60°). Minimal rotation or deviation.		
Capsule	Surrounds joints	Weak stabilizer
Proper collateral	B/w adjacent phalanges	Similar to PIPJ, constant tension, no "cam effect"
Accessory collateral	Volar to collateral ligaments	Similar to PIPJ, less prone to contracture than PIPJ
Volar (palmar) **plate**	Volarly b/w phalanges	Primary restraint to hyperextension; can be injured
OTHER STRUCTURES		
Grayson's ligament	From flexor sheath to skin; volar to neurovascular bundle	Stabilizes skin & neurovascular bundle Involved in Dupuytren's disease/nodules
Cleland's ligament	From periosteum to skin	Stabilizes skin during flexion/extension; dorsal to NV bundle

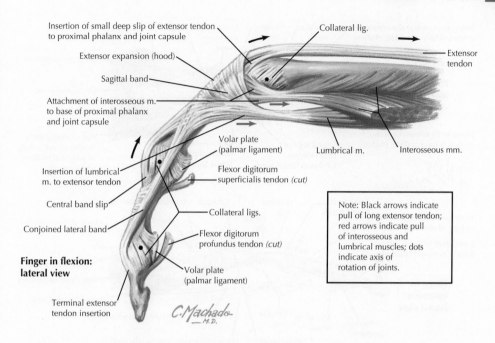

Insertion of small deep slip of extensor tendon to proximal phalanx and joint capsule

Collateral lig.

Extensor tendon

Extensor expansion (hood)

Sagittal band

Attachment of interosseous m. to base of proximal phalanx and joint capsule

Volar plate (palmar ligament)

Lumbrical m.

Interosseous mm.

Insertion of lumbrical m. to extensor tendon

Flexor digitorum superficialis tendon (cut)

Central band slip

Collateral ligs.

Conjoined lateral band

Flexor digitorum profundus tendon (cut)

Finger in flexion: lateral view

Volar plate (palmar ligament)

Terminal extensor tendon insertion

C. Machado — M.D.

Note: Black arrows indicate pull of long extensor tendon; red arrows indicate pull of interosseous and lumbrical muscles; dots indicate axis of rotation of joints.

MOTION	STRUCTURE	COMMENT
	**JOINT MOTION**	
	**Metacarpophalangeal Joint**	
Flexion	Interosseous muscles	Insert on proximal phalanx and lateral band (volar to rotation axis)
	Lumbricals	Inserts on radial lateral band (volar to axis of rotation of MCPJ)
Extension	EDC via sagittal bands	Sagittal bands insert on volar plate, creating a "lasso" around proximal phalanx base and extend joint through the lasso. EDC has minimal attachment to P1 (which does not extend the joint) but extends joints via the sagittal bands.
	**Proximal Interphalangeal Joint**	
Flexion	Flexor digitorum superficialis (FDS)	Primary PIPJ flexor via insertion on middle phalanx volar base
	Flexor digitorum profundus (FDP)	Secondary PIPJ flexor
Extension	EDC via the central slip (band)	Central slip of EDC inserts on dorsal P2 base to extend PIPJ
	Lumbricals via lateral bands	Has attachment to radial lateral band (dorsal to rotation axis)
	**Distal Interphalangeal Joint**	
Flexion	Flexor digitorum profundus (FDP)	Tendon attaches at P3 volar base, pulls through tendon sheath
Extension	EDC via terminal extensor tendon	Lateral bands converge at terminal insertion on dorsal P3 base
	Oblique retinacular ligament (ORL)	Links PIPJ & DIPJ extension; extends DIPJ as PIPJ is extended

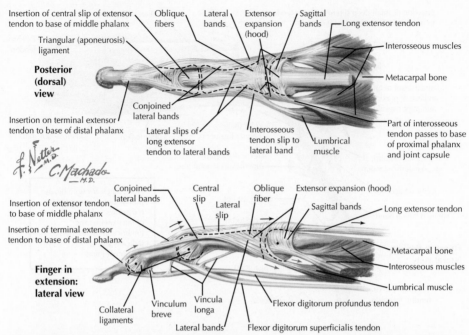

Insertion of central slip of extensor tendon to base of middle phalanx
Oblique fibers
Lateral bands
Extensor expansion (hood)
Sagittal bands
Long extensor tendon
Triangular (aponeurosis) ligament
Interosseous muscles
Posterior (dorsal) view
Metacarpal bone
Conjoined lateral bands
Insertion on terminal extensor tendon to base of distal phalanx
Lateral slips of long extensor tendon to lateral bands
Interosseous tendon slip to lateral band
Lumbrical muscle
Part of interosseous tendon passes to base of proximal phalanx and joint capsule

Conjoined lateral bands
Central slip
Oblique fiber
Extensor expansion (hood)
Insertion of extensor tendon to base of middle phalanx
Lateral slip
Sagittal bands
Long extensor tendon
Insertion of terminal extensor tendon to base of distal phalanx
Metacarpal bone
Interosseous muscles
Finger in extension: lateral view
Lumbrical muscle
Collateral ligaments
Vinculum breve
Vincula longa
Flexor digitorum profundus tendon
Lateral bands
Flexor digitorum superficialis tendon

STRUCTURE	DESCRIPTION	COMMENT
INTRINSIC APPARATUS		
• **Dorsal Extensor Aponeurosis** (also called dorsal expansion, dorsal hood, extensor hood)		
○ Sagittal band	Inserts on volar plate (P1); extensor tendon (EDC) glides under it	Extends MCPJ via "lasso" around P1 base; radial sagittal bands are weaker, may rupture
○ Oblique fibers	Covers MCPJ and base of proximal phalanx	Holds EDC centered over MCPJ
○ Lateral bands	Lateral hood fibers join tendinous portion of interossei/lumbricals to form lateral bands	Volar to MCPJ axis: flexes MCPJ Dorsal to PIPJ axis: extends PIPJ
• **Extrinsic Extensor Tendon (EDC)** glides under the dorsal hood (to extend MCP) before trifurcating at prox. phalanx		
○ Lateral slip	EDC trifurcates over P1 giving two lateral slips	These slips conjoin with lateral bands
○ Central slip	Central slip of trifurcation; inserts base of P2	Extends PIPJ; torn in boutonniere injury
○ Terminal extensor tendon	Confluence of two conjoined lateral bands on dorsal base of distal phalanx (P3)	Extends DIPJ via insertion on dorsal base of P3; avulsed in mallet finger injury
• Conjoined lateral band	Confluence of EDC lateral slips and lateral bands from extensor aponeurosis	Both join distally to make terminal extensor tendon
• Transverse retinacular ligaments	From PIPJ volar plate and flexor sheath to both conjoined lateral bands	Prevents conjoined lateral band dorsal sub-luxation during PIPJ extension
• Triangular ligament (aponeurosis)	Transverse bands over P2, connects both conjoined lateral bands and terminal tendon	Prevents lateral band volar subluxation in PIPJ flexion; torn in boutonniere injury
• Oblique retinacular ligament (ORL)	From volar P1 to dorsal P3/terminal tendon	Extends DIPJ when PIPJ is extended
OTHER STRUCTURES		
Junctura tendinae	Tendinous connections between ECD tendons to adjacent fingers proximal to MCPJ	Prevents full extension of finger when adjacent digit is flexed (see page 155)

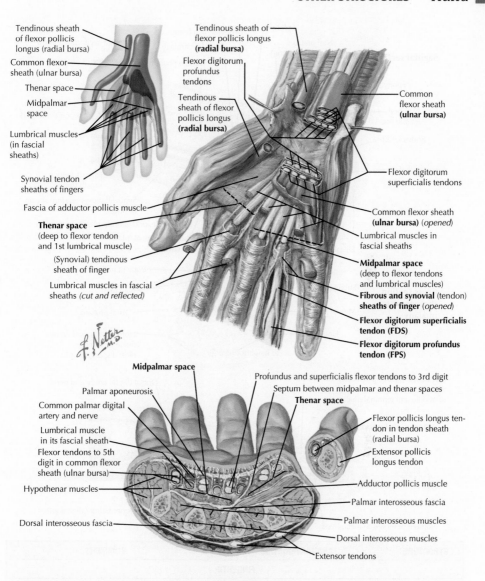

Tendinous sheath of flexor pollicis longus (radial bursa)

Common flexor sheath (ulnar bursa)

Thenar space

Midpalmar space

Lumbrical muscles (in fascial sheaths)

Synovial tendon sheaths of fingers

Fascia of adductor pollicis muscle

Thenar space (deep to flexor tendon and 1st lumbrical muscle)

(Synovial) tendinous sheath of finger

Lumbrical muscles in fascial sheaths (cut and reflected)

Tendinous sheath of flexor pollicis longus **(radial bursa)**

Flexor digitorum profundus tendons

Tendinous sheath of flexor pollicis longus **(radial bursa)**

Common flexor sheath **(ulnar bursa)**

Flexor digitorum superficialis tendons

Common flexor sheath **(ulnar bursa)** (opened)

Lumbrical muscles in fascial sheaths

Midpalmar space (deep to flexor tendons and lumbrical muscles)

Fibrous and synovial (tendon) **sheaths of finger** (opened)

Flexor digitorum superficialis tendon (FDS)

Flexor digitorum profundus tendon (FPS)

Midpalmar space

Palmar aponeurosis

Common palmar digital artery and nerve

Lumbrical muscle in its fascial sheath

Flexor tendons to 5th digit in common flexor sheath (ulnar bursa)

Hypothenar muscles

Dorsal interosseous fascia

Profundus and superficialis flexor tendons to 3rd digit

Septum between midpalmar and thenar spaces

Thenar space

Flexor pollicis longus tendon in tendon sheath (radial bursa)

Extensor pollicis longus tendon

Adductor pollicis muscle

Palmar interosseous fascia

Palmar interosseous muscles

Dorsal interosseous muscles

Extensor tendons

HAND SPACES		
STRUCTURE	**CHARACTERISTICS**	**COMMENT**
Thenar space	Between flexor tendons and adductor pollicis	Potential space: site of possible infection
Midpalmar space	Between flexor tendons and metacarpals	Potential space: site of possible infection
Parona's space	Between flexor tendons and pronator quadratus. Thumb and SF flexor sheaths communicate here	Potential space: "horseshoe" abscess can occur here as infection tracks proximally
Radial bursa	Proximal extension of FPL sheath	Infection can track proximally
Ulnar bursa	Communicates with SF FDS/FDP flexor tendon sheath	Flexor sheath infection can track proximally into bursa

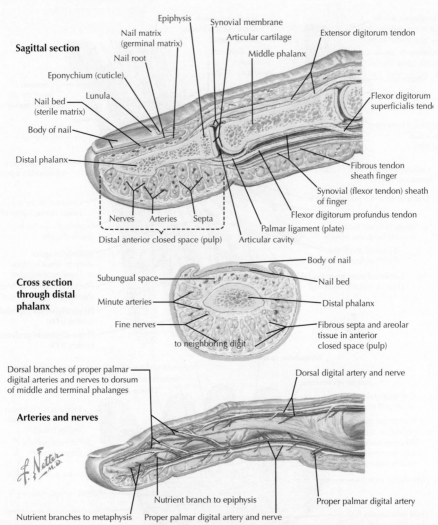

Sagittal section

Epiphysis
Nail matrix (germinal matrix)
Synovial membrane
Articular cartilage
Extensor digitorum tendon
Middle phalanx
Nail root
Eponychium (cuticle)
Lunula
Nail bed (sterile matrix)
Body of nail
Distal phalanx
Flexor digitorum superficialis tendon
Fibrous tendon sheath finger
Synovial (flexor tendon) sheath of finger
Flexor digitorum profundus tendon
Nerves Arteries Septa
Palmar ligament (plate)
Distal anterior closed space (pulp) Articular cavity

Cross section through distal phalanx

Subungual space
Minute arteries
Fine nerves
to neighboring digit
Body of nail
Nail bed
Distal phalanx
Fibrous septa and areolar tissue in anterior closed space (pulp)

Dorsal branches of proper palmar digital arteries and nerves to dorsum of middle and terminal phalanges
Dorsal digital artery and nerve

Arteries and nerves

Nutrient branch to epiphysis
Proper palmar digital artery
Nutrient branches to metaphysis
Proper palmar digital artery and nerve

STRUCTURE	CHARACTERISTICS	COMMENT
FINGERTIP		
Nail	Cornified epithelium	If completely avulsed, consider replacing to prevent eponychium and matrix adhesions
Nail bed/matrix Germinal	Under eponychium and nail to edge of lunula	Where nail grows (1mm a week), must be intact (repaired) for normal nail growth
Sterile	Under nail, distal to lunula	Adheres to nail. Repair may prevent nail deformity.
Pulp	Multiple septa, nerves, arteries	Felon is an infection of the pulp
Paronychia	Radial and ulnar nail folds	Common site of infection
Eponychia	Proximal nail fold	Common site of infection
• The digital artery is superficial/volar to the nerve proximally but runs dorsal to the nerve in the finger. • Volar neurovascular bundle supplies the distal finger and fingertip.		

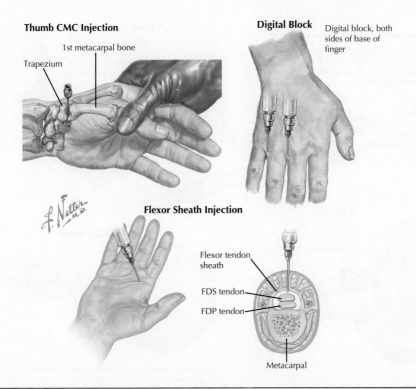

Thumb CMC Injection

1st metacarpal bone

Trapezium

Digital Block

Digital block, both
sides of base of
finger

Flexor Sheath Injection

Flexor tendon
sheath

FDS tendon

FDP tendon

Metacarpal

STEPS
INJECTION OF THUMB CMC JOINT

1. Ask patient about allergies
2. Palpate thumb CMC joint on volar radial aspect
3. Prepare skin over CMC joint (iodine/antiseptic soap)
4. Anesthetize skin locally (quarter size spot)
5. Palpate base of thumb MC, pull axial distraction on thumb with slight flexion to open joint. Use 22 gauge or smaller needle, and insert into joint (if available use an image intensifier to confirm needle is in joint). Aspirate to ensure needle is not in a vessel. Inject 1-2 ml of 1:1 local (without epinephrine) /corticosteroid preparation into CMC joint. (The fluid should flow easily if needle is in joint)
6. Dress injection site

FLEXOR TENDON SHEATH BLOCK

1. Ask patient about allergies
2. Palpate the flexor tendon at the distal palmar crease over metacarpal head/A1 pulley.
3. Prepare skin over palm (iodine/antiseptic soap)
4. Insert 25 gauge needle into flexor tendon at the level of the distal palmar crease. Withdraw needle very slightly so that it is just outside tendon, but inside sheath. Inject 2-3ml of local anesthetic without epinephrine. (Add corticosteroid if injecting for trigger finger).
5. Dress injection site

DIGITAL/METACARPAL BLOCK

1. Prepare skin over dorsal proximal finger web space (iodine/antiseptic soap)
2. Insert 25 gauge needle between metacarpal necks (metacarpal block) or on either side of proximal phalanx (digital block) in digital web space. Aspirate to ensure that needle is not in a vessel. Inject 1-2ml of local anesthetic (without epinephrine) on both sides of the bones. Consider injecting local anesthetic dorsally over the bone as well.
3. Care should be taken not to inject too much fluid into the closed space of the proximal digit.
4. Dress injection site

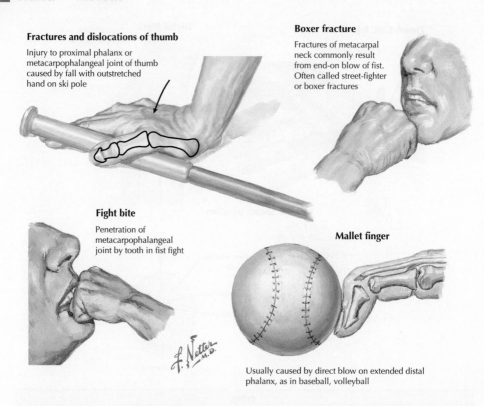

Fractures and dislocations of thumb

Injury to proximal phalanx or metacarpophalangeal joint of thumb caused by fall with outstretched hand on ski pole

Boxer fracture

Fractures of metacarpal neck commonly result from end-on blow of fist. Often called street-fighter or boxer fractures

Fight bite

Penetration of metacarpophalangeal joint by tooth in fist fight

Mallet finger

Usually caused by direct blow on extended distal phalanx, as in baseball, volleyball

QUESTION	ANSWER	CLINICAL APPLICATION
1. Hand dominance	Right or left	Dominant hand injured more often
2. Age	Young Middle age-elderly	Trauma, infection Arthritis, nerve entrapments

3. Pain
  a. Onset
 	
  b. Location
	
	Acute
	Chronic
	CMC (thumb)
	Joints (MCPs, IPs)
	Volar (fingers)
		
		Trauma, infection
		Arthritis
		Arthritis (OA) especially in women
		Arthritis (osteoarthritis, rheumatoid)
		Purulent tenosynovitis (+ Kanavel signs)

4. Stiffness	In AM, "catching" Catching/clicking	Rheumatoid arthritis Trigger finger
5. Swelling	After trauma No trauma	Infection (e.g., purulent tenosynovitis, felon, paronychia) Trigger finger, arthritides, gout, tendinitis
6. Mass		Ganglion, Dupuytren's contracture, giant cell tumor
7. Trauma	Fall, sports injury Open wound	Fracture, dislocation, tendon avulsion, ligament injury Infection
8. Activity	Sports, mechanical	Trauma (e.g., fracture, dislocation, tendon or ligament injury)
9. Neurologic symptoms	Pain, numbness, tingling Weakness	Nerve entrapment (e.g., carpal tunnel), thoracic outlet syndrome, radiculopathy (cervical) Nerve entrapment (usually in wrist or more proximal)
10. History of arthritides	Multiple joints involved	Rheumatoid arthritis, Reiter's syndrome, etc.

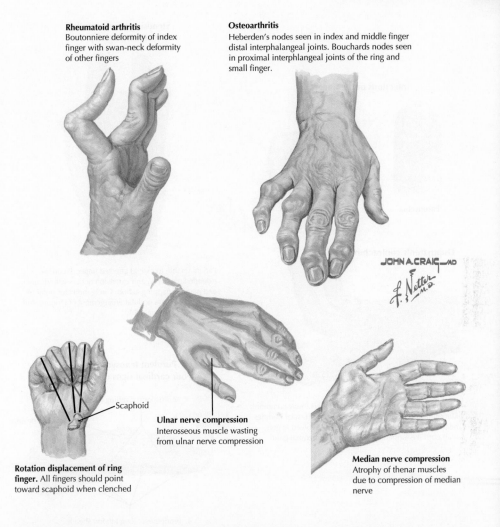

Rheumatoid arthritis
Boutonniere deformity of index finger with swan-neck deformity of other fingers

Osteoarthritis
Heberden's nodes seen in index and middle finger distal interphalangeal joints. Bouchards nodes seen in proximal interphlangeal joints of the ring and small finger.

JOHN A.CRAIG—AD

Scaphoid

Ulnar nerve compression
Interosseous muscle wasting from ulnar nerve compression

Rotation displacement of ring finger. All fingers should point toward scaphoid when clenched

Median nerve compression
Atrophy of thenar muscles due to compression of median nerve

EXAMINATION	TECHNIQUE	CLINICAL APPLICATION
INSPECTION		
Gross deformity	Ulnar drift/swan neck, boutonniere	Rheumatoid arthritis
	Rotational or angular deformity	Fracture
Finger position	Flexion	Dupuytren's contracture, purulent tenosynovitis
	Rotation of digit	Fracture (acute), fracture malunion
Skin, hair, nail changes	Cool, hairless, spoon, etc	Neurovascular disorders: Raynaud's, diabetes, nerve injury
Swelling	DIPs	Osteoarthritis: Heberden's nodes (at DIPs: #1),
	PIPs	Bouchard's nodes (at PIPs)
	MCPs	Rheumatoid arthritis
	Fusiform shape finger	Purulent tenosynovitis
Muscle wasting	Thenar eminence	Median nerve injury, CTS, C8/T1 pathology
	Hypothenar eminence/intrinsics	Ulnar nerve injury (e.g., cubital tunnel syndrome)

Infections of the fingers

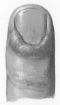

Paronychia

Felon

Stenosing tenosynovitis (trigger finger)

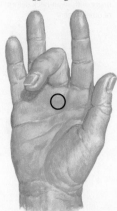

Dupuytren's contracture

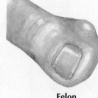

Patient unable to extend affected finger. It can be extended passively, and extension occurs with distinct and painful snapping action. Circle indicates point of tenderness where nodular enlargement of tendons and sheath is usually palpable

Flexion contracture of 4th and 5th fingers (most common). Dimpling and puckering of skin. Palpable fascial nodules near flexion crease of palm at base of involved fingers with cordlike formations extending to proximal palm

Purulent tenosynovitis. Four cardinal signs of Kanavel

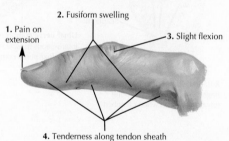

2. Fusiform swelling

1. Pain on extension

3. Slight flexion

4. Tenderness along tendon sheath

EXAMINATION	TECHNIQUE	CLINICAL APPLICATION
PALPATION		
Skin	Warm, red Cool, dry	Infection Neurovascular compromise
Metacarpals	Each along its length	Tenderness may indicate fracture
Phalanges and finger joints	Each separately	Tenderness: fracture, arthritis Swelling: arthritis
Soft tissues	Thenar eminence Hypothenar eminence Palm (palmar fascia) Flexor tendons: along volar finger All aspects of finger tip	Wasting indicates median nerve injury Wasting indicates ulnar nerve injury Nodules: Dupuytren's contracture; snapping A1 pulley with finger extension: trigger finger Tenderness suggests purulent tenosynovitis Tenderness: paronychia or felon

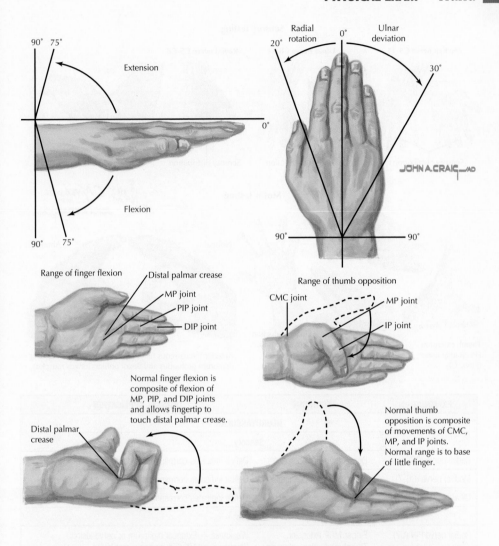

Extension

90° 75°

0°

Flexion

90° 75°

Radial rotation 0° Ulnar deviation

20° 30°

90° 90°

JOHN A.CRAIG—AD

Range of finger flexion — Distal palmar crease

MP joint
PIP joint
DIP joint

Normal finger flexion is composite of flexion of MP, PIP, and DIP joints and allows fingertip to touch distal palmar crease.

Distal palmar crease

Range of thumb opposition

CMC joint — MP joint
IP joint

Normal thumb opposition is composite of movements of CMC, MP, and IP joints. Normal range is to base of little finger.

EXAMINATION	TECHNIQUE	CLINICAL APPLICATION
RANGE OF MOTION		
Finger		
MCP joint	Flex 90°, extend 0°, adduct/abduct 0-20°	Decreased flexion if casted in extension (collateral ligaments shorten)
PIP joint	Flex 110°, extend 0°	Hyperextension leads to swan neck
DIP joint	Flex 80°, extend 10°	All fingers should point to scaphoid at full flexion
Thumb		
CMC joint	Radial abduction: flex 50°, extend 50°	Motion is in plane of palm
	Palmar abduction: abduct 70, adduct 0°	Motion is perpendicular to plane of the palm
MCP joint	In plane of palm: flex 50°, extend 0°	
IP joint	In plane of palm: flex 75°, extend 10°	
Opposition	Touch thumb to small finger base	Motion is mostly at CMC joint

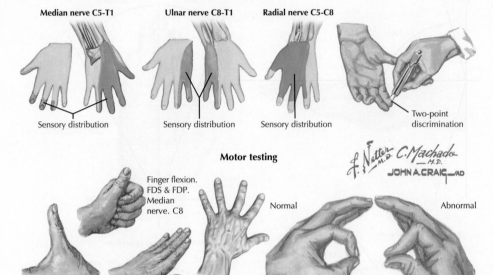

Sensory testing

Median nerve C5-T1 Ulnar nerve C8-T1 Radial nerve C5-C8

Sensory distribution Sensory distribution Sensory distribution Two-point discrimination

Motor testing

Finger flexion. FDS & FDP. Median nerve. C8

Normal Abnormal

Thumb extension. EPL. Radial nerve (PIN). C7

Finger extension. EDC. Radial nerve (PIN). C7

Finger abduction. Interosseous m. Ulnar n. T1

Anterior interosseous nerve dysfunction (paresis of flexor digitorum profundus and flexor pollicis longus muscles).

EXAMINATION	TECHNIQUE	CLINICAL APPLICATION
NEUROVASCULAR		
Sensory		
Radial nerve (C6)	Dorsal thumb, web space	Deficit indicates corresponding nerve/root lesion
Median nerve (C6-7)	Radial border, index finger	Deficit indicates corresponding nerve/root lesion
Ulnar nerve (C8)	Ulnar border, small finger	Deficit indicates corresponding nerve/root lesion
Motor		
Radial nerve/PIN (C7)	Finger MCP extension	Weakness = Extensor digitorum or nerve lesion
	Thumb abduction/extension	Weakness = APL/EPL or nerve/root lesion
Median nerve (C8)	Finger PIP flexion	Weakness = FDS or corresponding nerve/root lesion
AIN	Index finger DIP flexion	Weakness = FDP or AIN nerve lesion
	Thumb IP flexion	Weakness = FPL or corresponding nerve/root lesion
Motor recurrent branch	Thumb opposition	Weakness = APB, OP, 1/2 FPB or nerve lesion; (CTS)
Ulnar nerve (deep branch) (T1)	Finger abduction	Weakness = Dorsal/volar interosseous or nerve lesion
	Thumb adduction	Weakness = Adductor pollicis or nerve/root lesion
Reflex		
Hoffman's	Flick MF DIPJ into flexion	Pathologic if thumb IPJ flexes: myelopathy
Vascular		
Capillary refill	Squeeze finger tip	Color (blood) should return in less than 2 seconds
Allen's test	Occlude both radial & ulnar arteries, then release one	Hand should "pink up" if artery that was released AND arches are patent. Failure to "pink up" = arterial injury
Doppler	Arches, digital borders	Use if presence of pulses/patent vessels is in question

Positive Froment's sign

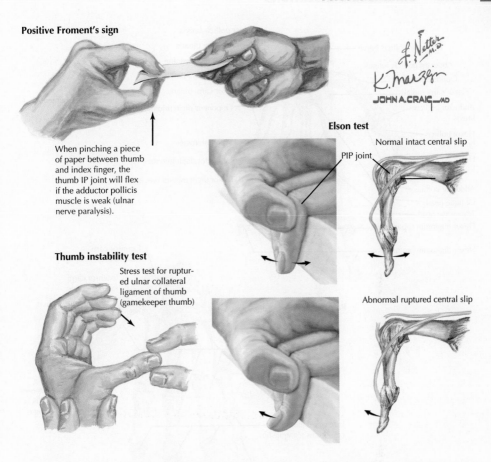

When pinching a piece of paper between thumb and index finger, the thumb IP joint will flex if the adductor pollicis muscle is weak (ulnar nerve paralysis).

Thumb instability test

Stress test for ruptured ulnar collateral ligament of thumb (gamekeeper thumb)

JOHN A. CRAIG—AD

Elson test

PIP joint   Normal intact central slip

Abnormal ruptured central slip

EXAMINATION	TECHNIQUE	CLINICAL APPLICATION
SPECIAL TESTS		
Profundus test	Stabilize PIPJ in extension, flex DIPJ only	Inability to flex DIP alone indicates FDP pathology
Sublimus test	Extend all fingers, flex a single finger at PIPJ	Inability to flex PIP of isolated finger indicates FDS pathology
Froment's sign	Hold paper with thumb and index finger, pull paper	If thumb IP flexion is positive, suggest adductor pollicis weakness and/or ulnar nerve palsy
CMC grind test	Axial compress and rotate CMC joint	Pain indicates arthritis at CMC joint of thumb
Finger instability test	Stabilize proximal joint, apply varus and valgus stress	Laxity indicates collateral ligament injury
Thumb instability test	Stabilize MCP, apply valgus stress in extension and 30° of flexion	Laxity at 30°: ulnar collateral ligament injury Laxity in extension: accessory collateral ligament and/or volar plate injury
Bunnell-Littler test	Extend MCPJ, passively flex PIPJ	Tight or inability to flex PIPJ, improved with MCPJ flexion indicates tight intrinsic muscles
Elson test	Flex PIPJ 90° over table edge, resist P2 extension	DIPJ rigidly extending (via lateral bands) indicates central slip injury (boutonnière)

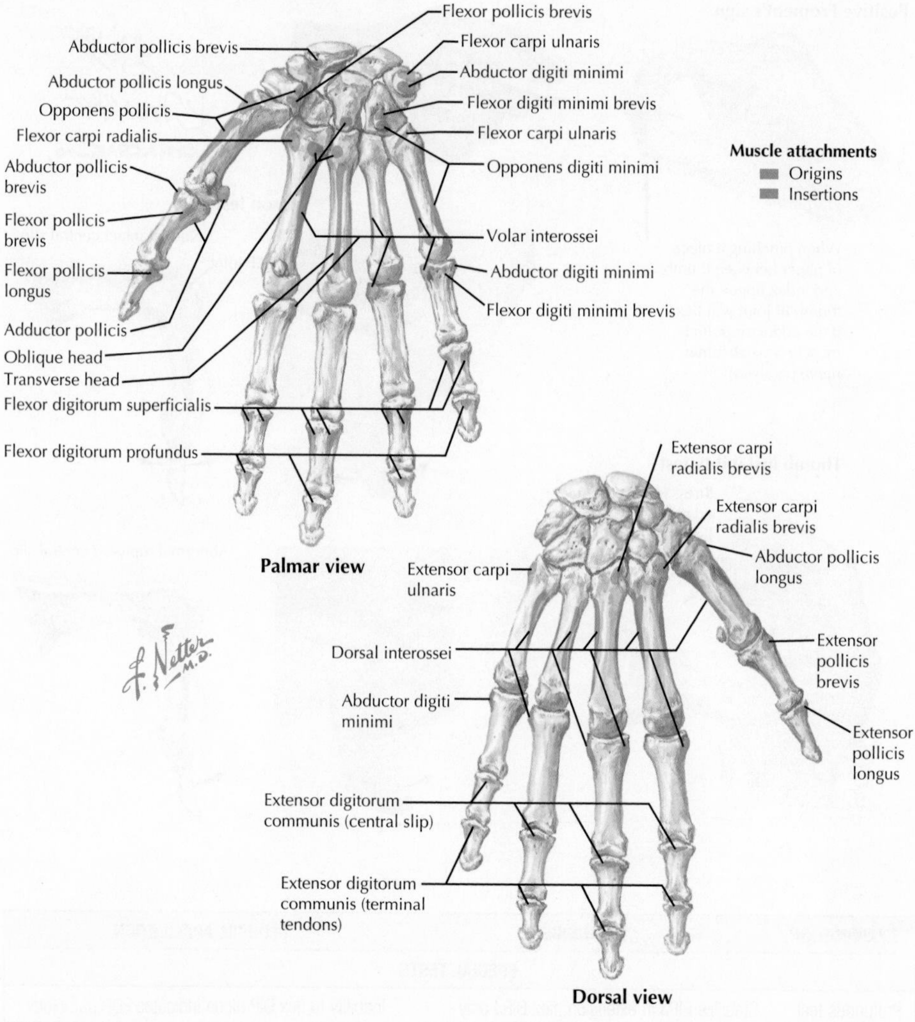

Muscle attachments
■ Origins
■ Insertions

Palmar view

f. Netter M.D.

Dorsal view

CARPUS	METACARPAL	PHALANGES—DORSAL	PHALANGES—PLANTAR
Trapezium	Dorsal interosseous	**Proximal phalanx**	**Proximal phalanx**
Abductor pollicis brevis	Palmar interosseous	Ext. pollicis brevis (thumb)	Abductor pollicis brevis (thumb)
Flexor pollicis brevis	Adductor pollicis	Dorsal interossei	Flexor pollicis brevis (thumb)
Opponens pollicis	Abd. pollicis longus	Abductor digiti minimi	Adductor pollicis (thumb)
Capitate	Opponens pollicis	**Middle phalanx**	Palmar interossei
Adductor pollicis	Opp. digiti minimi	Extensor digitorum com-	Flexor digiti minimi brevis
Hamate	Flexor carpi radialis	munis (central slip)	Abductor digiti minimi
Flex. digiti minimi brevis	Flexor carpi ulnaris	**Distal phalanx**	**Middle phalanx**
Opponens digiti minimi	Ext. carpi rad. longus	Ext. pollicis longus	Flexor digitorum superficialis
Pisiform	Ext. carpi rad. brevis	(thumb)	**Distal phalanx**
Abductor digiti minimi	Extensor carpi ulnaris	Extensor digitorum com-	Flexor pollicis longus (thumb)
		munis (terminal tendon)	Flexor digitorum profundus

Lumbricals originate on flexor digitorum profundus [FDP] tendon and insert on the radial lateral bands

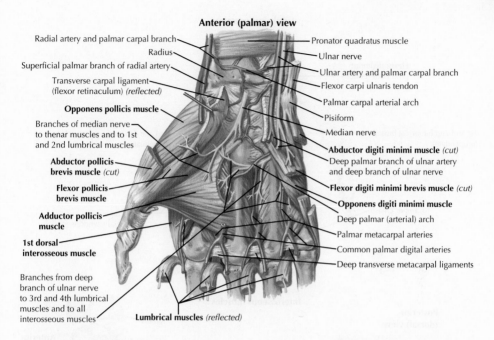

Anterior (palmar) view

Radial artery and palmar carpal branch
Radius
Superficial palmar branch of radial artery
Transverse carpal ligament (flexor retinaculum) *(reflected)*
Opponens pollicis muscle
Branches of median nerve to thenar muscles and to 1st and 2nd lumbrical muscles
Abductor pollicis brevis muscle *(cut)*
Flexor pollicis brevis muscle
Adductor pollicis muscle
1st dorsal interosseous muscle
Branches from deep branch of ulnar nerve to 3rd and 4th lumbrical muscles and to all interosseous muscles
Lumbrical muscles *(reflected)*

Pronator quadratus muscle
Ulnar nerve
Ulnar artery and palmar carpal branch
Flexor carpi ulnaris tendon
Palmar carpal arterial arch
Pisiform
Median nerve
Abductor digiti minimi muscle *(cut)*
Deep palmar branch of ulnar artery and deep branch of ulnar nerve
Flexor digiti minimi brevis muscle *(cut)*
Opponens digiti minimi muscle
Deep palmar (arterial) arch
Palmar metacarpal arteries
Common palmar digital arteries
Deep transverse metacarpal ligaments

MUSCLE	ORIGIN	INSERTION	NERVE	ACTION	COMMENT
THENAR COMPARTMENT					
Abductor pollicis brevis (APB)	Scaphoid, trapezium	Lateral prox. phalanx (thumb)	Median	Palmar pronation	Primary muscle in opposition
Flexor pollicis brevis 1. Superficial head 2. Deep head	Trans. carpal lig. Trapezium	Base of thumb Proximal phalanx	Median Ulnar	Thumb MPC flexion	Muscle has dual innervations
Opponens pollicis	Trapezium	Lateral thumb MC	Median	Oppose (flex/ abduct) thumb	Pronates/stabilizes thumb MC
ADDUCTOR COMPARTMENT					
Adductor pollicis 1. Oblique head 2. Transverse head	1. Capitate, 2nd and 3rd MC 2. 3rd metacarpal	Ulnar base of proximal pha- lanx of thumb	Ulnar	Thumb adduc- tion and thumb MCP flexion	Test function with Froment's test
HYPOTHENAR COMPARTMENT					
Palmaris brevis [PB]	Transverse carpal ligament [TCL]	Skin on medial palm	Ulnar	Wrinkles skin	Protects ulnar nerve
Abductor digiti minimi [ADQ]	Pisiform (FCU tendon)	Ulnar base of prox. phalanx	Ulnar	SF abduction	Ulnar nerve and artery under it
Flexor digiti minimi brevis [FDMB]	Hamate, TCL	Base of proximal phalanx of SF	Ulnar	SF MCP flexion	Deep to ADQ and nerve
Opponens digiti min- imi [ODQ]	Hamate, TCL	Ulnar side 5th metacarpal	Ulnar	Oppose (flex and supinate) SF	Deep to other muscles

- Abductor muscles are superficial; opponens muscles are deep
- Motor recurrent branch of median innervates thenar muscle and radial 2 lumbricals
- Deep branch at ulnar nerve innervates hypothenar, adductor pollicis, interossei, and ulnar 2 lumbricals

Lumbrical muscles

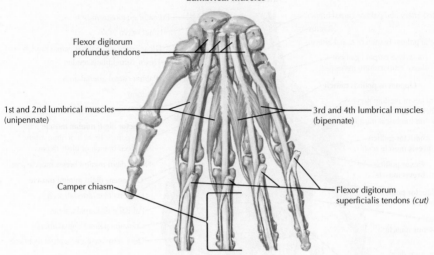

Flexor digitorum profundus tendons

1st and 2nd lumbrical muscles (unipennate)

3rd and 4th lumbrical muscles (bipennate)

Camper chiasm

Flexor digitorum superficialis tendons *(cut)*

Interosseous muscles

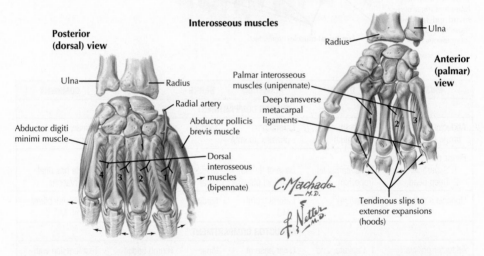

Posterior (dorsal) view

Ulna
Radius
Radial artery
Abductor pollicis brevis muscle
Abductor digiti minimi muscle
Dorsal interosseous muscles (bipennate)

Anterior (palmar) view

Ulna
Radius
Palmar interosseous muscles (unipennate)
Deep transverse metacarpal ligaments
Tendinous slips to extensor expansions (hoods)

C. Machado M.D.
F. Netter M.D.

MUSCLE	ORIGIN	INSERTION	NERVE	ACTION	COMMENT
INTRINSICS					
Lumbricals 1 & 2	FDP tendons (radial 2)	Radial lateral bands	Median	Extend PIP, flex MCP	Only muscles in body to insert on their own antagonist (FDP). Palmar to deep transverse MC ligaments.
Lumbricals 3 & 4	FDP tendons (medial 3)	Radial lateral bands	Ulnar	Extend PIP, flex MCP	
Interosseous: dorsal (DIO)	Adjacent metacarpals	Proximal phalanx and extensor expansion (lateral bands)	Ulnar	Digit abduction MCP flexion	DAB: Dorsal ABduct Bipennate: each belly has separate insertion
Interosseous: palmar (PIO)	Adjacent metacarpals	Extensor expansion (lateral bands)	Ulnar	Digit adduction	PAD: Palmar ADduct Unipennate

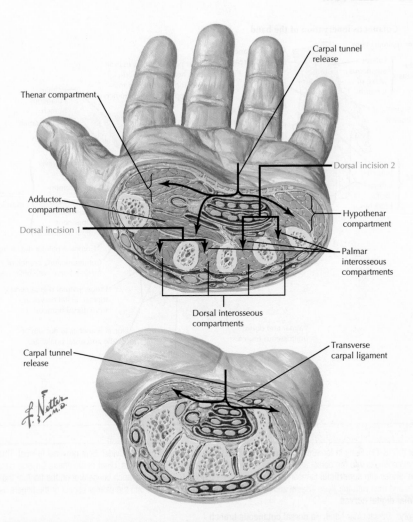

Thenar compartment

Carpal tunnel release

Dorsal incision 2

Adductor compartment

Dorsal incision 1

Hypothenar compartment

Palmar interosseous compartments

Dorsal interosseous compartments

Carpal tunnel release

Transverse carpal ligament

CONTENTS	COMPARTMENT
COMPARTMENTS (10)	
Thenar	Abductor pollicis brevis, flexor pollicis brevis, opponens pollicis
Hypothenar	Abductor digiti minimi, flexor digiti minimi brevis, opponens digiti minimi
Adductor	Adductor pollicis
Palmar interosseous (3)	Palmar interosseous muscles
Dorsal interosseous (4)	Dorsal interosseous muscles
FASCIOTOMIES	
Incisions	3 incisions (2 dorsal and 1 carpal tunnel release) can release all compartments.
Dorsal (1)	Over 2nd metacarpal, dissect on both sides: release radial 2 interosseous (2 dorsal, 1 palmar)
Dorsal (2)	Over 4th metacarpal, dissect on both sides: release ulnar 4 interosseous (2 dorsal, 2 palmar)
Medial	Release transverse carpal ligament, then thenar, hypothenar, & adductor compartments

Cutaneous innervation of the hand

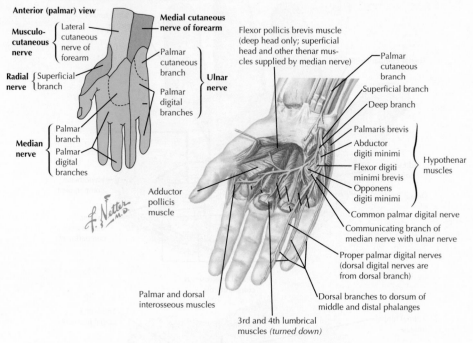

Anterior (palmar) view

Musculo-cutaneous nerve { Lateral cutaneous nerve of forearm

Radial nerve { Superficial branch

Median nerve { Palmar branch, Palmar digital branches

Medial cutaneous nerve of forearm

Palmar cutaneous branch

Ulnar nerve { Palmar digital branches

Flexor pollicis brevis muscle (deep head only; superficial head and other thenar muscles supplied by median nerve)

Palmar cutaneous branch

Superficial branch

Deep branch

Palmaris brevis

Abductor digiti minimi

Flexor digiti minimi brevis

Opponens digiti minimi

} Hypothenar muscles

Adductor pollicis muscle

Common palmar digital nerve

Communicating branch of median nerve with ulnar nerve

Proper palmar digital nerves (dorsal digital nerves are from dorsal branch)

Palmar and dorsal interosseous muscles

Dorsal branches to dorsum of middle and distal phalanges

3rd and 4th lumbrical muscles *(turned down)*

BRACHIAL PLEXUS
Medial Cord

Ulnar (C[7]8-T1): Runs in forearm under FCU, on FDP. **Dorsal cutaneous branch** divides 5cm proximal to wrist. This nerve continues into the dorsal aspect of the ulnar digits as **dorsal digital nerves**. Ulnar nerve enters Guyon's canal, then divides into **superficial** (sensory) and **deep** (motor) branches. The deep branch bends around the hook of the hamate and runs with the deep arterial arch. The superficial branch continues into the palmar aspect of the fingers as the **palmar digital nerves**.

Sensory: Dorsal ulnar hand: via **dorsal cutaneous branch**
Dorsal small & ring fingers: via **dorsal digital branches**
Ulnar proximal palm: via **palmar cutaneous branch**
Ulnar distal palm: via **common palmar digital branches**
Palmar small & ring fingers: via **proper palmar digital branches**

Motor: **Superficial (sensory) branch**
  ○ Palmaris brevis—only muscle innervated by this branch
  Deep (motor) branch: travels with deep arterial arch
  • Hypothenar compartment
    ○ Abductor digiti minimi (ADM)
    ○ Flexor digiti minimi brevis (FDMB)
    ○ Opponens digiti minimi (ODM)
  • Adductor compartment
    ○ Adductor pollicis
  • Intrinsic muscles
    ○ Lumbricals (ulnar two [3,4])
    ○ Dorsal interossei (DIO)
    ○ Palmar (volar) interossei (VIO)
  • Thenar compartment
    ○ Flexor pollicis brevis (FPB)—deep head only

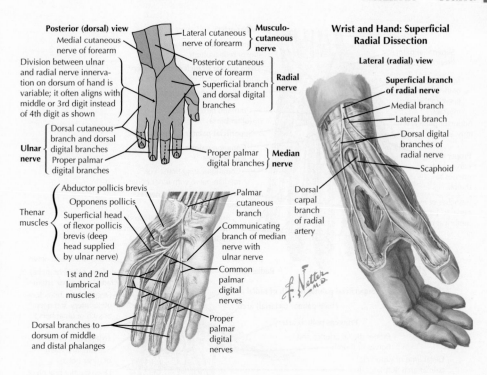

Posterior (dorsal) view

Medial cutaneous nerve of forearm

Lateral cutaneous nerve of forearm } Musculo-cutaneous nerve

Division between ulnar and radial nerve innervation on dorsum of hand is variable; it often aligns with middle or 3rd digit instead of 4th digit as shown

Posterior cutaneous nerve of forearm

Superficial branch and dorsal digital branches } Radial nerve

Ulnar nerve {
Dorsal cutaneous branch and dorsal digital branches
Proper palmar digital branches
}

Proper palmar digital branches } Median nerve

Thenar muscles {
Abductor pollicis brevis
Opponens pollicis
Superficial head of flexor pollicis brevis (deep head supplied by ulnar nerve)
}

Palmar cutaneous branch

Communicating branch of median nerve with ulnar nerve

Common palmar digital nerves

Proper palmar digital nerves

1st and 2nd lumbrical muscles

Dorsal branches to dorsum of middle and distal phalanges

Wrist and Hand: Superficial Radial Dissection

Lateral (radial) view

Superficial branch of radial nerve
Medial branch
Lateral branch
Dorsal digital branches of radial nerve
Scaphoid

Dorsal carpal branch of radial artery

BRACHIAL PLEXUS
Medial and Lateral Cords

Median (C[5]8-T1): Runs in forearm on FDP. **Palmar cutaneous branch** branches proximal to the carpal tunnel. The median nerve enters the carpal tunnel. The **motor recurrent branch** exits distal to transverse carpal ligament (TCL) and supplies the thenar muscles. Anatomic variants include exit through (at risk in carpal tunnel release) or under the TCL. The remainder of the nerve is sensory and supplies the palmar radial 3½ digits.

Sensory: Palm of hand: via **palmar cutaneous branch**
Volar thumb, IF, MF, radial RF: via **palmar digital branches**
Dorsal distal thumb, IF, MF, radial RF: via **proper palmar digital branch**

Motor: **Motor (recurrent) branch**
• Thenar compartment
  ◦ Abductor pollicis brevis (APB)
  ◦ Opponens pollicis
  ◦ Flexor pollicis brevis (FPB)—superficial head only
• Intrinsic muscles
  ◦ Lumbricals (radial two [1,2])

Posterior Cord

Radial (C5-T1): Superficial branch runs under brachioradialis to wrist, then bifurcates in medial & lateral branches that supply the dorsal hand & thumb web space. They continue as **dorsal digital branches** to the dorsal fingers.

Sensory: Dorsal radial hand: via **superficial branch**
Dorsal proximal thumb, IF, MF, radial RF: via **dorsal digital branches**
Motor: None (in hand)

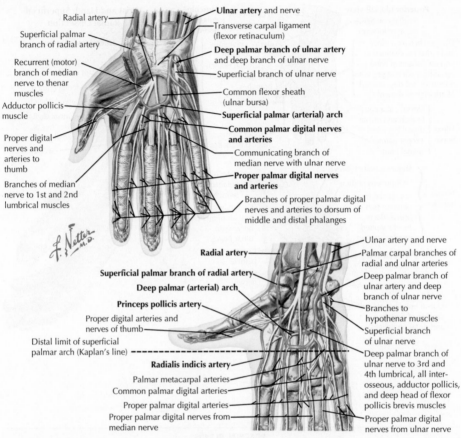

Radial artery
Superficial palmar branch of radial artery
Recurrent (motor) branch of median nerve to thenar muscles
Adductor pollicis muscle
Proper digital nerves and arteries to thumb
Branches of median nerve to 1st and 2nd lumbrical muscles

Ulnar artery and nerve
Transverse carpal ligament (flexor retinaculum)
Deep palmar branch of ulnar artery and deep branch of ulnar nerve
Superficial branch of ulnar nerve
Common flexor sheath (ulnar bursa)
Superficial palmar (arterial) arch
Common palmar digital nerves and arteries
Communicating branch of median nerve with ulnar nerve
Proper palmar digital nerves and arteries
Branches of proper palmar digital nerves and arteries to dorsum of middle and distal phalanges

Radial artery
Superficial palmar branch of radial artery
Deep palmar (arterial) arch
Princeps pollicis artery
Proper digital arteries and nerves of thumb
Distal limit of superficial palmar arch (Kaplan's line) - - - - -
Radialis indicis artery
Palmar metacarpal arteries
Common palmar digital arteries
Proper palmar digital arteries
Proper palmar digital nerves from median nerve

Ulnar artery and nerve
Palmar carpal branches of radial and ulnar arteries
Deep palmar branch of ulnar artery and deep branch of ulnar nerve
Branches to hypothenar muscles
Superficial branch of ulnar nerve
Deep palmar branch of ulnar nerve to 3rd and 4th lumbrical, all inter-osseous, adductor pollicis, and deep head of flexor pollicis brevis muscles
Proper palmar digital nerves from ulnar nerve

COURSE	BRANCHES	COMMENT/SUPPLY
• **Radial artery:** divides at wrist into **superficial branch,** which anastomoses with the superficial palmar arch. The **deep branch** runs thru the bellies of the 1st dorsal interosseous muscle & terminates as the **deep palmar arch.** • **Ulnar artery:** divides at wrist into a **deep branch,** which anastomoses with the deep palmar arch. The **superficial branch** terminates as the **superficial palmar arch.**		
DEEP PALMAR ARCH		
Runs volar to the bases of the metacarpals. It is proximal to the superficial arch.	Princeps pollicis Radialis indicis Proper digital arteries of thumb (2) Palmar metacarpal (3)	Continuation of deep branch of radial artery Supplies radial IF; may branch from deep arch Two terminal branches of bifurcated princeps pollicis Anastomoses with common digital arteries
SUPERFICIAL PALMAR ARCH		
Located at Kaplan's line; distal to the deep arch	Proper palmar digital artery to SF Common palmar digital (3) Proper palmar digital	First branch off arch; supplies ulnar small finger In 2nd-4th web spaces, each bifurcates Runs on radial & ulnar borders of digits
• Superficial arch supplies most of the hand/fingers. It is dominant ⅔ of the time. This arch is complete 80% of the time. • Deep arch supplies the thumb (& radial IF). It is usually the nondominant arch. This arch is complete 98% of the time. • The arches are codominant ⅓ of the time. Allen's test determines if arch is complete (but not which is dominant). • Arteries are volar to the nerves in the palm, but cross to become dorsal to the nerves in the fingers.		

Osteoarthritis

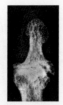

Section through distal interphalangeal joint shows irregular, hyperplastic bony nodules (Heberden's nodes) at articular margins of distal phalanx. Cartilage eroded and joint space narrowed

Radiograph of distal interphalangeal joint reveals late-stage degenerative changes. Cartilage destruction and marginal osteophytes (Heberden's nodes)

Rheumatoid arthritis

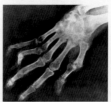

Radiograph shows cartilage thinning at proximal interphalangeal joints, erosion of carpus and wrist joint, osteoporosis, and finger deformities

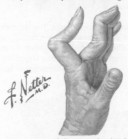

Late-stage degenerative changes in carpometacarpal articulation of thumb

Boutonniere deformity of index finger with swan-neck deformity of other fingers

DESCRIPTION	Hx & PE	WORKUP/FINDINGS	TREATMENT
OSTEOARTHRITIS			
• Loss of articular cartilage • Due to wear or posttraumatic • DIPJ #1 (Heberden's nodes) • PIPJ #2 (Bouchard's nodes)	**Hx:** Elderly or hx of injury Pain: worse w/activity **PE:** Nodule/deformity, tenderness, decreased ROM	**XR:** OA findings: joint space loss, osteophytes, sclerosis, subchondral cysts	1. NSAIDs 2. Steroid injection 3. Arthrodesis/fusion 4. Arthroplasty
MUCOUS CYST			
• Ganglion cyst from arthritic joint (DIPJ #1)	**Hx:** Mass near a joint **PE:** Mass, +/− tenderness	**XR:** Joint arthritis	1. Excision of cyst and associated osteophyte
RHEUMATOID ARTHRITIS			
• Autoimmune disease attacks synovium and destroys joints • MCPJ #1 • Multiple deformities develop	**HX:** Pain and stiffness (worse in AM) **PE:** Deformities (ulnar drift, swan neck, boutonniere)	**XR:** Joint destruction **LABS:** RF, ANA, ESR, CBC, uric acid	1. Medical management 2. Synovectomy (1 joint) 3. Tendon transfer/repair 4. Arthrodesis/arthroplasty
SWAN NECK DEFORMITY			
• FDS insertion/volar plate injury • Traumatic or assoc. with RA • Lateral bands subluxate dorsally, hyperextends PIPJ	**Hx:** Injury or RA **PE:** Deformity: flexed DIPJ, injury hyperextended PIPJ	**XR:** Shows bony deformity	1. Early: splint 2. Late: surgical release and reconstruction 3. Arthrodesis
BOUTONNIERE DEFORMITY			
• Central slip (EDC) and triangular ligament injury • Traumatic or assoc. with RA • Lateral bands subluxate volarly, hyperflexes PIPJ	**Hx:** Traumatic injury or RA **PE:** Deformity: flexed PIPJ, + Elson's test (inability to extend the flexed PIPJ)	**XR:** Shows bony deformity	1. Early: splint PIPJ in extension 2. Reconstruct lateral bands and central slip 3. Arthrodesis/arthroplasty

Tenosynovitis

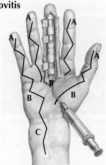

Tenosynovitis of the middle finger. Treated with zigzag volar incision. Tendon sheath opened by reflecting cruciate pulleys. Fine plastic catheter inserted for irrigation. Lines of incision indicated for tendon sheaths of other fingers (A); radial and ulnar bursae (B); and Parona's subtendinous space (C)

Paronychia infection

Eponychium elevated from nail surface

Sporotrichosis

Begins as small nodule and spreads to hand, wrist, forearm (even systemically).

Horseshoe abscess

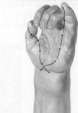

From focus in thumb spreads through radial and ulnar bursae and tendon sheath of little finger, with rupture into Parona's subtendinous space

Felon

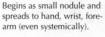

Cross section shows division of septum in finger pulp

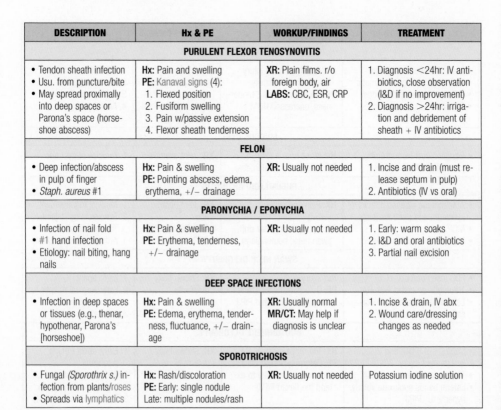

DESCRIPTION	Hx & PE	WORKUP/FINDINGS	TREATMENT
PURULENT FLEXOR TENOSYNOVITIS			
• Tendon sheath infection • Usu. from puncture/bite • May spread proximally into deep spaces or Parona's space (horseshoe abscess)	**Hx:** Pain and swelling **PE:** Kanaval signs (4): 1. Flexed position 2. Fusiform swelling 3. Pain w/passive extension 4. Flexor sheath tenderness	**XR:** Plain films. r/o foreign body, air **LABS:** CBC, ESR, CRP	1. Diagnosis <24hr: IV antibiotics, close observation (I&D if no improvement) 2. Diagnosis >24hr: irrigation and debridement of sheath + IV antibiotics
FELON			
• Deep infection/abscess in pulp of finger • *Staph. aureus* #1	**Hx:** Pain & swelling **PE:** Pointing abscess, edema, erythema, +/− drainage	**XR:** Usually not needed	1. Incise and drain (must release septum in pulp) 2. Antibiotics (IV vs oral)
PARONYCHIA / EPONYCHIA			
• Infection of nail fold • #1 hand infection • Etiology: nail biting, hang nails	**Hx:** Pain & swelling **PE:** Erythema, tenderness, +/− drainage	**XR:** Usually not needed	1. Early: warm soaks 2. I&D and oral antibiotics 3. Partial nail excision
DEEP SPACE INFECTIONS			
• Infection in deep spaces or tissues (e.g., thenar, hypothenar, Parona's [horseshoe])	**Hx:** Pain & swelling **PE:** Edema, erythema, tenderness, fluctuance, +/− drainage	**XR:** Usually normal **MR/CT:** May help if diagnosis is unclear	1. Incise & drain, IV abx 2. Wound care/dressing changes as needed
SPOROTRICHOSIS			
• Fungal *(Sporothrix s.)* infection from plants/roses • Spreads via lymphatics	**Hx:** Rash/discoloration **PE:** Early: single nodule Late: multiple nodules/rash	**XR:** Usually not needed	Potassium iodine solution

Deep space infections

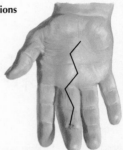

Infection of midpalmar space secondary to tenosynovitis of middle finger. Focus is infected puncture wound at distal crease. Line of incision indicated

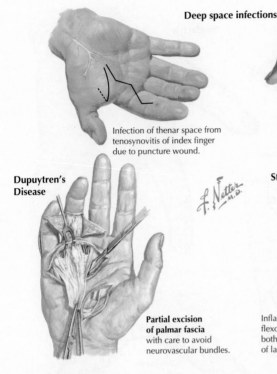

Infection of thenar space from tenosynovitis of index finger due to puncture wound.

Dupuytren's Disease

Partial excision of palmar fascia with care to avoid neurovascular bundles.

Stenosing Tenosynovitis (Trigger Finger)

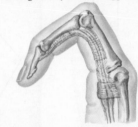

Inflammatory thickening of fibrous sheath (pulley) of flexor tendons with fusiform nodular enlargement of both tendons. Broken line indicates line for incision of lateral aspect of pulley

DESCRIPTION	Hx & PE	WORKUP/FINDINGS	TREATMENT
BITES: HUMAN/ANIMAL			

• Usually dominant hand
• "Fight bite" = fist to mouth #1
• Bacteria: *Strep., Staph. a.*
    Human: *Eikenella corr.*
    Animal: *Pasteurella mult.*
	Hx: Bite, pain & swelling
	PE: Puncture wound or laceration, edema, +/– drainage, erythema (local or tracking proximally)
		XR: Hand series: rule out foreign body (e.g., tooth) or air in tissues/joint
		LABS: CBC, ESR, CRP
			1. Td & rabies prophylaxis if indicated
			2. I&D, wound care
			3. IV antibiotics (ampicillin/sulbactam)

STENOSING TENOSYNOVITIS (TRIGGER FINGER)			
• Tight/thickened A1 pulley en-traps flexor tendon • Associated with DM, RA, age • Congenital form in pediatrics	**Hx:** 40+, pain, snapping or locking (esp. in AM) **PE:** Tender flexor sheath, snapping with flex./ext.	**XR:** Usually normal **MR:** Not needed, PE is diagnostic	1. Splint, occupational rx 2. Corticosteroid injection into tendon sheath 3. A1 pulley release
DUPUYTREN'S DISEASE			
• Contracture of palmar fascia • Myofibroblasts create thick cords of type III collagen • Associated with northern Europeans (AD), DM, EtOH	**Hx:** Usually male, 40+, c/o hand mass **PE:** Nodule in palm, +/– contracture of MCPJ or PIPJ	**XR:** Usually normal **MR:** Not needed if diagnosis is clear. May be useful if etiology of mass is unclear.	1. Early (mass, no contrac-ture): reassurance 2. Late (contracture): surgi-cal excision of cords
RETINACULAR CYST			
• Ganglion-type cyst of the flexor tendon sheath • Most common hand mass	**Hx:** Small volar mass **PE:** Firm, "pea"-size nod-ule, does not move w/tendon	**XR:** Usually normal **MR:** Not needed	1. Aspiration/puncture 2. Surgical excision if recurrent

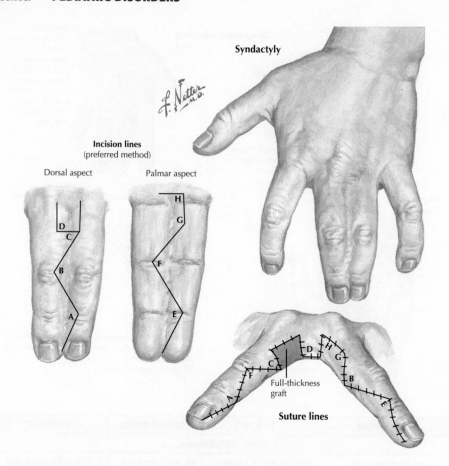

Syndactyly

F. Netter M.D.

Incision lines
(preferred method)

Dorsal aspect   Palmar aspect

Full-thickness graft

Suture lines

DESCRIPTION	EVALUATION	TREATMENT
SYNDACTYLY		
• Failure of differentiation of finger tissue • Most common congenital hand anomaly • Complete (to finger tip) vs incomplete • Simple (soft tissue) vs complex (bone)	**Hx:** Fingers are connected **PE:** Fingers are connected either to tip or incompletely down the finger **XR:** Will determine if bones are fused (complex)	1. Should wait approximately 1yr, then surgically separate fingers 2. Careful incision planning and skin grafts improve results
CAMPTODACTYLY		
• Congenital finger flexion anomaly • Usually PIPJ of small finger • Type 1 (infants), type 2 (adolescents) • Etiology: abnormal lumbrical or FDS insertion	**Hx:** Finger flexed. Noticed at birth or during adolescent growth **PE:** Inability to fully extend joint **XR:** Shows flexion, bones typically normal	1. Nonoperative: stretching, splint 2. Functionally debilitating contracture: surgical release/tendon transfer
CLINODACTYLY		
• Deviation of finger in coronal plane • Radial deviation of small finger #1 • Etio: delta-shaped middle phalanx	**Hx/PE:** Deviation of finger, cosmetic and functional complaints **XR:** Shows delta-shaped middle phalanx	1. Mild: no treatment 2. Functional deficit: surgical correction/realignment osteotomy

Polydactyly

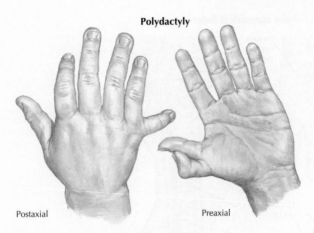

Postaxial   Preaxial

Congenital constriction band syndrome

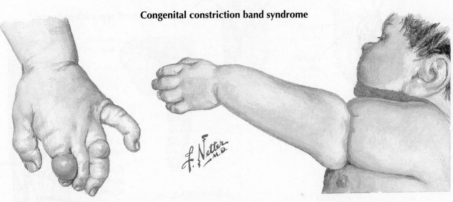

DESCRIPTION	EVALUATION	TREATMENT
DUPLICATE THUMB (PREAXIAL POLYDACTYLY)		
• An extra thumb or portion thereof • Wassel classification (7 types): Type 4 is most common • Autosomal dominant or sporadic • Associated with some syndromes	**Hx/PE:** Extra thumb or portion of thumb **XR:** Will show bifid or extra phalanges depending on which type of duplication	1. Surgical reconstruction to obtain stable thumb. Generally, retain ulnar thumb/ structures & reconstruct radial side (e.g., type 4)
THUMB HYPOPLASIA		
• Partial or complete absence of thumb • Blauth classification: Types I– V • Treatment based on presence of CMC joint • Associated with some syndromes	**Hx/PE:** Small to completely absent thumb **XR:** Range of small, shortened, or absent bones (phalanges, metacarpal, trapezium). Evaluate for presence of the CMC joint	1. Type I: Small thumb: no treatment 2. Types II-IIIA: Reconstruction 3. Types IIIB-V (no CMCJ): amputation & pollicization
CONSTRICTION BAND SYNDROME		
• Constrictive bands lead to digit necrosis or diminished growth/ development. • Nonhereditary	**Hx/PE:** Short/truncated fingers with bands at level of diminished growth **XR:** Small, shortened, or absent phalanges	1. Complete amputations if needed 2. Release/excise bands, Z-plasty as needed for skin coverage

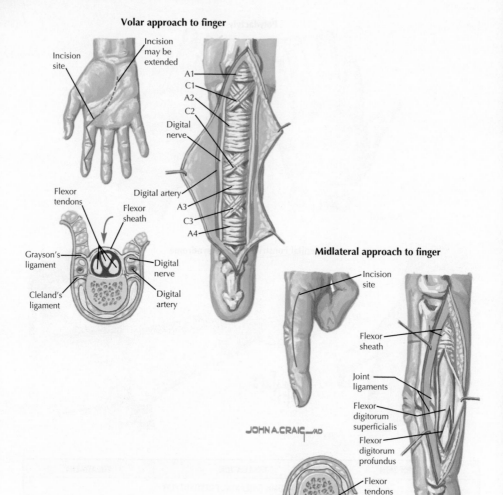

Volar approach to finger

Incision site

Incision may be extended

Incision site

A1
C1
A2
C2
Digital nerve

Digital artery
A3
C3
A4

Flexor tendons

Flexor sheath

Grayson's ligament

Cleland's ligament

Digital nerve

Digital artery

Midlateral approach to finger

Incision site

Flexor sheath

Joint ligaments

Flexor digitorum superficialis

Flexor digitorum profundus

Flexor tendons

Digital nerve

Digital artery

JOHN A. CRAIG—AD

USES	INTERNERVOUS PLANE	DANGERS	COMMENT
FINGER: VOLAR APPROACH			
• Flexor tendons (repair/explore) • Digital nerves • Soft tissue releases • Infection drainage	No planes	• Digital artery • Digital nerve • Flexor tendon	• Make a "zigzag" incision connecting finger creases • Neurovascular bundle is lateral to the tendon sheath.
FINGER: MID-LATERAL APPROACH			
• Phalangeal fractures	No planes	• Digital nerve • Digital artery	• Soft tissues are thin; capsule can be incised if care is not taken.

CHAPTER 7
Pelvis

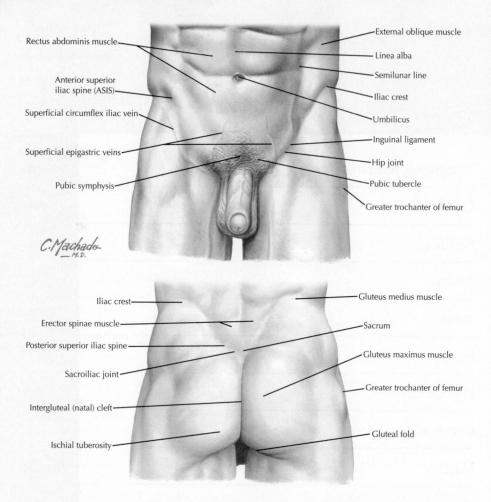

STRUCTURE	CLINICAL APPLICATION
Iliac crest	Site for contusion of lilac crest ("hip pointers") Common site for autologous bone graft harvest
Anterior superior iliac spine	Origin of sartorius muscle. An avulsion fracture can occur here. Lateral femoral cutaneous nerve (LFCN) courses here and can be entrapped. Landmark used for measuring the "Q" angle of the knee
Symphysis pubis	Site of osteitis pubis; uncommon cause of anterior pelvic pain
Inguinal ligament	External iliac artery becomes femoral artery here; femoral pulse can be palpated just inferior to the ligament in the femoral triangle.
Greater trochanter	Tenderness can indicate trochanteric bursitis.
Erector spinae muscles	Overuse and spasm are common causes of lower back pain (LBP).
Posterior superior iliac spine	Site of bone graft harvest in posterior spinal procedures.
Sacroiliac joint	Degeneration of joint can cause lower back pain (LBP).
Ischial tuberosity	Avulsion fracture (hamstring muscles) or bursitis can occur here.

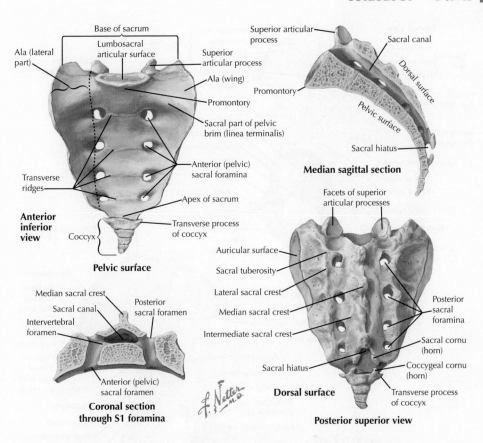

Base of sacrum
Lumbosacral articular surface
Ala (lateral part)
Superior articular process
Ala (wing)
Promontory
Sacral part of pelvic brim (linea terminalis)
Anterior (pelvic) sacral foramina
Transverse ridges
Apex of sacrum
Anterior inferior view
Coccyx
Transverse process of coccyx

Pelvic surface

Superior articular process
Sacral canal
Dorsal surface
Promontory
Pelvic surface
Sacral hiatus
Median sagittal section

Median sacral crest
Sacral canal
Posterior sacral foramen
Intervertebral foramen
Anterior (pelvic) sacral foramen
Coronal section through S1 foramina

Facets of superior articular processes
Auricular surface
Sacral tuberosity
Lateral sacral crest
Median sacral crest
Intermediate sacral crest
Posterior sacral foramina
Sacral cornu (horn)
Coccygeal cornu (horn)
Sacral hiatus
Transverse process of coccyx
Dorsal surface
Posterior superior view

CHARACTERISTICS	OSSIFY	FUSE	COMMENTS
PELVIS			

• Combination of 3 bones (two innominate bones & sacrum) and 3 joints (two sacroiliac joints & symphysis pubis)
• The pelvis has no inherent stability. It requires ligamentous support for its stability.
• Two portions of pelvis divided by pelvic brim/iliopectineal line
  ○ False (greater) pelvis—above the brim, bordered by the sacral ala and iliac wings
  ○ True (lesser) pelvis—below the brim, bordered by the ischium and pubis			

SACRUM			
• 5 vertebra are fused • 4 pairs of foramina (left and right) • Ala (wing) expands laterally • Sacral canal opens to hiatus distally • Kyphotic (approx. 25°), the apex is at S3	**Primary** Body Arches Costal elements **Secondary** 11-14yr	8wk (fetal) 2-8yr 2-8yr 2-8yr 20yr	• Transmits weight from spine to pelvis • Nerves exit through the sacral foramina (anterior & posterior) • Ala is common site for sacral fractures • Sacral canal narrows distally before opening to sacral hiatus • Segments fuse to each other at puberty
COCCYX			
• 4 vertebrae are fused • Lack features of typical vertebrae	Primary arch Body	7-8wk (fetal) 1-2yr 7-10yr	• Is attached to gluteus maximus and coccygeal m. • Common site for "tailbone" fracture

Lateral view

Gluteal lines
{ Anterior
  Inferior
  Posterior }

Intermediate zone
Tuberculum } Iliac crest
Outer lip

Wing (ala) of ilium (gluteal surface)

Anterior superior iliac spine

Anterior inferior iliac spine

Acetabulum

Lunate surface

Margin (limbus) of acetabulum

Acetabular notch/condyloid fossa

Superior pubic ramus

Pubic tubercle

Obturator crest

Inferior pubic ramus

Obturator foramen

Posterior superior iliac spine

Posterior inferior iliac spine

Greater sciatic notch

Body of ilium

Ischial spine

Lesser sciatic notch

Body of ischium

Ischial tuberosity

Ramus of ischium

Ilium
Ischium
Pubis

Intermediate zone } Iliac crest
Inner lip

Iliac tuberosity

Posterior superior iliac spine

Auricular surface (for sacrum)

Posterior inferior iliac spine

Greater sciatic notch

Ischial spine

Body of ilium

Lesser sciatic notch

Body of ischium

Ischial tuberosity

Ramus of ischium

Obturator foramen

Anterior superior iliac spine

Wing (ala) of ilium (iliac fossa)

Anterior inferior iliac spine

Arcuate line

Iliopubic eminence

Superior pubic ramus

Pecten pubis (pectineal line)

Pubic tubercle

Symphyseal surface

Obturator groove

Inferior pubic ramus

Coxal bone
{ Ilium (8th week)
  Ischium (16th week)
  Pubis (16th week) }

Triradiate cartilage

CHARACTERISTICS	OSSIFY		FUSE		COMMENTS
INNOMINATE BONE					
• 3 bones (ilium, ischium, pubis) fuse to become one bone at triradiate cartilage in acetabulum • Ilium: body, ala (wing) • Pubis: inferior & superior rami • Ischium: body & tuberosity • Acetabulum: "socket" of hip joint, has 2 walls (anterior & posterior) & notch/condyloid fossa inferiorly. Articular cartilage is horseshoe shaped	**Primary** (one in each body) **Secondary** Iliac crest Triradiate Ischial tuberosity AIIS Pubis	2-6mo 15yr	to acetabulum 15yr All fuse	 20yr	• Iliac crest is common site for both tricortical and cancellous bone graft harvest • Contusion to iliac crest known as "hip pointer" • Iliac crest ossification used to determine skeletal maturity (Risser stage) • Multiple iliac spines serve as anatomic landmarks & muscle insertion sites (ASIS, AIIS, PSIS, PIIS) • Acetabulum: 45° oblique orientation, 15° anteverted

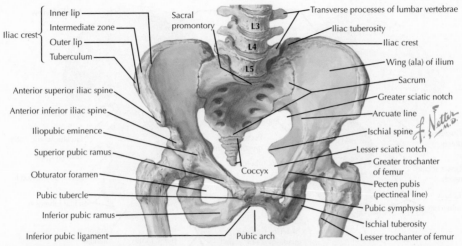

Iliac crest:
- Inner lip
- Intermediate zone
- Outer lip
- Tuberculum

Anterior superior iliac spine
Anterior inferior iliac spine
Iliopubic eminence
Superior pubic ramus
Obturator foramen
Pubic tubercle
Inferior pubic ramus
Inferior pubic ligament

Sacral promontory
L3
L4
L5
Coccyx
Pubic arch

Transverse processes of lumbar vertebrae
Iliac tuberosity
Iliac crest
Wing (ala) of ilium
Sacrum
Greater sciatic notch
Arcuate line
Ischial spine
Lesser sciatic notch
Greater trochanter of femur
Pecten pubis (pectineal line)
Pubic symphysis
Ischial tuberosity
Lesser trochanter of femur

STRUCTURE	ATTACHMENTS/RELATED STRUCTURES	COMMENT
LANDMARKS AND OTHER STRUCTURES OF THE PELVIS		
Anterior superior iliac spine (ASIS)	Sartorius Inguinal ligament Transverse & int. oblique abdominal m.	• LFCN crosses the ASIS & can be compressed there • Sartorius can avulse from it (avulsion fx) • Landmark to measure Q angle of the knee
Anterior inferior iliac spine (AIIS)	Rectus femoris Tensor fasciae latae Iliofemoral ligament (hip capsule)	• Rectus femoris can avulse from it (avulsion fx)
Posterior superior iliac spine (PSIS)	Posterior SI ligaments Marked by skin dimple	• Excellent bone graft site
Arcuate line	Pectineus	• Aka pectineal line. Strong, weight-bearing region
Gluteal lines	3 lines: anterior, inferior, posterior	• Separate origins of gluteal muscles
Gtr. trochanter	SEE ORIGINS/INSERTIONS	• Tender with trochanteric bursitis
Lesser trochanter	Iliacus/psoas muscle	• Tendon can snap over trochanter ("snapping hip")
Ischial tuberosity	SEE ORIGINS/INSERTIONS Sacrotuberous ligaments	• Excessive friction = bursitis (weaver's bottom) • Hamstrings can avulse (avulsion fx)
Ischial spine	Coccygeus & levator ani attach Sacrospinous ligaments	

Lesser sciatic foramen	Short external rotators exit:
	  Obturator externus
	  Obturator internus
		• Obturator internus is landmark to posterior column
		• Obt. externus not seen in posterior approach

Greater sciatic foramen	Structures that exit:
	  1. Superior gluteal nerve
	  2. Superior gluteal artery
	  3. Piriformis muscle
	  4. Pudendal nerve
	  5. Inferior pudendal artery
	  6. Nerve to the Obturator internus
	  7. Posterior Cutaneous nerve of thigh
	  8. Sciatic nerve
	  9. Inferior gluteal nerve
	  10. Inferior gluteal artery
	  11. Nerve to Quadratus femoris
		• Piriformis muscle is the reference point
		• Superior gluteal nerve and artery exit superior to the piriformis
		• **POP'S IQ** is a mnemonic for the nerves (structures) that exit inferior to the piriformis (medial to lateral) (see page 243)
		• Sciatic nerve (especially peroneal division) may exit pelvis above or through the piriformis as an anatomic variation

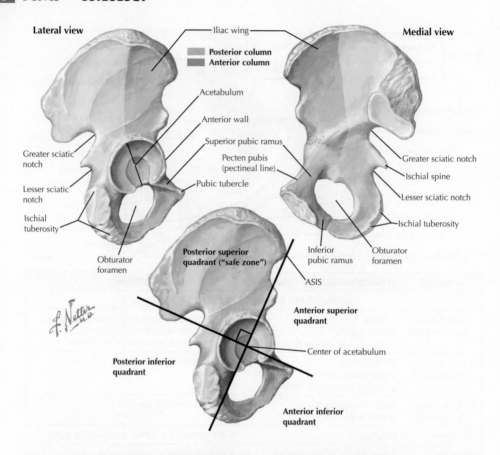

STRUCTURE	RELATED STRUCTURES	COMMENT
ACETABULAR COLUMNS		
Anterior (iliopubic)	1. Superior pubic ramus 2. Anterior acetabular wall 3. Anterior iliac wing 4. Pelvic brim	Involved in several different fracture patterns
Posterior (ilioischial)	1. Ischial tuberosity 2. Posterior acetabular wall 3. Greater & lesser sciatic notches	Involved in several different fracture patterns
ACETABULAR ZONES		
Zones defined by 2 lines: 1. ASIS to center of acetabulum, 2. perpendicular to line 1 Structures can be injured when screws are placed in these zones (e.g., acetabular cups)		
Anterior superior	External iliac artery & vein	Do not put screws in this zone
Anterior inferior	Obturator nerve, artery, vein	Do not put screws in this zone
Posterior superior	Sciatic nerve Superior gluteal nerve, artery, vein	This is the safe zone
Posterior inferior	Sciatic nerve Inferior gluteal nerve, artery, vein Internal pudendal nerve, artery, vein	This is a secondary safe zone. Safe screw placement can be achieved with care if necessary.

Radiograph, AP pelvis

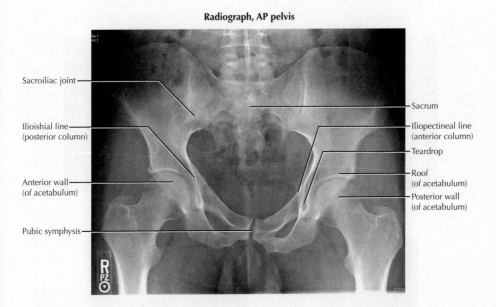

Sacroiliac joint

Sacrum

Ilioishial line (posterior column)

Iliopectineal line (anterior column)

Teardrop

Anterior wall (of acetabulum)

Roof (of acetabulum)

Posterior wall (of acetabulum)

Pubic symphysis

RADIOGRAPH	TECHNIQUE	FINDINGS	CLINICAL APPLICATION
AP (anteroposterior)	AP, IR feet 15°, beam directed at midpelvis	6 radiographic lines: 1. Iliopectineal (ant. column) 2. Ilioischial (post. column) 3. Radiographic "teardrop" 4. Acetabular roof ("dome") 5. Ant. acetabulum rim/wall 6. Post. acetabulum rim/wall	Screening for fractures (sacral, pelvic acetabular, proximal femur), use ATLS protocol; dysplasia, degenerative joint disease/arthritis
Pelvic inlet view	AP, beam 45° caudal	Sacroiliac joints, pelvic brim/pubic rami, sacrum	Pelvic ring fractures: shows posterior displacement or symphysis widening
Pelvic outlet view	AP, beam 45° cephalad	Iliac crest, symphysis pubis, sacral foramina	Pelvic ring fractures: shows superior displacement of hemipelvis
Oblique/Judet views Obturator oblique	Beam at affected hip: Elevate affected hip 45°	Obturator foramen	Acetabulum fx: anterior column, posterior wall
Iliac oblique	Elevate unaffected hip 45°	Iliac crest, sciatic notches	Acetabulum fx: posterior column, anterior wall
OTHER STUDIES			
CT	Axial, coronal, & sagittal	Articular congruity, fx fragments	Fractures, especially sacrum & acetabulum
MRI	Sequence protocols	Soft tissues: muscles, cartilage	Labral tears, tumors, stress fx
Bone scan		All bones evaluated	Tumors, infection

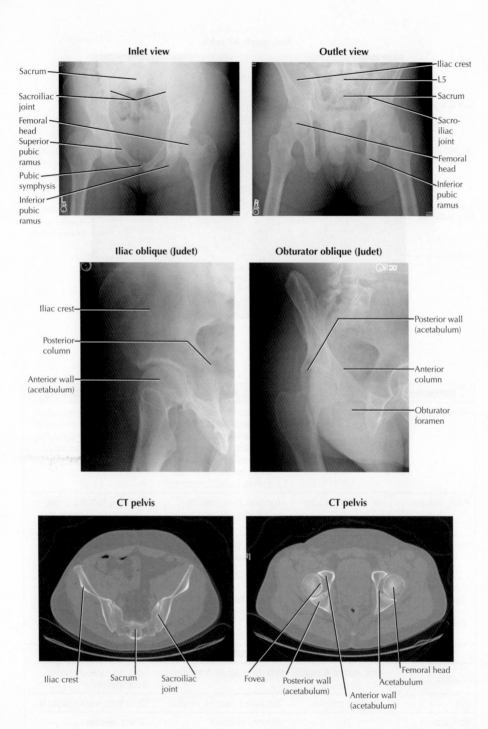

Inlet view

Sacrum
Sacroiliac joint
Femoral head
Superior pubic ramus
Pubic symphysis
Inferior pubic ramus

Outlet view

Iliac crest
L5
Sacrum
Sacroiliac joint
Femoral head
Inferior pubic ramus

Iliac oblique (Judet)

Iliac crest
Posterior column
Anterior wall (acetabulum)

Obturator oblique (Judet)

Posterior wall (acetabulum)
Anterior column
Obturator foramen

CT pelvis

Iliac crest
Sacrum
Sacroiliac joint

CT pelvis

Fovea
Posterior wall (acetabulum)
Anterior wall (acetabulum)
Femoral head
Acetabulum

Vertical sacral fracture, Denis classification

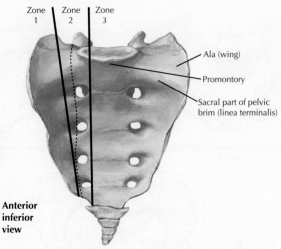

Zone 1   Zone 2   Zone 3

Ala (wing)

Promontory

Sacral part of pelvic brim (linea terminalis)

Anterior inferior view

Pelvic surface

Sacral fractures

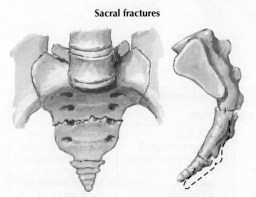

Transverse fracture of the sacrum that is minimally displaced

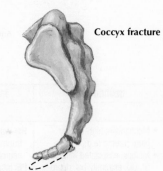

Coccyx fracture

Fracture usually requires no treatment other than care in sitting; inflatable ring helpful. Pain may persist for a long time.

DESCRIPTION	EVALUATION	CLASSIFICATION	TREATMENT
SACRAL FRACTURE			

• Mechanism: elderly—fall; young—high energy (e.g., MVA)
• Isolated injuries rare, usually assoc. w/pelvis or spine fx
• Nerve root injury very common
• Plain XR identifies <50% of fractures
• Easily missed & difficult to treat, can lead to chronic pain
	Hx: Trauma (fall or accident), pain +/− neurologic sx
	PE: Palpate spine & sacrum. Complete neuro exam including rectal exam.
	XR: AP pelvis, lateral sacrum
	CT: Necessary for diagnosis & preop planning
		By direction of fracture
		• Vertical. Denis:
		  ○ Zone 1: lateral to foramina
		  ○ Zone 2: through foramina
		  ○ Zone 3: medial to foramina
		• II. Transverse
		• III. Oblique
		• Complex: "U" or "H" shape
			• Minimally displaced/stable:
			  ○ Nonoperative
			• Displaced/unstable:
			  ○ Closed reduction and percutaneous fixation
			  ○ Open reduction, internal fixation
			• Nerve injury: decompression

COMPLICATIONS: Nerve root injury & cauda equina syndrome, esp. zone 3 fractures; nonunion/malunion, chronic pain			

Classification of pelvic fractures (Young and Burgess)

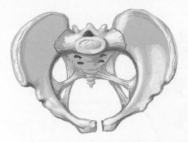

Anteroposterior Compression Type I
(APC-I)

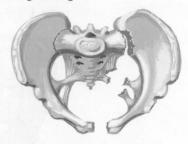

Anteroposterior Compression Type II
(APC-II)

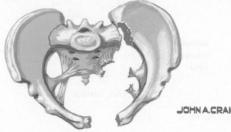

JOHN A.CRAIG—AD

Anteroposterior Compression Type III
(APC-III)

DESCRIPTION	EVALUATION	CLASSIFICATION	TREATMENT
PELVIC RING FRACTURE			

• Mechanism: high-energy blunt trauma (e.g., MVA)
• Multiple associated injuries: GI, GU, extremity fxs, neurologic, vascular, head (LC)
• Very high morbidity, usually due to uncontrolled hemorrhage (venous>arterial bleeding) esp. w/ APC3 ("open book") fxs
• Open fracture has higher morbidity and complication rate.
• Stability of fx based on ligament disruption (esp. ST, SS, posterior SI)
• Avulsion of iliolumbar ligament/L5 transverse process suggests unstable fx
• Lateral compression most common
  ◦ LC1: posterior-directed force
  ◦ LC2: anterior-directed force
	Hx: High-energy trauma, pain +/− neurologic sx
	PE: Inspect perineum for open injury. LE may be malrotated. Pelvic "rock." Rectal & vaginal exams for associated injuries. Complete neuro exam incl. rectal tone & bulbocavernosus reflexes.
	XR: AP pelvis, inlet and outlet views are essential.
	CT: Especially useful to define sacral/SIJ injury
	AGRAM: If hemodynamically unstable after pelvic stabilization; consider embolization of artery
		Young & Burgess:
		AP Compression (APC)
		I. <2.5cm pubic diastasis + 1 or 2 pubic rami fractures
		II. >2.5cm diastasis + anterior SI injury, but vertically stable
		III. Complete ant. (symphysis) & post. (SIJ) disruption. Unstable
		Lateral Compression (LC)
		I. Sacral compression + ipsilateral rami fracture
		II. LC1 + iliac wing fx or post. SIJ injury. Vertically stable
		III. LC 2 with contralateral APC3 ("windswept" pelvis)
		Vertical Shear
		SIJ & ST/SS ligament disruption + rami fxs. Vertically unstable
			• ATLS protocol. Treat life-threatening injuries
			• Pelvic hemorrhage: pelvis compression (e.g., sheet) or external fixation to reduce pelvic volume
			• Diverting colostomy for open injury or any communication w/open bowel
			• Nonoperative: WBAT for LC1, APC1, ramus fx
			• Operative for LC2 & 3; APC 2 & 3, vertical stress
			  ◦ Anterior: ORIF of symphysis
			  ◦ Post: 1. ORIF of iliac wing and sacral fractures; 2. SI screws for dislocated SIJ

COMPLICATIONS: Hemorrhage (venous>arterial [internal pudendal a. > superior gluteal a.]), neurologic injuries (L5 root at risk w/SI screws), malunion/nonunion, chronic pain (esp. at SIJ) and functional disability, infection, thromboembolism			

Classification of Pelvic Fractures (Young and Burgess)

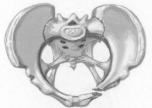

Lateral Compression Type I
(LC-I)

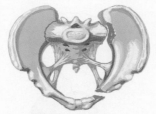

Lateral Compression Type II
(LC-II)

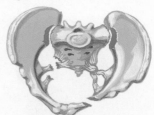

Lateral Compression Type III
(LC-III)

Vertical shear

Pelvic rami fractures

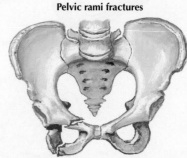

Fracture of ipsilateral pubic and ischial ramus requires only symptomatic treatment with short-term bed rest and limited activity with walker- or crutch-assisted ambulation for 4 to 6 weeks.

Fracture of pelvis without disruption of pelvic ring

Avulsions

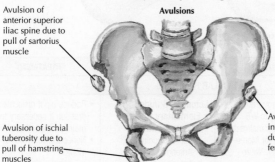

Avulsion of anterior superior iliac spine due to pull of sartorius muscle

Avulsion of ischial tuberosity due to pull of hamstring muscles

Avulsion of anterior inferior iliac spine due to pull of rectus femoris muscle

JOHN A.CRAIG—MD

DESCRIPTION	EVALUATION	CLASSIFICATION	TREATMENT
PELVIC FRACTURE—OTHER			
• Mechanism: Low-energy trauma (fall, sports injury, etc) • Stable isolated fractures, pelvic ring not disrupted • Can occur in osteopenic bone	**Hx:** Pain, esp. with WB **PE:** TTP at bony site **XR:** AP, inlet/outlet views **CT:** Often not needed, can determine displacement	**Isolated fxs:** Inferior or superior pubic rami, iliac wing/crest **Avulsions:** ASIS (sartorius), AIIS (rectus femoris), ischial tuberosity (hamstrings)	• Isolated fxs: treat with limited rest, WBAT • Avulsion fx: most treated nonoperatively. Reattach if widely displaced.
COMPLICATIONS: Malunion/nonunion, chronic pain/disability, thromboembolism			

Acetabulum—Elementary Fractures

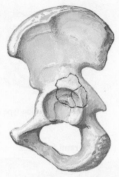

Fracture of posterior wall

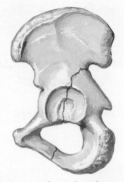

Fracture of posterior column

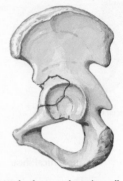

Wedge fracture of anterior wall

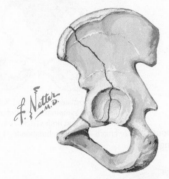

Fracture of anterior column

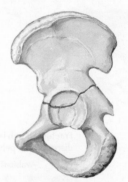

Transverse fracture

DESCRIPTION	EVALUATION	CLASSIFICATION	TREATMENT
ACETABULAR FRACTURE			

• Mechanism: high-energy blunt trauma (e.g., MVA); fem. head into acetabulum
• Fracture pattern determined by force vector & position of femoral head at impact
• Multiple associated injuries: GI, GU, extremity fractures
• Surgical approaches:
  ○ Kocher-Langenbeck: posterior fxs (PW, PC, transverse, T type)
  ○ Ilioinguinal: anterior fxs (AW, AC/HT, both columns)
	Hx: High-energy trauma, pain, inability to WB
	PE: LE may be malrotated. Inspect skin for Morel-Lavalle lesion. Neuro exam.
	XR: AP pelvis, obturator & iliac obliques (Judet views) are essential. Roof arc angle to fx (<45° is WB)
	CT: Essential to accurately define fx (size, impaction, articular involvement, LB) & do preop planning
		Letournel & Judet:
		• **Elementary fractures**
		  ○ Posterior wall
		  ○ Posterior column
		  ○ Anterior wall
		  ○ Anterior column
		  ○ Transverse
		• **Associated fractures**
		  ○ Post. column & post. wall
		  ○ Transverse & post. wall
		  ○ T type
		  ○ Ant. column and post. hemitransverse
		  ○ Both columns
			• Reduce hip if dislocated (traction if necessary to maintain reduction)
			• Nonoperative: NWB for 12wk
			  ○ <2mm articular displacement
			  ○ Roof arc angle >45°
			  ○ Posterior wall fx <20-30%
			• Operative: ORIF, NWB 12wk
			  ○ 2mm articular displacement
			  ○ Posterior wall >40%
			  ○ Irreducible fx/dx
			  ○ Marginal impaction
			  ○ Loose bodies in hip joint
			• XRT for HO prophylaxis

COMPLICATIONS: Posttraumatic arthritis, nerve injury (sciatic nerve), postsurgical (heterotopic ossification [HO], sciatic nerve injury, bleeding), malunion/nonunion, infection (assoc. with Morel-Lavalle lesion), thromboembolism			

Acetabulum—Associated Fractures

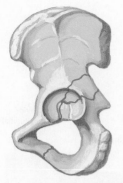

Posterior column/posterior wall

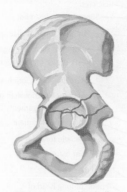

Transverse/posterior wall

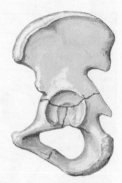

T-shaped fracture

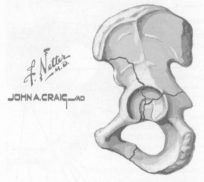

Anterior column/posterior hemi transverse

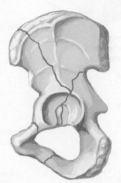

Both columns

Open reduction internal fixation acetabular fracture

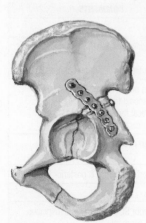

Posterior column fracture.
Repair with plate and lag screw

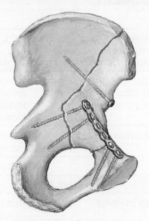

Anterior column fracture.
Repair with plate and long screws

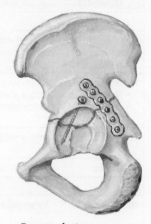

Transverse fracture.
Repair with plate and lag screw

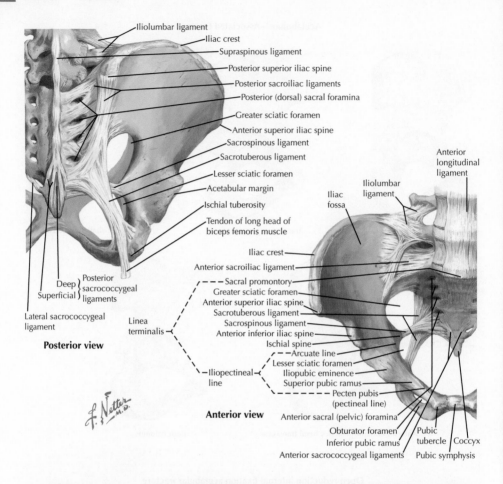

Iliolumbar ligament
Iliac crest
Supraspinous ligament
Posterior superior iliac spine
Posterior sacroiliac ligaments
Posterior (dorsal) sacral foramina
Greater sciatic foramen
Anterior superior iliac spine
Sacrospinous ligament
Sacrotuberous ligament
Lesser sciatic foramen
Acetabular margin
Ischial tuberosity
Tendon of long head of biceps femoris muscle

Anterior longitudinal ligament
Iliolumbar ligament
Iliac fossa
Iliac crest
Anterior sacroiliac ligament

Deep / Superficial } Posterior sacrococcygeal ligaments
Lateral sacrococcygeal ligament
Linea terminalis

Posterior view

Sacral promontory
Greater sciatic foramen
Anterior superior iliac spine
Sacrotuberous ligament
Sacrospinous ligament
Anterior inferior iliac spine
Ischial spine
Arcuate line
Lesser sciatic foramen
Iliopubic eminence
Superior pubic ramus
Pecten pubis (pectineal line)

Iliopectineal line

Anterior view

Anterior sacral (pelvic) foramina
Obturator foramen
Inferior pubic ramus
Anterior sacrococcygeal ligaments

Pubic tubercle
Pubic symphysis
Coccyx

LIGAMENTS	ATTACHMENTS	COMMENTS
SACROILIAC		
• This is a gliding joint. It has minimal rotational motion during gait. There should be no vertical motion in the normal joint. • Vertical stability is essential; the body weight is transmitted through this joint. • Articular surface (located inferiorly in articulation) covered with: sacrum (articular cartilage), ilium (fibrocartilage)		
Posterior sacroiliac ∘ Short sacroiliac ∘ Long sacroiliac	Posterolateral sacrum to posteromedial ilium Oblique orientation: sacrum to PSIS & PIIS Vertical orientation: sacrum to PSIS	Strongest in pelvis: key to vertical stability Resists rotational forces Resists vertical forces. Blends with sacrotuberous ligament
Anterior sacroiliac	Anterior sacrum to anterior ilium	Weaker than posterior; resists rotational forces
Interosseous	Sacrum to ilium	Adds support to anterior & posterior ligaments
PELVIC STABILITY		
Rotational stability	Tranverse/horizontal orientation	Short posterior SI, anterior SI, sacrospinous, iliolumbar ligaments
Vertical stability	Longitudinal/vertical orientation	Long posterior SI, sacrotuberous, lumbosacral ligaments

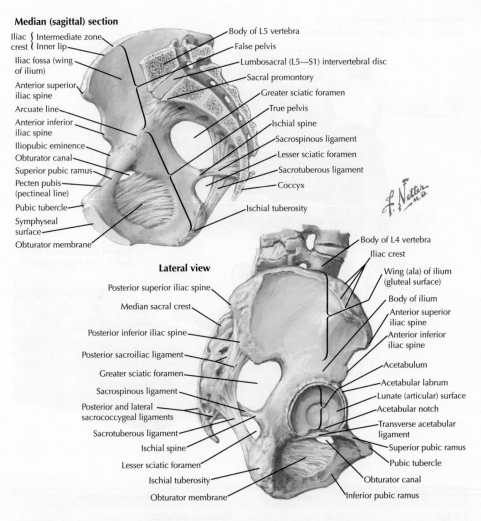

Median (sagittal) section

Iliac { Intermediate zone
crest { Inner lip
Iliac fossa (wing of ilium)
Anterior superior iliac spine
Arcuate line
Anterior inferior iliac spine
Iliopubic eminence
Obturator canal
Superior pubic ramus
Pecten pubis (pectineal line)
Pubic tubercle
Symphyseal surface
Obturator membrane

Body of L5 vertebra
False pelvis
Lumbosacral (L5—S1) intervertebral disc
Sacral promontory
Greater sciatic foramen
True pelvis
Ischial spine
Sacrospinous ligament
Lesser sciatic foramen
Sacrotuberous ligament
Coccyx
Ischial tuberosity

Lateral view

Posterior superior iliac spine
Median sacral crest
Posterior inferior iliac spine
Posterior sacroiliac ligament
Greater sciatic foramen
Sacrospinous ligament
Posterior and lateral sacrococcygeal ligaments
Sacrotuberous ligament
Ischial spine
Lesser sciatic foramen
Ischial tuberosity
Obturator membrane

Body of L4 vertebra
Iliac crest
Wing (ala) of ilium (gluteal surface)
Body of ilium
Anterior superior iliac spine
Anterior inferior iliac spine
Acetabulum
Acetabular labrum
Lunate (articular) surface
Acetabular notch
Transverse acetabular ligament
Superior pubic ramus
Pubic tubercle
Obturator canal
Inferior pubic ramus

LIGAMENTS	ATTACHMENTS	COMMENTS
PUBIC SYMPHYSIS		
• Anterior articulation of two hemipelves. Articulating surfaces are covered with hyaline cartilage. • Fibrocartilage disc between two pubic bones in the joint		
Superior pubic	Both pubic bones superiorly (& anteriorly)	Strongest supporting ligament
Arcuate pubic	Both pubic bones inferiorly	Muscle attachments also support inferiorly
OTHER LIGAMENTS		
Sacrospinous	Anterolateral sacrum to spinous process	Resists rotation, divides sciatic notches
Sacrotuberous	Posterolateral sacrum to ischial tuberosity	Resists vertical forces, provides vertical stability
Iliolumbar	L4 & L5 transverse process to posterior iliac crest	Avulsion fracture sign of unstable pelvic ring injury
Lumbosacral	L5 transverse process to sacral ala	Anterior support, assists in providing vertical stability

Anteroposterior compression pelvic fracture of pelvis (open book fracture)

Forceful frontal impact causes anteroposterior compression of pelvis

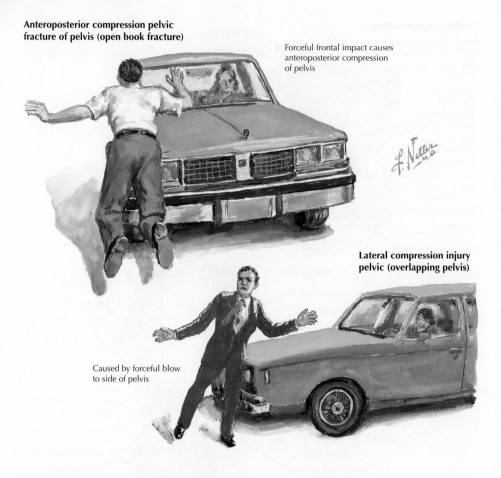

Lateral compression injury pelvic (overlapping pelvis)

Caused by forceful blow to side of pelvis

QUESTION	ANSWER	CLINICAL APPLICATION
1. Age	Young	Ankylosing spondylitis
	Middle aged–elderly	Sacroiliitis, decreased mobility
2. Pain		
a. Onset	Acute	Trauma: fracture, dislocation, contusion
	Chronic	Systemic inflammatory, degenerative disorder
b. Character	Deep, non-specific	Sacroiliac etiology, infection, tumor
	Radiating	To thigh or buttock, SI joint, L-spine
c. Occurrence	In/out of bed, on stairs	Sacroiliac etiology
	Adducting legs	Symphysis pubis etiology
3. PMHx	Pregnancy	Laxity of ligament in SI joint causes pain
4. Trauma	Fall on buttock, twist injury	Sacroiliac joint injury
	High velocity: MVA, fall	Fracture, pelvic ring disruption
5. Activity/work	Twisting, stand on one-leg	Sacroiliac etiology
6. Neurologic symptoms	Pain, numbness, tingling	Spine etiology, sacroiliac etiology
7. History of arthritides	Multiple joints involved	SI involvement of RA, Reiter's syndrome, ankylosing spondylitis, etc

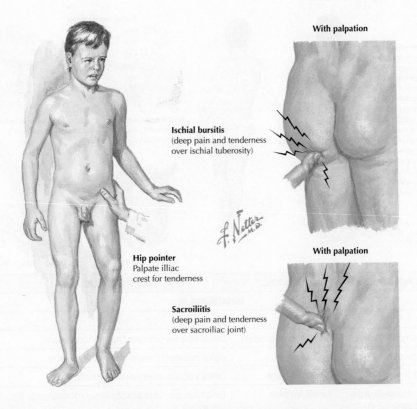

With palpation

Ischial bursitis
(deep pain and tenderness
over ischial tuberosity)

Hip pointer
Palpate iliac
crest for tenderness

Sacroiliitis
(deep pain and tenderness
over sacroiliac joint)

With palpation

EXAM/OBSERVATION	TECHNIQUE	CLINICAL APPLICATION
INSPECTION		
Skin	Discoloration, wounds	Recent trauma
ASIS's/iliac crests	Both level (same plane)	If on different plane: leg length discrepancy, sacral torsion
Lumbar curvature	Increased lordosis Decreased lordosis	Flexion contracture Paraspinal muscle spasm
PALPATION		

Bony structures	Standing: ASIS, pubic &
	  iliac tubercles, PSIS
	Lying: iliac crest,
	  ischial tuberosity
		Unequal side to side = pelvic obliquity: leg length discrepancy
		
		"Hip pointer"/contusion, fractures
		Ischial bursitis ("weaver's bottom"), avulsion fx

Soft tissues	Sacroiliac joint Inguinal ligament Femoral pulse & nodes Muscle groups	Sacroiliitis Protruding mass: hernia Diminished pulse: vascular injury; palpable nodes: infection Each group should be symmetric bilaterally
RANGE OF MOTION		
Forward flexion	Standing: bend forward	PSISs should elevate slightly (equally)
Extension	Standing: lean backward	PSISs should depress (equally)
Hip flexion	Standing: knee to chest	PSIS should drop but will elevate in hypomobile SI joint Ischial tuberosity should move laterally; will elevate in hypomobile SI joint

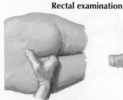

Rectal examination

Trendelenburg test
Left: patient demon-
strates negative
Trendelenburg test
of normal right hip.
Right: positive test
of involved left hip.
When weight is on
affected side, normal
hip drops, indicat-
ing weakness of left
gluteus medius
muscle. Trunk shifts
left as patient attempts
to maintain balance

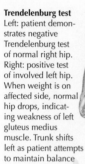

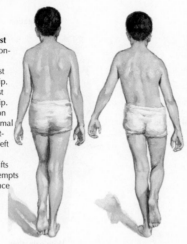

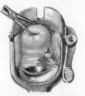

Rectal examination for sphincter function and perianal
sensation. Gross blood indicates pelvic fracture
communicating with colon.

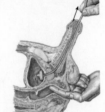

Vaginal examination   **Bulbcavernosus reflex test**

EXAM/OBSERVATION	TECHNIQUE	CLINICAL APPLICATION
NEUROVASCULAR		
Sensory		
Iliohypogastric nerve (L1)	Suprapubic, lat butt/thigh	Deficit indicates corresponding nerve/root lesion
Ilioinguinal nerve (L1)	Inguinal region	Deficit indicates corresponding nerve/root lesion
Genitofemoral nerve	Scrotum or mons	Deficit indicates corresponding nerve/root lesion
Lateral femoral cutane-ous nerve (L2-3)	Lateral hip/thigh	Deficit indicates corresponding nerve/root lesion (e.g., meralgia paresthetica)
Pudendal nerve (S2-4)	Perineum	Deficit indicates corresponding nerve/root lesion
Motor		
Femoral (L2-4)	Hip flexion	Weakness = iliopsoas or corresponding nerve/root lesion
Inferior gluteal nerve	External rotation	Weakness = gluteus maximus or nerve/root lesion
N. to quad. femoris	External rotation	Weakness = short rotators or corresponding nerve/root lesion
Superior gluteal nerve	Abduction	Weakness = glut. med./min or nerve/root lesion
Other		
Reflex	Bulbocavernosus	Finger in rectum, squeeze or pull penis (Foley)/clitoris; anal sphincter should contract
Pulses	Femoral pulse	Diminished pulse abnormal
SPECIAL TESTS		
Pelvic rock	Push both iliac crests	Instability/motion indicates pelvic ring injury
SI stress test	Press ASIS & iliac crests	Pain in SI could be SI ligament injury
Trendelenburg sign	Standing: lift one leg (flex hip)	Flexed side: pelvis should elevate; if pelvis falls, abductor or gluteus medius (superior gluteal n.) dysfunction
Patrick (FABER)	Flex, **Ab**duct, **ER** hip, then abduct more	Positive if pain or LE will not continue to abduct below other leg; SI joint pathology
Meralgia	Pressure medial to ASIS	Reproduction to pain, burning, numbness = LFCN entrapment
Rectal and vaginal	Especially after trauma	Gross blood indicates trauma communicating with those organs

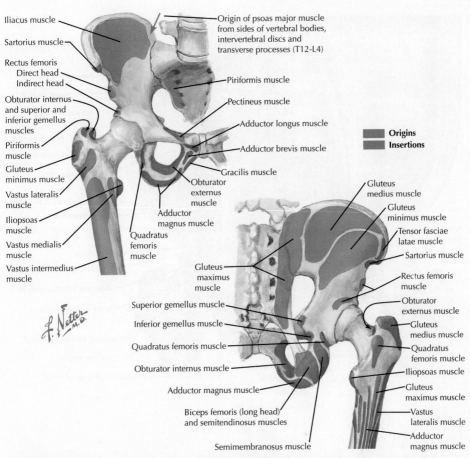

Iliacus muscle

Sartorius muscle

Rectus femoris
Direct head
Indirect head

Obturator internus
and superior and
inferior gemellus
muscles

Piriformis
muscle

Gluteus
minimus muscle

Vastus lateralis
muscle

Iliopsoas
muscle

Vastus medialis
muscle

Vastus intermedius
muscle

Origin of psoas major muscle
from sides of vertebral bodies,
intervertebral discs and
transverse processes (T12-L4)

Piriformis muscle

Pectineus muscle

Adductor longus muscle

Adductor brevis muscle

Gracilis muscle

Obturator
externus
muscle

Adductor
magnus muscle

Quadratus
femoris
muscle

Origins
Insertions

Gluteus
medius muscle

Gluteus
minimus muscle

Tensor fasciae
latae muscle

Sartorius muscle

Rectus femoris
muscle

Obturator
externus muscle

Gluteus
medius muscle

Quadratus
femoris muscle

Iliopsoas muscle

Gluteus
maximus muscle

Vastus
lateralis muscle

Adductor
magnus muscle

Gluteus
maximus
muscle

Superior gemellus muscle

Inferior gemellus muscle

Quadratus femoris muscle

Obturator internus muscle

Adductor magnus muscle

Biceps femoris (long head)
and semitendinosus muscles

Semimembranosus muscle

PUBIC RAMI	GREATER TROCHANTER	ISCHIAL TUBEROSITY	LINEA ASPERA
ORIGINS			

Pectineus
Adductor longus
Adductor brevis
Adductor magnus*
Gracilis
Obturator internus
Obturator externus
		Semimembranosus
		Semitendinosus
		Biceps femoris (LH)
		Adductor magnus*
		ISCHIUM
		    Quadratus femoris
		    Inferior gemellus
			Vastus lateralis
			Vastus intermedius
			Vastus medialis
			Biceps femoris (SH)

INSERTIONS			

	Gluteus medius (posterior)
	Gluteus minimus (anterior)
	Quadratus femoris (inferior)
	Obturator externus (fossa)
	SHORT EXTERNAL ROTATORS
	    Piriformis
	    Superior gemellus
	    Obturator internus
	    Inferior gemellus
			Gluteus maximus
			Adductor magnus
			Adductor brevis
			Adductor longus
			Pectineus

*Has two origins			

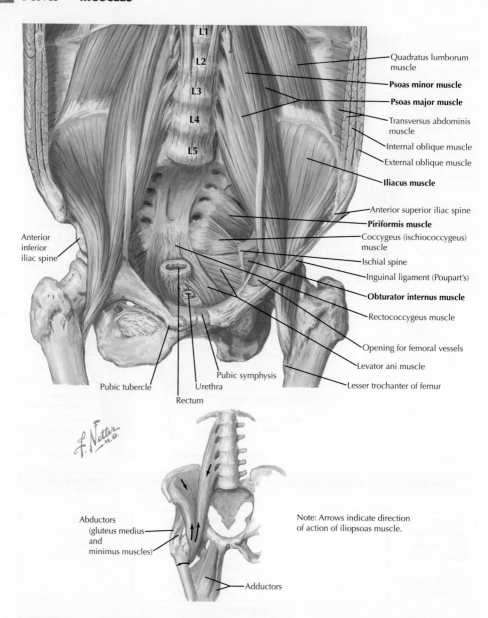

Quadratus lumborum muscle
Psoas minor muscle
Psoas major muscle
Transversus abdominis muscle
Internal oblique muscle
External oblique muscle
Iliacus muscle
Anterior superior iliac spine
Piriformis muscle
Coccygeus (ischiococcygeus) muscle
Ischial spine
Inguinal ligament (Poupart's)
Obturator internus muscle
Rectococcygeus muscle
Opening for femoral vessels
Levator ani muscle
Lesser trochanter of femur

L1
L2
L3
L4
L5

Anterior inferior iliac spine

Pubic tubercle
Urethra
Rectum
Pubic symphysis

Abductors (gluteus medius and minimus muscles)

Adductors

Note: Arrows indicate direction of action of iliopsoas muscle.

MUSCLE	ORIGIN	INSERTION	NERVE	ACTION	COMMENT
HIP FLEXORS					
Psoas major	T12-L5 vertebrae	Lesser trochanter	Femoral	Flex hip	Covers lumbar plexus
Psoas minor	T12-L1 vertebrae	Iliopubic eminence	L1-ventral ramus	Assists in hip flexion	Weak—present in 50% of people
Iliacus	Iliac fossa/sacral ala	Lesser trochanter	Femoral	Flex hip	Covers ant. ilium
Also see muscles of the thigh/hip in Chapter 8.					

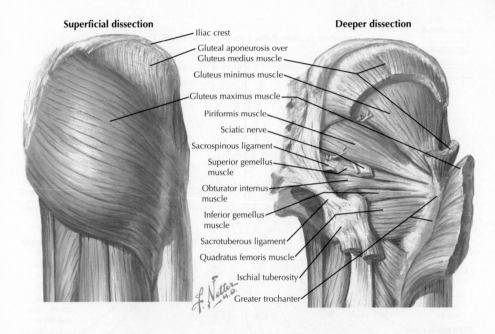

Superficial dissection — Deeper dissection

Iliac crest
Gluteal aponeurosis over Gluteus medius muscle
Gluteus minimus muscle
Gluteus maximus muscle
Piriformis muscle
Sciatic nerve
Sacrospinous ligament
Superior gemellus muscle
Obturator internus muscle
Inferior gemellus muscle
Sacrotuberous ligament
Quadratus femoris muscle
Ischial tuberosity
Greater trochanter

MUSCLE	ORIGIN	INSERTION	NERVE	ACTION	COMMENT
HIP ABDUCTORS					
Tensor fasciae latae	Iliac crest, ASIS	Iliotibial band/proximal tibia	Superior gluteal	Abducts, flex, IR thigh	A plane in anterior approach to hip
Gluteus medius	Ilium b/w ant. and post. gluteal lines	Greater trochanter (posterior)	Superior gluteal	Abducts, IR thigh	Trendelenburg gait if muscle is out
Gluteus minimus	Ilium b/w ant. and inf. gluteal lines	Greater trochanter (anterior)	Superior gluteal	Abducts, IR thigh	Works in conjunction with medius
HIP EXTENSORS AND EXTERNAL ROTATORS					
Gluteus maximus	Ilium, dorsal sacrum	ITB, gluteal tuberosity (femur)	Inferior gluteal	Extend, ER thigh	Must be split in posterior approach to hip
Obturator externus	Ischiopubic rami, obturator membrane	Trochanteric fossa	Obturator	ER thigh	Inserts at start point for IM nail
Short External Rotators					
Piriformis	Anterior sacrum	Superior greater trochanter	N. to piriformis	ER thigh	Used as landmark for sciatic nerve
Superior gemellus	Ischial spine	Medial greater trochanter	N. to obturator internus	ER thigh	Detached in posterior approach to hip
Obturator internus	Ischiopubic rami, obturator mem.	Medial greater trochanter	N. to obturator internus	ER, abduct thigh	Exits through lesser sciatic foramen
Inferior gemellus	Ischial tuberosity	Medial greater trochanter	N. to quadratus femoris	ER thigh	Detached in posterior approach to hip
Quadratus femoris	Ischial tuberosity	Intertrochanteric crest	N. to quadratus femoris	ER thigh	Ascending br. medial circumflex artery under muscle

Transverse Section: Pubic Crest, Femoral Heads, Coccyx

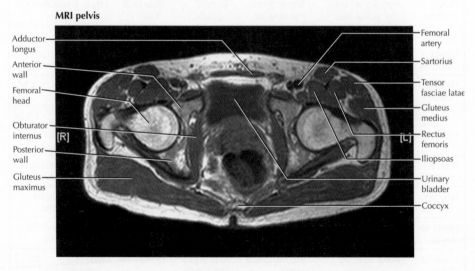

Superior portion of pubic symphysis

Spermatic cord

Beginning of urethra

Prostate gland with prostatic urethra

Psoas muscle and tendon

Iliacus muscle

Head of femur

Neck of femur

Gluteus medius muscle

Gluteus minimus tendon

Greater trochanter

Inferior gemellus muscle

Right sciatic nerve

Gluteus maximus muscle

Obturator internus muscle

Sacrotuberous ligament

Ejaculatory ducts

Perineal flexure (termination of rectum, beginning of anal canal)

Tip of coccyx

Interior of urinary bladder

Adductor longus muscle

Body of pubis

Pectineus muscle

Femoral vein

Femoral artery

Femoral nerve

Sartorius muscle

Iliopsoas muscl

Rectus femori muscle

Tensor fasciae lata muscle

Gluteus medius muscle

Obturator artery, vein, and nerve

Acetabular fossa

Lunate (articular) surface of acetabulum

Left sciatic nerve

Internal pudendal artery and vein

Pudendal nerve

Fat body of ischioanal fossa

Levator ani muscle (puborectalis)

C.Machado — M.D.

MRI pelvis

Adductor longus

Anterior wall

Femoral head

Obturator internus

Posterior wall

Gluteus maximus

[R]

[L]

Femoral artery

Sartorius

Tensor fasciae latae

Gluteus medius

Rectus femoris

Iliopsoas

Urinary bladder

Coccyx

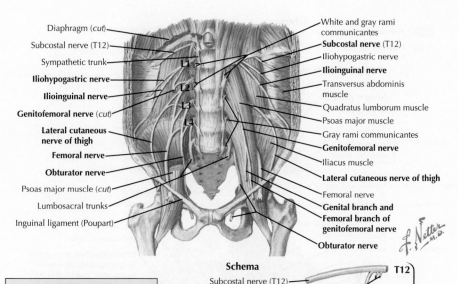

Schema

LUMBAR PLEXUS

Lumbar plexus comprises the ventral rami of L1-L4. Two divisions: anterior (innervates flexors), posterior (extensors). Plexus formed within the psoas muscle.

Anterior Division

Subcostal (T12): Inferior to 12th rib

Sensory:	Subxyphoid region
Motor:	None

Iliohypogastric (L1): Under psoas, pierces abdominal muscles

Sensory:	Above pubis
	Posterolateral buttocks
Motor:	Transversus abdominis
	Internal oblique

Ilioinguinal (L1): Under psoas, pierces abdominal muscles

Sensory:	Inguinal region, anterosuperior thigh
Motor:	None

Genitofemoral(L1-2): Pierces psoas lies on anterior surface of psoas muscle

Sensory	Scrotum or labia majora
Motor:	Cremaster

Obturator (L2-4): Exits via obturator canal, splits into ant. & post. division (can be injured by retractors placed behind the transverse acetabular ligament [TAL])

Sensory:	Inferomedial thigh via **cut. br. of obturator n.**
Motor:	External oblique
	Obturator externus (posterior division)

Accessory Obturator (L2-4): Inconsistent

Sensory:	None
Motor:	Psoas

Posterior Division

Lateral Femoral Cutaneous (FFCN) (L2-3): runs on iliacus, crosses inferior to ASIS (can be compressed there: meralgia paresthetica)

Sensory:	None (in pelvis)
Motor:	None

Femoral (L2-4): Lies between psoas major and iliacus

Sensory:	None (in pelvis)
Motor:	Psoas
	Iliacus
	Pectineus

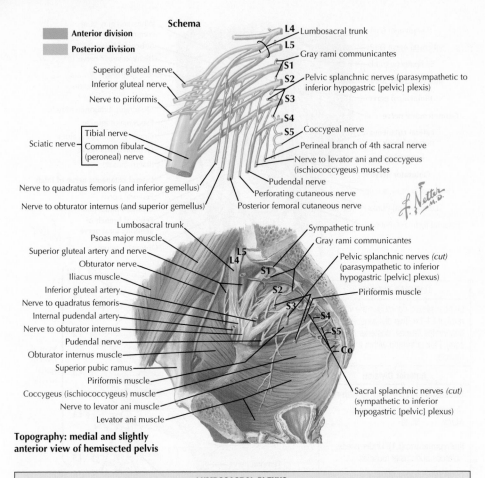

Schema

Anterior division
Posterior division

Superior gluteal nerve
Inferior gluteal nerve
Nerve to piriformis

Sciatic nerve — Tibial nerve
Common fibular (peroneal) nerve

Nerve to quadratus femoris (and inferior gemellus)
Nerve to obturator internus (and superior gemellus)

L4 Lumbosacral trunk
L5
Gray rami communicantes
S1
S2 Pelvic splanchnic nerves (parasympathetic to inferior hypogastric [pelvic] plexis)
S3
S4
S5 Coccygeal nerve
Perineal branch of 4th sacral nerve
Nerve to levator ani and coccygeus (ischiococcygeus) muscles
Pudendal nerve
Perforating cutaneous nerve
Posterior femoral cutaneous nerve

Lumbosacral trunk
Psoas major muscle
Superior gluteal artery and nerve
Obturator nerve
Iliacus muscle
Inferior gluteal artery
Nerve to quadratus femoris
Internal pudendal artery
Nerve to obturator internus
Pudendal nerve
Obturator internus muscle
Superior pubic ramus
Piriformis muscle
Coccygeus (ischiococcygeus) muscle
Nerve to levator ani muscle
Levator ani muscle

Sympathetic trunk
Gray rami communicantes
Pelvic splanchnic nerves (cut) (parasympathetic to inferior hypogastric [pelvic] plexus)
Piriformis muscle
L5
L4
S1
S2
S3
S4
S5
Co
Sacral splanchnic nerves (cut) (sympathetic to inferior hypogastric [pelvic] plexus)

Topography: medial and slightly anterior view of hemisected pelvis

LUMBOSACRAL PLEXUS
Lumbosacral plexus comprises the ventral rami of L4-S3(4). Two divisions: Anterior (innervates flexors), posterior (extensors). Plexus lies on anterior piriformis muscle.

Anterior Division	

Nerve to quadratus femoris (L4-S1): Exits greater sciatic foramen
 	
Sensory: None
Motor: Quadratus femoris
          Inferior gemelli
 	
Nerve to obturator internus (L5-S2): Exits greater sciatic foramen
 	
Sensory: None
Motor: Obturator internus
          Superior gemelli
	Pudendal (S2-4): Exits greater then re-enters pelvis through lesser sciatic foramen
	
	Sensory: Perineum:
	            via **perineal nerve** (scrotal/labial br.)
	            via **inferior rectal nerve**
	            via **dorsal nerve** to penis/clitoris
	Motor: Bulbospongiosus: **perineal nerve**
	           Ischiocavernosus: **perineal nerve**
	           Urethral sphincter: **perineal nerve**
	           Urogenital diaphragm: **perineal nerve**
	           Sphincter ani externus: **inferior rectal nerve**
	
	Nerve to coccygeus (S3-4): directly innervates muscle
	
	Sensory: None
	Motor: Coccygeus
	           Levator ani

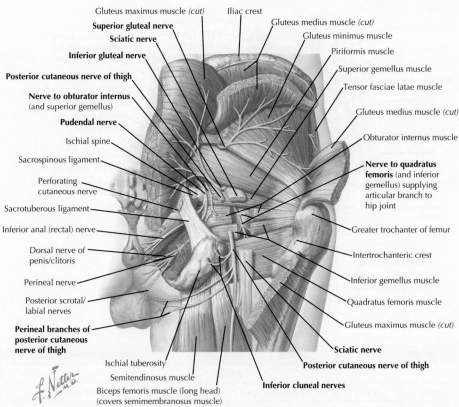

Gluteus maximus muscle *(cut)*
Iliac crest
Superior gluteal nerve
Gluteus medius muscle *(cut)*
Sciatic nerve
Gluteus minimus muscle
Piriformis muscle
Inferior gluteal nerve
Superior gemellus muscle
Posterior cutaneous nerve of thigh
Tensor fasciae latae muscle
Nerve to obturator internus
(and superior gemellus)
Gluteus medius muscle *(cut)*
Pudendal nerve
Obturator internus muscle
Ischial spine
Sacrospinous ligament
Nerve to quadratus femoris (and inferior gemellus) supplying articular branch to hip joint
Perforating cutaneous nerve
Sacrotuberous ligament
Greater trochanter of femur
Inferior anal (rectal) nerve
Intertrochanteric crest
Dorsal nerve of penis/clitoris
Inferior gemellus muscle
Perineal nerve
Quadratus femoris muscle
Posterior scrotal/ labial nerves
Gluteus maximus muscle *(cut)*
Perineal branches of posterior cutaneous nerve of thigh
Sciatic nerve
Ischial tuberosity
Posterior cutaneous nerve of thigh
Semitendinosus muscle
Inferior cluneal nerves
Biceps femoris muscle (long head) (covers semimembranosus muscle)

LUMBOSACRAL PLEXUS	
Posterior Division	**Both Divisions**
Superior Gluteal (L4-S1): Exits greater sciatic foramen above the piriformis *Sensory:* None *Motor:* Gluteus medius 　　　　Gluteus minimus 　　　　Tensor fasciae latae	**Posterior Femoral Cutaneous (S1-S3):** Exits via greater sciatic foramen, under piriformis, medial to sciatic nerve *Sensory:* Inferior buttocks: via **inferior cluneal nerves** 　　　　　Posterior perineum: **perineal branches** 　　　　　Posterior thigh (see Chapter 8) *Motor:* None
Inferior Gluteal (L5-S2): Exits greater sciatic foramen *Sensory:* None *Motor:* Gluteus maximus	**Sciatic (L4-S3):** Largest nerve in body. Two components: tibial (ant. division) and peroneal (post. division). Exits greater sciatic foramen under piriformis. Anatomic variants include exiting through or above piriformis. Reflecting short ERs will protect sciatic in posterior approach to hip.
Nerve to Piriformis (S2): Directly innervates muscle *Sensory:* None *Motor:* Piriformis	*Sensory:* None (in pelvis; see Chapters 8-10) *Motor:* None (in pelvis; see Chapters 8-10)
Other Nerves (Nonplexus)	
Superior Cluneal (L1-3): Branches of dorsal rami. *Sensory:* Superior ⅔ of buttocks	**Medial Cluneal (S1-3):** Branches of dorsal rami *Sensory:* Sacral and medial buttocks
• Piriformis muscle is the landmark in gluteal region. Most nerves exit inferior to it. **POP'S IQ** is a mnemonic: **P**udendal, **N**. to **O**bturator internus, **P**osterior cutaneous, **S**ciatic, **I**nferior gluteal, **N**. to **Q**uadratus femoris.	

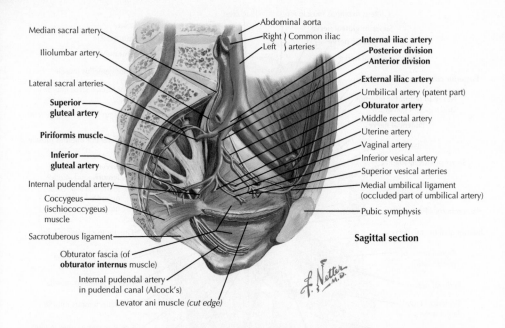

Median sacral artery

Iliolumbar artery

Lateral sacral arteries

Superior gluteal artery

Piriformis muscle

Inferior gluteal artery

Internal pudendal artery

Coccygeus (ischiococcygeus) muscle

Sacrotuberous ligament

Obturator fascia (of **obturator internus** muscle)

Internal pudendal artery in pudendal canal (Alcock's)

Levator ani muscle *(cut edge)*

Abdominal aorta

Right) Common iliac
Left) arteries

Internal iliac artery
Posterior division
Anterior division

External iliac artery
Umbilical artery (patent part)

Obturator artery
Middle rectal artery
Uterine artery
Vaginal artery
Inferior vesical artery
Superior vesical arteries

Medial umbilical ligament (occluded part of umbilical artery)

Pubic symphysis

Sagittal section

ARTERY	COURSE	COMMENT/SUPPLY
AORTA		
Common iliacs	Branch at L4, run along anterior spine	Blood supply to pelvis & lower extremities
Median sacral	Descends along anterior spine & sacrum	Anastomoses with lateral sacral arteries
COMMON ILIAC ARTERY		
Internal iliac	Under ureter toward sacrum, then divides	Supplies most of pelvis & pelvic organs Divides into anterior & posterior divisions
External iliac	On ant. surface of psoas to inguinal ligament	Does not supply much of the pelvis
INTERNAL ILIAC		
Anterior Division		
Obturator	Through obturator foramen w/obturator nerve	Fovea artery (ligamentum teres) branches
Inferior gluteal	Exits greater sciatic foramen under piriformis	Supplies gluteus maximus muscle
Multiple visceral branches	Umbilical Uterine/vaginal (females) Inferior vesical (males) Middle rectal Internal pudendal	Supplies bladder (via sup. vesical arteries) Supplies uterus & vagina (via vaginal br.) Supplies bladder, prostate, ductus deferens Anastomoses w/sup. & inf. rectal arteries Runs with pudendal nerve Inferior rectal art. branches from this artery
Posterior Division		
Superior gluteal	Exits greater sciatic foramen above piriformis	In sciatic notch, can be injured in posterior column fractures or pelvic ring injuries
Iliolumbar	Runs superiorly toward iliac fossa	Supplies ilium, iliacus, & psoas muscles
Lateral sacral	Run along sacrum, anterior to the sacral roots	Supplies sacrum/sacral muscles/nerves Anastomoses w/median sacral art. (aorta)

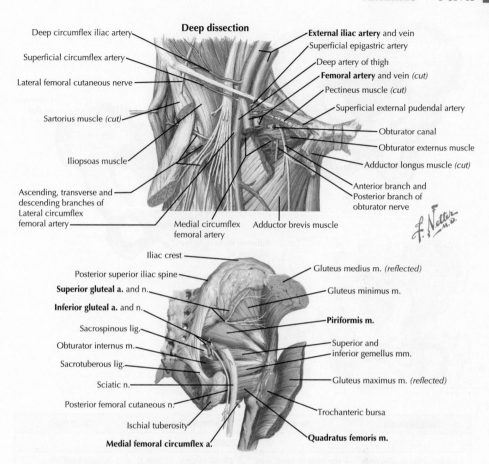

Deep dissection

Deep circumflex iliac artery

Superficial circumflex artery

Lateral femoral cutaneous nerve

Sartorius muscle *(cut)*

Iliopsoas muscle

Ascending, transverse and descending branches of Lateral circumflex femoral artery

Medial circumflex femoral artery

External iliac artery and vein

Superficial epigastric artery

Deep artery of thigh

Femoral artery and vein *(cut)*

Pectineus muscle *(cut)*

Superficial external pudendal artery

Obturator canal

Obturator externus muscle

Adductor longus muscle *(cut)*

Anterior branch and Posterior branch of obturator nerve

Adductor brevis muscle

Iliac crest

Posterior superior iliac spine

Superior gluteal a. and n.

Inferior gluteal a. and n.

Sacrospinous lig.

Obturator internus m.

Sacrotuberous lig.

Sciatic n.

Posterior femoral cutaneous n.

Ischial tuberosity

Medial femoral circumflex a.

Gluteus medius m. *(reflected)*

Gluteus minimus m.

Piriformis m.

Superior and inferior gemellus mm.

Gluteus maximus m. *(reflected)*

Trochanteric bursa

Quadratus femoris m.

ARTERY	COURSE	COMMENT/SUPPLY
EXTERNAL ILIAC ARTERY		
Deep circumflex iliac	Runs laterally under internal oblique to iliac crest	Supplies anterolateral abdominal wall muscles
Inferior epigastric	Runs superiorly in transversalis fascia	Supplies anterior abdominal wall muscles
Femoral artery	Continuation of EIA under inguinal ligament	Terminal branch of external iliac artery
FEMORAL ARTERY		
Superficial circumflex iliac	In subcutaneous tissues toward ASIS	Supplies superficial abdominal tissues
Superficial epigastric	In subcutaneous tissues toward umbilicus	Supplies superficial abdominal tissues
Superficial & deep external pudendal	Medially over the adductors & spermatic cord to inguinal and genital regions	Supplies subcutaneous tissues in the pubic region and the scrotum/labia majus
Profunda femoris (deep artery of thigh)	Between adductor longus & pectineus/adductor brevis	Gives off circumflex (2) & perforating branches
Medial circumflex femoral	B/w pectineus & psoas, then posterior to femoral neck under quadratus femoris	Runs under quadratus femoris; can be injured in posterior approach to hip
Lateral circumflex femoral	Runs laterally deep to sartorius & rectus	At risk in anterolateral approach to hip

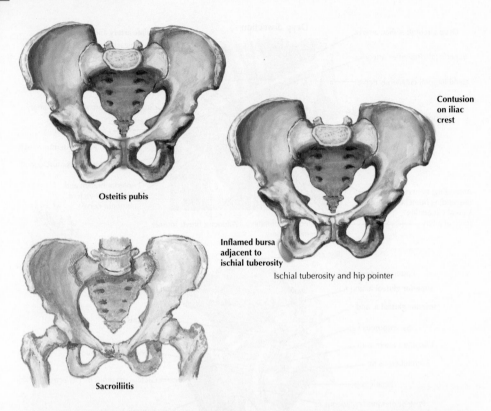

Osteitis pubis

Contusion on iliac crest

Inflamed bursa adjacent to ischial tuberosity

Ischial tuberosity and hip pointer

Sacroiliitis

DESCRIPTION	Hx & PE	WORKUP/FINDINGS	TREATMENT
OSTEITIS PUBIS			
• Inflammation or degeneration of pubic symphysis • Etiology: repetitive microtrauma (sports) or fracture	**Hx:** Anterior pelvic pain, sports or trauma **PE:** Symphysis pubis is tender to palpation	**XR:** AP pelvis (+/− inlet & outlet views) **CT/MR:** Not usually necessary for diagnosis	1. Activity modification 2. Rest, NSAIDs 3. Fusion if symptoms are refractory to conservative care
SACROILIITIS			
• Inflammation or degeneration of sacroiliac joint • Infection can also occur here • Assoc. w/Reiter's syndrome	**Hx:** Low back pain **PE:** SIJ tender to palpation, + FABER test; injection can help diagnosis	**XR/CT:** SI joints, +/− DJD **Bone Scan:** r/o infection **LABS:** CBC, ESR, CRP if infection is suspected	1. Rest, NSAIDs 2. Injection can be diagnostic & therapeutic (corticosteroid) 3. Fusion: rarely indicated
ISCHIAL BURSITIS			
• Inflammation of bursa of ischial tuberosity • Often from prolonged sitting • Aka "weaver's bottom" • Mimics hamstring injury	**Hx:** Buttocks pain, sitting **PE:** Ischial tuberosity tender to palpation; active hamstrings NOT painful	**XR:** Pelvis, r/o tuberosity avulsion **MR:** Can evaluate/ r/o hamstring insertion injury	1. Rest 2. NSAIDs 3. Activity modification: decrease sitting or increase cushion
ILIAC CREST CONTUSION (HIP POINTER)			
• Direct trauma to iliac crest • Common in contact sports (e.g., football, hockey, etc)	**Hx:** Trauma, "hip" pain **PE:** Iliac crest tender to palpation	**XR:** Pelvis, r/o fracture **MR/CT:** Usually not necessary for diagnosis	1. Rest, NSAIDs 2. Padding to iliac crest 3. Corticosteroid injection

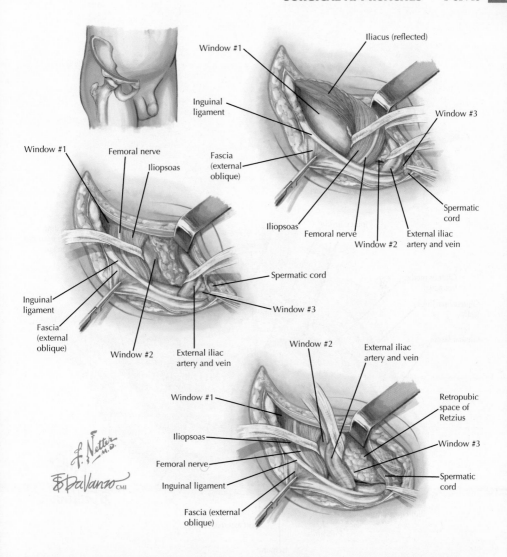

Iliacus (reflected)

Window #1

Inguinal ligament

Window #3

Fascia (external oblique)

Window #1

Femoral nerve

Iliopsoas

Spermatic cord

Iliopsoas

Femoral nerve

External iliac artery and vein

Window #2

Spermatic cord

Inguinal ligament

Window #3

Fascia (external oblique)

Window #2

External iliac artery and vein

Window #1

External iliac artery and vein

Window #2

Retropubic space of Retzius

Iliopsoas

Window #3

Femoral nerve

Inguinal ligament

Spermatic cord

Fascia (external oblique)

USES	INTERNERVOUS PLANE	DANGERS	COMMENT
ILIOINGUINAL APPROACH			
• Open reduction, internal fixation of acetabular fractures involving anterior column of acetabulum	3 windows—interval (access): 1. Lateral to iliopsoas & femoral nerve (anterior, SIJ, iliac fossa, pelvic brim) 2. Between iliopsoas/femoral nerve & external iliac artery (pelvic brim, lateral superior pubic ramus) 3. Medial to external iliac artery & spermatic cord (quadrilateral plate & retropubic space [of Retzius])	• Ext. iliac (EI) vessels • Corona mortis (vessel from obt. art. to EI art.) • Femoral nerve • Lateral femoral cutaneous nerve • Inferior epigastric artery • Spermatic cord • Bladder (use a Foley)	• Good knowledge of abdominal & pelvic anatomy essential to perform this approach • Must detach pelvic insertion of abdominal muscles & iliacus muscle for exposure • Use rubber drains around iliopsoas/femoral n. & external iliac vessels to access windows

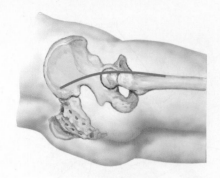

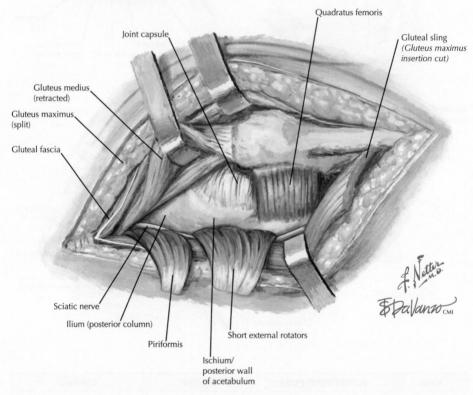

Quadratus femoris

Joint capsule

Gluteal sling
(*Gluteus maximus
insertion cut*)

Gluteus medius
(retracted)

Gluteus maximus
(split)

Gluteal fascia

Sciatic nerve

Ilium (posterior column)

Piriformis

Short external rotators

Ischium/
posterior wall
of acetabulum

USES	INTERNERVOUS PLANE	DANGERS	COMMENT
KOCHER-LANGENBECK APPROACH			
• Open reduction, internal fixation of acetabular fractures involving posterior column of acetabulum	No internervous plane • Gluteus maximus (inf. gluteal n.) fascia is split in line with its fibers; inferior gluteal nerve is limit to the split. • Tensor fasciae latae also split in line with its fibers	• Sciatic nerve • Inferior gluteal artery • Superior gluteal vessels & nerve (esp. w/excessive retraction)	• Heterotopic ossification is common, prophylaxis (e.g., XRT) is often needed. • Do not take down quadratus femoris due to vascular risk

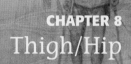

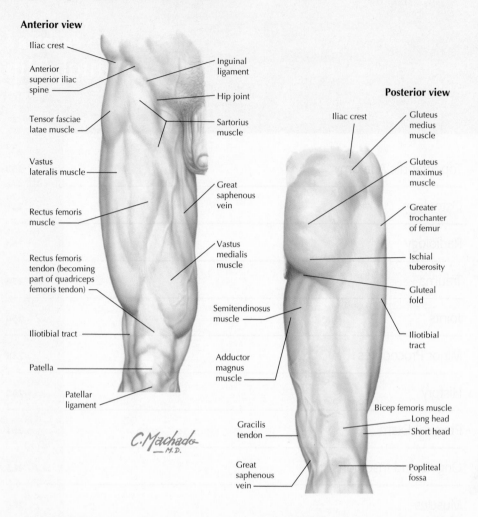

Anterior view

Iliac crest
Anterior superior iliac spine
Tensor fasciae latae muscle
Vastus lateralis muscle
Rectus femoris muscle
Rectus femoris tendon (becoming part of quadriceps femoris tendon)
Iliotibial tract
Patella
Patellar ligament

Inguinal ligament
Hip joint
Sartorius muscle
Great saphenous vein
Vastus medialis muscle
Semitendinosus muscle
Adductor magnus muscle
Gracilis tendon
Great saphenous vein

C. Machado M.D.

Posterior view

Iliac crest
Gluteus medius muscle
Gluteus maximus muscle
Greater trochanter of femur
Ischial tuberosity
Gluteal fold
Iliotibial tract
Bicep femoris muscle
Long head
Short head
Popliteal fossa

STRUCTURE	CLINICAL APPLICATION
Iliac crest	Site for "hip pointers"/contusion of iliac crest Common site for autologous bone graft harvest
Greater trochanter	Tenderness can indicate trochanteric bursitis.
Ischial tuberosity	Avulsion fracture (hamstrings) or bursitis can occur here.
Iliotibial tract (band)	Can snap over greater trochanter of femur, creating "snapping hip" syndrome. Tightness can cause lateral knee and/or thigh pain.
Quadriceps muscle • Vastus lateralis • Vastus medialis • Rectus femoris • Vastus intermedius (not shown)	Atrophy can indicate an injury and/or contribute to knee pain.
Quadriceps tendon	Can rupture with eccentric loading. Defect is felt here.
Popliteal fossa	Popliteal artery pulse can be palpated here.

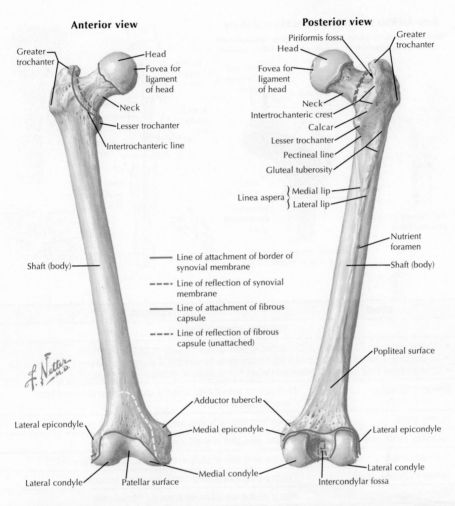

Anterior view

Greater trochanter
Head
Fovea for ligament of head
Neck
Lesser trochanter
Intertrochanteric line
Shaft (body)

Line of attachment of border of synovial membrane
Line of reflection of synovial membrane
Line of attachment of fibrous capsule
Line of reflection of fibrous capsule (unattached)

Lateral epicondyle
Adductor tubercle
Medial epicondyle
Medial condyle
Lateral condyle
Patellar surface

Posterior view

Piriformis fossa
Greater trochanter
Head
Fovea for ligament of head
Neck
Intertrochanteric crest
Calcar
Lesser trochanter
Pectineal line
Gluteal tuberosity
Linea aspera { Medial lip / Lateral lip }
Nutrient foramen
Shaft (body)
Popliteal surface
Lateral epicondyle
Lateral condyle
Intercondylar fossa

f. Netter M.D.

CHARACTERISTICS	OSSIFY	FUSE	COMMENTS
FEMUR			

• Long bone characteristics
• Proximal femur
  ○ Head: nearly spherical (⅔)
  ○ Neck: anteverted from shaft
  ○ Greater trochanter: lateral
  ○ Lesser trochanter: postero-medial
• Shaft: tubular, bows anteriorly
  ○ Linea aspera posterior: insertion of fascia and muscles
• Distal femur: 2 condyles
  ○ Medial: larger, more posterior
  ○ Lateral: more anterior & proximal
  ○ Trochlea: anterior articular depression between condyles
	Primary
	(Shaft)
	
	Secondary
	Distal physis
	Head
	Gtr troch
	Lsr troch
		7-8wk
		(fetal)
		
		birth
		1yr
		4-5yr
		10yr
			16-18yr
			
			19yr
			18yr
			16yr
			16yr
				• Blood supply
				  ○ Head/neck: primarily medial femoral circumflex artery (also lateral FCA and of ligamentum teres artery)
				  ○ Shaft: nutrient artery (from profunda fem.)
				• Head vascularity is susceptible to disruption in fracture or dislocation—leads to AVN
				• Proximal femur bone density decreases with age, making it more susceptible to fracture
				• Calcar femorale—vertically oriented dense bone in posteromedial aspect of prox. femur
				• Piriformis fossa—posteromedial base of gtr trochanter: starting point for femoral nails
				• Neck/shaft angle: 120-135°
				• Femoral anteversion: 10-15°
				• Distal femur physis: grows approx. 7mm/yr

Bone Architecture in Relation to Physical Stress

Wolff's law. Bony structures orient themselves in form and mass to best resist extrinsic forces (ie, form and mass follow function)

Trabecular configuration in proximal femur

Trabecular groups confirm to lines of stress in weight bearing

Labels: Principal compressive group; Principal tensile group; Load; Greater trochanteric group; Secondary tensile group; Ward's triangle; Secondary compressive group; Femoral anatomic axis; Femoral mechanical axis; Vertical axis; Knee axis; Tibial mechanical axis; Calcar femorale; 6°; 3°; 81°; 87°; 87°

GROUP	COMMENT
PROXIMAL FEMUR OSTEOLOGY	
• Proximal femur comprises several distinct trabecular bone groups that support the head and neck. • The presence or absence of these groups helps to determine the presence & degree of osteopenia in the prox. femur. • Malalignment of bone groups determines the fracture type in displaced femoral neck fractures.	
Primary compressive	From superior femoral head to medial neck, strongest cancellous bone, supports body weight
Primary tensile	From inferior femoral head to lateral cortex
Secondary compressive	Oriented along lines of stress in proximal femur
Secondary tensile	Oriented along lines of stress in lateral proximal femur
Greater trochanteric group	Oriented along lines of stress within the greater trochanter
Ward's triangle	Area of relative few trabeculae within the femoral neck
LOWER EXTREMITY ALIGNMENT	
Definitions	
Anatomic axis	Line drawn along the axis of the femur
Mechanical axis	Line drawn between center of femoral head and intercondylar notch
Knee axis	Line drawn along the inferior aspect of both femoral condyles
Vertical axis	Vertical line, perpendicular to the ground
Lateral femoral angle	Angle formed between the knee axis and the femoral axis
Relationships	
Knee axis	Parallel to the ground and perpendicular to vertical axis
Mechanical axis	Average of 6° from anatomic axis Approximately 3° from the vertical axis
Lateral femoral angle	81° with respect to femoral anatomic axis 87° with respect to femoral mechanical axis

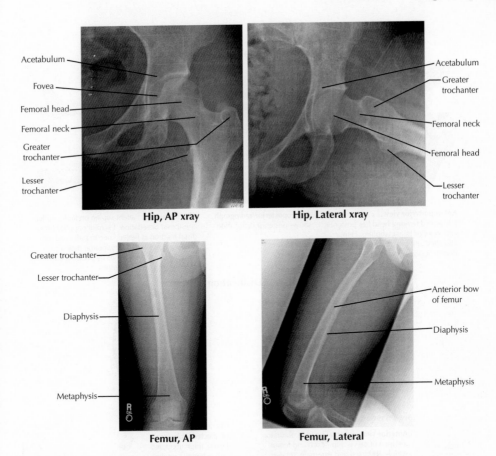

Hip, AP xray

Hip, Lateral xray

Femur, AP

Femur, Lateral

RADIOGRAPH	TECHNIQUE	FINDINGS	CLINICAL APPLICATION
AP pelvis	Supine, beam at symphysis	Both hips and pelvis	Fractures, dislocations, arthritis
AP hip	Beam aimed at proximal femur	Femoral head, acetabulum	Fractures, arthritis
Lateral (frog leg)	Flex, abd. ER hip, beam at hip	Fem. neck, head, acetab. rim	Fractures, arthritis
Lateral (cross-table)	Flex contralateral hip to remove it; aim beam across table at hip	Femoral neck, head, acetabular rim. Ant & post. cortices seen well on lateral	Often needed for preop fx films Used intraop (fluoro) for ORIF
AP femur	Supine, beam at mid femur	Femur, soft tissues	Fractures, tumors
Lateral femur	Beam laterally at mid femur	Femur, soft tissues	Fractures, tumors
See Chapter 7, Pelvis, for views of acetabulum.			
OTHER STUDIES			
CT	Axial, coronal, & sagittal views	Articular congruity, fracture fragments	Intraarticular acetabulum or neck fractures
MRI	Sequence protocols vary	Labrum, cartilage, cancellous bone	Labral tears, AVN, stress fractures
Bone scan	Radioisotope	All bones evaluated	Stress fractures, infection, tumor

Posterior Dislocation

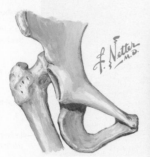

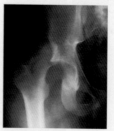

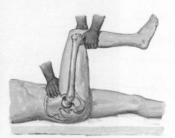

Anteroposterior view.
Dislocated femoral head lies posterior
and superior to acetabulum. Femur
adducted and internally rotated; hip
flexed. Sciatic nerve may be stretched

Anteroposterior radiograph
shows posterior dislocation

Allis maneuver. Patient supine on table, under
anesthesia or sedation. Examiner applies firm
distal traction at flexed knee to pull head into
acetabulum; slight rotary motion may also
help. Assistant fixes pelvis by pressing on
anterior superior iliac spines

Anterior Dislocation

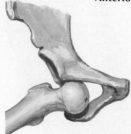

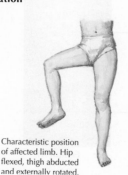

Anterior view. Femoral head in obturator
foramen of pelvis; hip flexed and femur
widely abducted and externally rotated

Characteristic position
of affected limb. Hip
flexed, thigh abducted
and externally rotated.

DESCRIPTION	EVALUATION	CLASSIFICATION	TREATMENT
HIP DISLOCATION			

• High-energy trauma (esp. MVA, dashboard injury) or significant fall
• Orthopaedic emergency; risk of femoral head AVN increases with late/de-layed reduction
• Multiple associated inju-ries +/– fractures (e.g., femoral head/neck, acetabulum)
• Posterior most common (85%)
	Hx: Trauma, severe pain, cannot move thigh/hip
	PE: Thigh position:
	• Post.: adducted, flexed, IR
	• Ant.: abducted, flexed, ER
	• Pain (esp. with motion), good neurovascular exam (sciatic n.)
	XR: AP pelvis, frog lateral (femoral head appears of different size), femur and knee series
	CT: R/o fx or bony fragments/ loose bodies (postreduction)
		Posterior: Thompson:
		I: No or minor post. wall fx
		II: Large posterior wall fx
		III: Comminuted acetabular fx
		IV: Acetabular floor fx
		V: Femoral head fx
		
		Anterior: Epstein:
		I (A, B, C): Superior
		II (A, B, C): Inferior
		  A: No associated fx
		  B: Femoral head fx
		  C: Acetabular fx
			Early reduction essential (<6 hr), then repeat XR & neuro exam
			Posterior:
			I: Closed reduction and abduction pillow
			II-V:
			1. Closed reduction (open if irreducible)
			2. ORIF(fracture or ex-cise fragment/LB)
			Anterior:
			Closed reduction, ORIF if necessary

COMPLICATIONS: Posttraumatic osteonecrosis (AVN) (reduced risk with early reduction); sciatic nerve injury (posterior dislocations); femoral artery/nerve injury (anterior dislocations); osteoarthritis; heterotopic ossification			

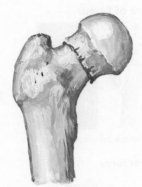

Type I. Impacted fracture

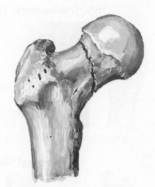

Type II. Nondisplaced fracture

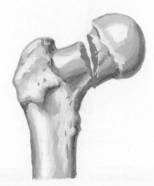

Type III. Partially displaced

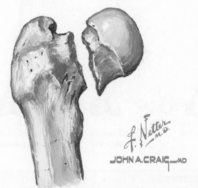

Type IV. Displaced fracture. vertical fracture line generally suggests poorer prognosis

DESCRIPTION	EVALUATION	CLASSIFICATION	TREATMENT
FEMORAL NECK FRACTURE			

• Mechanism
  ○ Fall by elderly person most common
  ○ High-energy injury in young adults (e.g., MVA)
• Intracapsular fractures
• Femoral head vascularity at risk in displaced fractures
• Associated with osteoporosis
• High morbidity & complication rates
	Hx: Fall, pain, inability to bear weight/walk
	PE: LE shortened, abducted, externally rotated. Pain w/"rolling"/log roll extremity
	XR: AP pelvis, cross-table lateral
	MR: If symptomatic with negative XR (i.e., rule out occult fracture)
		Garden (4 types):
		I: Incomplete fracture; valgus impaction
		II: Complete fracture; nondisplaced
		III: Complete fracture, partial displacement (varus)
		IV: Complete fracture, total displacement
			Young (high-energy)
			• Urgent reduction (CR vs OR)
			• ORIF (3 parallel screws)
			
			Elderly
			• Early medical evaluation
			• Types I & II: ORIF (3 screws)
			• Types III & IV: hemiarthroplasty
			• Medically unstable, nonoperative

COMPLICATIONS: Osteonecrosis (AVN): incidence increases with fx type (displacement) +/– late segmental collapse; nonunion; hardware failure

Intertrochanteric Fracture of Femur

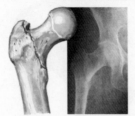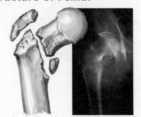

I. Nondisplaced fracture   III. Comminuted displaced fracture

Femoral Shaft Fractures

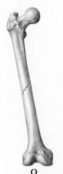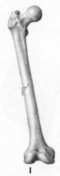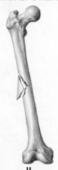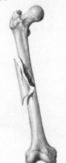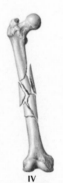

O	I	II	III	IV
Comminution	Small cortical discontinuity	Butterfly 50% contact of cortex	Large butterfly (zero rotational control)	Severe comminution

DESCRIPTION	EVALUATION	CLASSIFICATION	TREATMENT
INTERTROCHANTERIC FRACTURE			

• Fall by an elderly person most common
• Assoc. w/osteoporosis
• Occurs along or below intertrochanteric line
• Extracapsular fractures
• Stable vascularity
• Most heal well with proper fixation
	Hx: Fall, pain, inability to bear weight/walk
	PE: LE shortened, ER. Pain w/"log rolling" of leg
	XR: AP pelvis/hip cross-table
	MR: If symptomatic with negative XR (r/o occult fracture)
		Evans/Jensen:
		• Type IA: Nondisplaced
		• Type IB: 2 part displaced
		• Type IIA: 3 part, GT fragment
		• Type IIB: 3 part, LT fragment
		• Type III: 4 part
		Reverse obliquity
			• Early medical evaluation
			• Early (<48hr) ORIF
			  ○ Sliding hip screw/plate
			  ○ Cephalomedullary nail
			• Reverse obliquity
			  ○ Blade plate
			  ○ Cephalomedullary nail
			• Nonoperative; medically unstable patient

COMPLICATIONS: Nonunion/malunion, decr. ambulatory status, hardware failure, mortality (20% in 1st 6 mo)			
FEMORAL SHAFT FRACTURE			

• Orthopaedic emergency
• High-energy injury (e.g., MVA, fall)
• Associated injuries (common)
• Potential source of significant blood loss
• Compartment syndrome can occur
• Transport patient in traction
	Hx: Trauma, pain, swelling deformity, inability to walk/bear weight
	PE: Deformity, +/– open wound & soft tissue injury; check distal pulses
	XR: AP/lateral femur; Knee: trauma series Hip: r/o ipsilateral femoral neck fx
		Winquist/Hansen (5 types):
		Stable
		0: No comminution
		I: Minimal comminution
		II: Comminuted: >50% of cortices intact
		Unstable
		III: Comminuted: <50% of cortices intact
		IV: Complete comminution, no intact cortex
			Operative: within 24hr
			• Antegrade, reamed, locked IM nail
			• Retrograde nail if needed
			• External fixation
			  ○ Medically unstable
			  ○ High-grade open fx
			Traction—if surgery delayed, medically unstable patient

COMPLICATIONS: Neurovascular injury/hemorrhagic shock, nonunion/malunion, hardware failure, knee injury (5%)			

Distal Femur Fracture

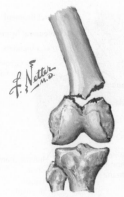 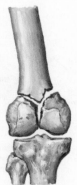 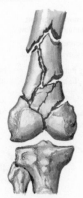 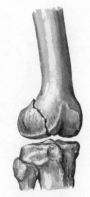

| Transverse supra-condylar fracture | Intercondylar (T or Y) fracture | Comminuted fracture extending into shaft | Fracture of single condyle (may occur in frontal or oblique plane) |

DESCRIPTION	EVALUATION	CLASSIFICATION	TREATMENT
SUBTROCHANTERIC FRACTURE			

• Within 5cm of lesser tro-chanter (LT)
• Mechanism:
  ○ Low-energy fall: elderly, pathologic fx
  ○ High-energy: younger (e.g., MVA)
• Vascularity is tenuous, can compromise healing
• Rule out pathologic fx if fracture occurs with minimal/no trauma
• High biomechanical stresses
	Hx: Trauma, pain, inability to bear weight
	PE: Shortened, rotated LE. No ROM (pain), check neurovascular status
	XR: AP & lateral of femur. Also, AP pelvis, hip (AP & cross-table lateral), & knee series
	CT: Usually not needed
		Russell-Taylor:
		Type I: no piriformis fossa extension/in-volvement
		A: intact LT
		B: detached LT
		Type II: fracture in-volves piriformis fossa
		A: intact LT
		B: detached LT
			By type:
			IA: standard IM nail
			IB: cephalomedullary nail
			IIA: cephalomedullary nail with trochanteric start point
			IIB: 95° blade plate or cephalo-medullary nail with trochanteric start point

COMPLICATIONS: Nonunion, malunion, loss of fixation/implant failure, loss of some ambulatory function (esp. in elderly)			
DISTAL FEMUR FRACTURE			

• Mechanism: direct impact
  ○ Young: high energy
  ○ Elderly: low energy (fall)
• Articular congruity needed for normal knee function
• Many associated injuries (e.g., tibia fx, knee ligament injury)
• Vascular injuries possible
• Quads/hamstrings: shorten fx. Gastroc: displace fx pos-teriorly
	Hx: Trauma, pain, inability to bear weight
	PE: Swollen, +/– gross deformity. Careful pulse evaluation (Doppler exam if needed)
	XR: AP & lateral knee, fe-mur, tibia
	CT: Evaluate intraarticular involvement & preop plan
		AO/Muller:
		A: Extraarticular subtypes 1, 2, 3
		B: Unicondylar subtypes 1, 2, 3
		C: Bicondylar subtypes 1, 2, 3
			• Nondisplaced/stable:
			  ○ Cast, immobilizer, brace
			• Displaced/unstable:
			  ○ Extraarticular: plate or nail
			  ○ Intraarticular: anatomic re-duction of articular surface & locking plate/blade plate
			• External fixation: temporarily in open fx, severely swollen soft tissues, unstable patient

COMPLICATIONS: Posttraumatic arthritis, nonunion/malunion, knee stiffness/loss of ROM			

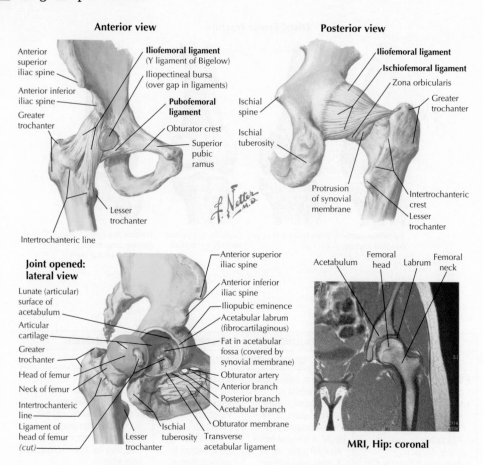

Anterior view

Anterior superior iliac spine

Iliofemoral ligament (Y ligament of Bigelow)

Iliopectineal bursa (over gap in ligaments)

Anterior inferior iliac spine

Pubofemoral ligament

Greater trochanter

Obturator crest

Superior pubic ramus

Lesser trochanter

Intertrochanteric line

Posterior view

Iliofemoral ligament

Ischiofemoral ligament

Zona orbicularis

Greater trochanter

Ischial spine

Ischial tuberosity

Protrusion of synovial membrane

Intertrochanteric crest

Lesser trochanter

Joint opened: lateral view

Lunate (articular) surface of acetabulum

Articular cartilage

Greater trochanter

Head of femur

Neck of femur

Intertrochanteric line

Ligament of head of femur (cut)

Lesser trochanter

Ischial tuberosity

Anterior superior iliac spine

Anterior inferior iliac spine

Iliopubic eminence

Acetabular labrum (fibrocartilaginous)

Fat in acetabular fossa (covered by synovial membrane)

Obturator artery

Anterior branch

Posterior branch

Acetabular branch

Obturator membrane

Transverse acetabular ligament

Acetabulum

Femoral head

Labrum

Femoral neck

MRI, Hip: coronal

LIGAMENTS	ATTACHMENTS	COMMENTS
HIP		
• The hip is a spheroidal (ball & socket) joint. It has intrinsic stability from osseous, ligamentous, & muscular structures.		
Labrum	Along acetabular rim except inferiorly	Deepens socket, increases femoral head coverage; can be torn (cause of hip pain)
Transverse acetabular	Anteroinferior to posteroinferior acetabulum	Covers cotyloid notch in inferior central acetabulum
Ligamentum teres	Fovea (femoral head) to cotyloid notch	Small artery to femoral head within this ligament
Capsule ○ Iliofemoral (2 bands) ○ Pubofemoral ○ Ischiofemoral	Acetabulum to femoral neck Superior: ASIS/ilium to greater trochanter Inferior: Ilium to intertrochanteric line/LT Anterior pubic ramus to intertroch. line Posterior acetabulum to superior femoral neck	Has some discrete thickenings (ligaments) Aka "Y ligament of Bigelow"; provides strong anterior support, resists extension Prevents hyperextension of hip, inferior joint support Broad, relatively weak ligament (minimal posterior support). Does not provide complete post. joint coverage, so lateral post. neck is extracapsular

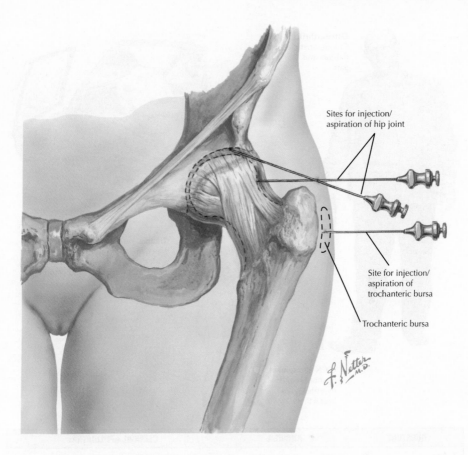

Sites for injection/
aspiration of hip joint

Site for injection/
aspiration of
trochanteric bursa

Trochanteric bursa

STEPS
HIP INJECTION/ASPIRATION

1. Ask patient about allergies
2. Place patient supine, palpate the greater trochanter
3. Prep skin over insertion site (iodine/antiseptic soap)
4. Anesthetize skin locally (quarter size spot)
5. **Anterior:** Find the point of intersection b/w a vertical line below ASIS and horizontal line from greater trochanter. Insert 20-gauge (3in) spinal needle upward/slightly medial direction at that point.
   Lateral: Insert a 20-gauge (3in) spinal needle superior and medial to greater trochanter until it hits the bone (the needle should be within the capsule, which extends down the femoral neck). Can "walk" needle up neck into joint.
6. Inject (or aspirate) local or local/steroid preparation into joint. (The fluid should flow easily if needle is in joint.)
7. Dress injection site

TROCHANTERIC BURSA INJECTION

1. Ask patient about allergies
2. Place patient in lateral decubitus position, palpate the greater trochanter
3. Prep skin over lateral thigh (iodine/antiseptic soap)
4. Insert 20-gauge needle (at least 1½ in; 3in in larger patients) into thigh to the bone at the point of most tenderness. Withdraw needle (1-2mm) so it is just off the bone and in the bursa. Aspirate to ensure needle is not in a vessel.
5. Inject local or local/corticosteroid preparation into bursa. May redirect needle slightly to inject a septated bursa
6. Dress injection site

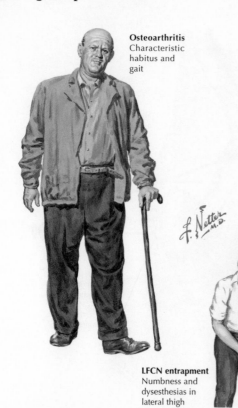

Osteoarthritis
Characteristic
habitus and
gait

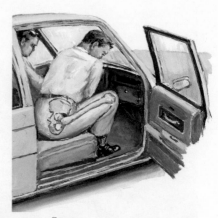

Trauma
Mechanism of injury often by impact
with dashboard, which drives femoral
head backward, out of acetabulum

LFCN entrapment
Numbness and
dysesthesias in
lateral thigh

QUESTION	ANSWER	CLINICAL APPLICATION
1. Age	Young	Trauma, developmental disorders
	Middle age–elderly	Arthritis, fractures
2. Pain		
a. Onset	Acute	Trauma, (fracture, dislocation), infection
	Chronic	Arthritis, labral tear
b. Location	Lateral hip/thigh	Bursitis, LFCN entrapment, snapping hip syndrome
	Buttocks/posterior thigh	Consider spine etiology
	Groin/medial thigh	Hip joint or acetabular etiology (likely not from spine)
	Anterior thigh	Proximal femur pathology
c. Occurrence	Ambulation/WB/motion	Hip joint etiology (i.e., not pelvis/spine)
	At night	Tumor, infection
3. Snapping	With ambulation	Snapping hip syndrome, loose bodies, arthritis
4. Assisted ambulation	Cane/crutch/walker	Use (and frequency) indicates severity of pain and condition
5. Activity tolerance	Walk distance and activity cessation	Less distance walked and fewer activities no longer performed = more severe
6. Trauma	Fall, MVA	Fracture, dislocation, labral tear
7. Activity/work	Repetitive use	Femoral stress fracture
8. Neurologic symptoms	Pain, numbness, tingling	LFCN entrapment, spine etiology (e.g., radiculopathy)
9. History of arthritides	Multiple joints involved	Systemic inflammatory disease

Femoral neck fracture

Typical deformity
of injured limb in shortened,
externally rotated position

Posterior hip dislocation

Typical deformity
injured limb
adducted, internally
rotated and flexed
at hip and knee,
with knee resting
on opposite thigh

Anterior hip dislocation

Characteristic position
of affected limb. Hip
flexed, thigh abducted
and externally rotated.

Flexion contracture of hip joint

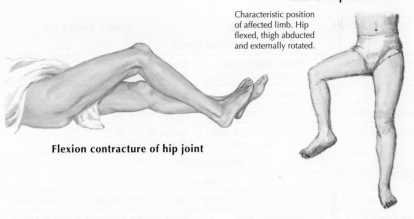

EXAM/OBSERVATION	TECHNIQUE	CLINICAL APPLICATION
INSPECTION		
Skin	Discoloration, wounds	Trauma
	Gross deformity	Fracture, dislocation
Position	Shortened, ER	Femoral neck fracture; intertrochanteric fracture
	Adducted, IR	Posterior dislocation
	Abducted, ER	Anterior dislocation
	Flexed	Hip flexion contracture
Gait		
Antalgic (painful)	Decreased stance phase	Knee, ankle, heel (spur), midfoot, toe pain
Lurch (Trendelenburg)	Lean laterally (on WB side)	Gluteus medius weakness
Lurch	Lean posteriorly (keep hip ext)	Gluteus maximus weakness
PALPATION		
Bony structures	Greater trochanter/bursa	Pain/palpable bursa: infection/bursitis, gluteus medius tendinitis
		Snapping—IT band may snap over GT
	Lesser trochanter	Snapping— Psoas tendon may snap over LT

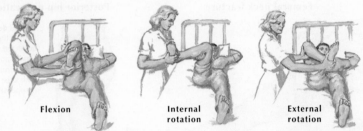

Flexion   **Internal rotation**   **External rotation**

Hip flexion-rotation exercises with patient supine. Hip and knee passively flexed, then limb rotated laterally and medially as pain permits

JOHN A.CRAIG___AD

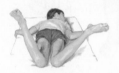

Internal rotation
Limitation of internal rotation of left hip. Hip rotation best assessed with patient in prone position because any restriction can be detected and measured easily

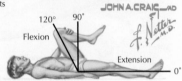

EXAM/OBSERVATION	TECHNIQUE	CLINICAL APPLICATION
RANGE OF MOTION		
Flexion	Supine: knee to chest Thomas test	Normal: 120-135° Rule out flexion contracture (see Special Tests, p. 263)
Extension	Prone: lift leg off table	Normal: 20-30°
Abduction/adduction	Supine: leg lateral/medial	Normal: Abd: 40-50°, Add: 20-30°
Internal/external rotation	Seated: foot lateral/medial Prone: flex knee leg in/out	Normal: IR: 30°, ER: 50° Normal: IR: 30°, ER: 50°
NEUROVASCULAR		
Sensory		
Genitofemoral nerve (L1-2)	Proximal anteromedial thigh	Deficit indicates corresponding nerve/root lesion
Obturator nerve (L2-4)	Inferomedial thigh	Deficit indicates corresponding nerve/root lesion
Lat. femoral cutaneous n. (L2-3)	Lateral thigh	Deficit indicates corresponding nerve/root lesion
Femoral nerve	Anteromedial thigh	Deficit indicates corresponding nerve/root lesion
Post. femoral cutaneous n. (S1-3)	Posterior thigh	Deficit indicates corresponding nerve/root lesion
Motor		
Obturator nerve (L2-4)	Thigh/hip adduction	Weakness = adductor muscle group or nerve/root lesion
Superior gluteal nerve L5)	Thigh abduction	Weakness = gluteus medius or nerve/root lesion
Femoral nerve (L2-4)	Hip flexion Knee extension	Weakness = iliopsoas or nerve/root lesion Weakness = quadriceps or nerve/root lesion
Inferior gluteal nerve (L5-S2)	Hip extension	Weakness = gluteus maximus or nerve/root lesion
Sciatic: Tibial portion (L4-S3) Peroneal portion (L4-S2)	Knee flexion Knee flexion	Weakness = biceps long head or nerve/root lesion Weakness = biceps short head or nerve/root lesion
Other		
Reflex	None	
Pulses	Femoral	

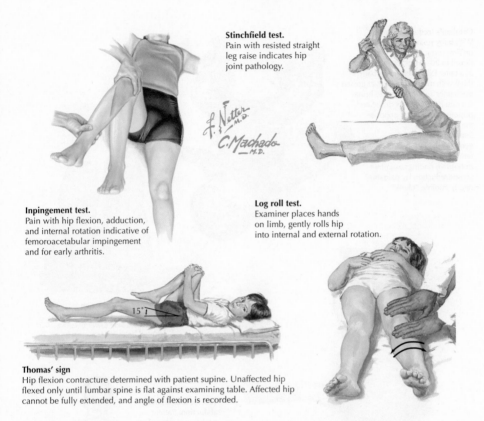

Stinchfield test.
Pain with resisted straight leg raise indicates hip joint pathology.

Inpingement test.
Pain with hip flexion, adduction, and internal rotation indicative of femoroacetabular impingement and for early arthritis.

Log roll test.
Examiner places hands on limb, gently rolls hip into internal and external rotation.

15°

Thomas' sign
Hip flexion contracture determined with patient supine. Unaffected hip flexed only until lumbar spine is flat against examining table. Affected hip cannot be fully extended, and angle of flexion is recorded.

EXAM/OBSERVATION	TECHNIQUE	CLINICAL APPLICATION
	SPECIAL TESTS	
Impingement	Supine: flex, adduct, IR hip	Pain may be indicative of femoral acetabular impingement.
FABER/Patrick	**F**lex, **AB**duct, **ER** hip, then abduct more (figure of 4)	Positive if painful. SI joint or hip pathology.
Log roll	Supine, hip extended: IR/ER	Pain in hip is consistent with arthritis.
Stinchfield	Resisted straight leg raise	Pain is positive test for hip pathology.
Thomas sign	Supine; one knee to chest	If opposite thigh elevates off table, flexion contracture.
Ober	On side: flex and abduct hip	Extend and adduct hip; if stays in abduction, ITB contracture.
Piriformis	On side: adduct hip	Pain in hip/pelvis indicates tight piriformis (compressing sciatic nerve).
90-90 straight leg	Flex hip & knee 90°, extend knee	>20° of flexion after full knee extension = tight hamstrings.
Ely's	Prone: passively flex knee	If hip flexes as knee is flexed, tight rectus femoris muscle.
Leg length	ASIS to medial malleolus	A measured difference of >1cm is positive.
Meralgia	Pressure medial to ASIS	Reproduction to pain, burning, numbness = LFCN entrapment.
See Chapter 7, Pelvis, for Trendelenburg test.		

Ortolani's (reduction) test
With baby relaxed and content on firm surface, hips and knees flexed to 90°. Hips examined one at a time. Examiner grasps baby's thigh with middle finger over greater trochanter and lifts thigh to bring femoral head from its dislocated posterior position to opposite the acetabulum. Simultaneously, thigh gently abducted, reducing femoral head into acetabulum. In positive finding, examiner senses reduction by palpable, nearly audible "clunk"

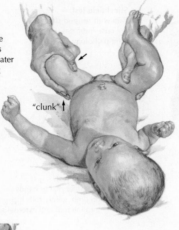

"clunk"

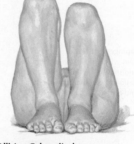

Allis' or Galeazzi's sign
With knees and hips flexed, knee on affected side lower because femoral head lies posterior to acetabulum in this position

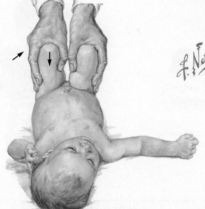

Test for limitation of abduction. Patient supine and relaxed on table. Legs gently and passively abducted to determine range of motion of each. Seen in Perthes disease.

Barlow's (dislocation) test
Reverse of Ortolani's test. If femoral head is in acetabulum at time of examination, Barlow's test is performed to discover any hip instability. Baby's thigh grasped as above and adducted with gentle downward pressure. Dislocation is palpable as femoral head slips out of acetabulum. Diagnosis confirmed with Ortolani's test

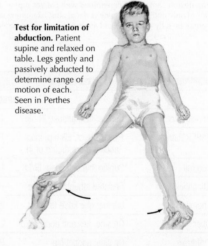

EXAM/OBSERVATION	TECHNIQUE	CLINICAL APPLICATION
SPECIAL TESTS		
Ortolani (peds)	Hips at 90°, abduct hips	A clunk indicates the hip(s) was dislocated and now reduced
Barlow (peds)	Hips at 90°, posterior force	A clunk indicates the hip(s) is now dislocated, should reduce with Ortolani
Galeazzi (peds)	Supine: flex hips & knees	Any discrepancy in knee height: 1. Dislocated hip, 2. Short femur

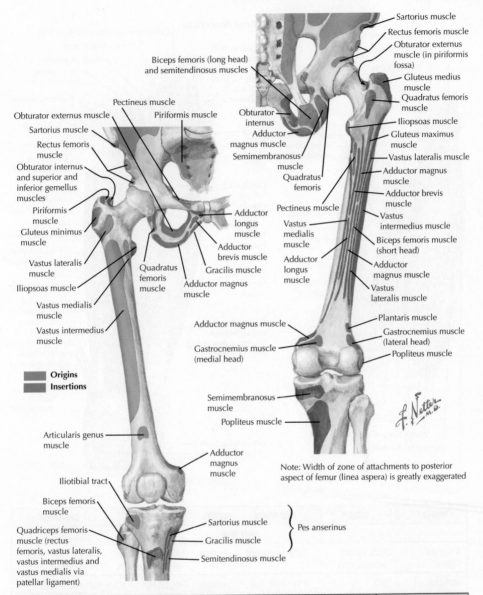

Sartorius muscle
Rectus femoris muscle
Obturator externus muscle (in piriformis fossa)
Gluteus medius muscle
Quadratus femoris muscle
Iliopsoas muscle
Gluteus maximus muscle
Vastus lateralis muscle
Adductor magnus muscle
Adductor brevis muscle
Vastus intermedius muscle
Biceps femoris muscle (short head)
Adductor magnus muscle
Vastus lateralis muscle
Plantaris muscle
Gastrocnemius muscle (lateral head)
Popliteus muscle

Biceps femoris (long head) and semitendinosus muscles
Pectineus muscle
Piriformis muscle
Obturator internus
Adductor magnus muscle
Semimembranosus muscle
Quadratus femoris

Obturator externus muscle
Sartorius muscle
Rectus femoris muscle
Obturator internus and superior and inferior gemellus muscles
Piriformis muscle
Gluteus minimus muscle
Vastus lateralis muscle
Iliopsoas muscle
Vastus medialis muscle
Vastus intermedius muscle

Quadratus femoris muscle
Adductor longus muscle
Adductor brevis muscle
Gracilis muscle
Adductor magnus muscle

Pectineus muscle
Vastus medialis muscle
Adductor longus muscle

Adductor magnus muscle
Gastrocnemius muscle (medial head)
Semimembranosus muscle
Popliteus muscle

Articularis genus muscle
Adductor magnus muscle

Iliotibial tract
Biceps femoris muscle
Quadriceps femoris muscle (rectus femoris, vastus lateralis, vastus intermedius and vastus medialis via patellar ligament)

Sartorius muscle
Gracilis muscle
Semitendinosus muscle
Pes anserinus

Origins
Insertions

Note: Width of zone of attachments to posterior aspect of femur (linea aspera) is greatly exaggerated

PUBIC RAMI (ASPECT)	GREATER TROCHANTER	ISCHIAL TUBEROSITY	LINEA ASPERA/ POSTERIOR FEMUR
Pectineus (pectineal line/sup)	Piriformis (anterior)	Inferior gemellus	Adductor magnus*
Adductor magnus (inferior)	Obturator internus (anterior)	Quadratus femoris	Adductor longus
Adductor longus (anterior)	Superior gemellus	Semimembranosus	Adductor brevis
Adductor brevis (inferior)	Gluteus medius (posterior)	Semitendinosus	Biceps femoris (SH)
Gracilis (inferior)	Gluteus minimus (anterior)	Biceps femoris (LH)	Pectineus
Psoas minor (superior)		Adductor magnus*	Gluteus maximus
			Vastus lateralis
			Vastus medialis

*Adductor magnus has two origins.

Superficial dissections

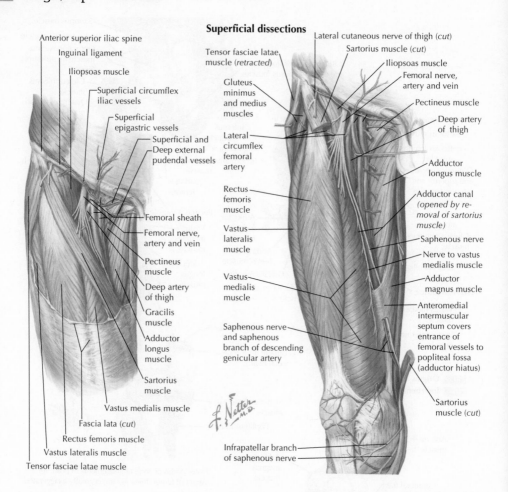

Anterior superior iliac spine
Inguinal ligament
Iliopsoas muscle
Superficial circumflex iliac vessels
Superficial epigastric vessels
Superficial and Deep external pudendal vessels
Femoral sheath
Femoral nerve, artery and vein
Pectineus muscle
Deep artery of thigh
Gracilis muscle
Adductor longus muscle
Sartorius muscle
Vastus medialis muscle
Fascia lata (cut)
Rectus femoris muscle
Vastus lateralis muscle
Tensor fasciae latae muscle

Tensor fasciae latae muscle (retracted)
Gluteus minimus and medius muscles
Lateral circumflex femoral artery
Rectus femoris muscle
Vastus lateralis muscle
Vastus medialis muscle
Saphenous nerve and saphenous branch of descending genicular artery
Infrapatellar branch of saphenous nerve

Lateral cutaneous nerve of thigh (cut)
Sartorius muscle (cut)
Iliopsoas muscle
Femoral nerve, artery and vein
Pectineus muscle
Deep artery of thigh
Adductor longus muscle
Adductor canal (opened by removal of sartorius muscle)
Saphenous nerve
Nerve to vastus medialis muscle
Adductor magnus muscle
Anteromedial intermuscular septum covers entrance of femoral vessels to popliteal fossa (adductor hiatus)
Sartorius muscle (cut)

MUSCLE	ORIGIN	INSERTION	NERVE	ACTION	COMMENT
ANTERIOR					
Articularis genus	Distal anterior femoral shaft	Synovial capsule	Femoral	Pulls capsule superiorly in extension	May join with vastus intermedialis
Sartorius	ASIS	Prox. med. tibia (pes anserinus)	Femoral	Flex, ER hip	Can avulse from ASIS (avulsion fracture)
Quadriceps					
Rectus femoris	1. AIIS 2. Sup. acetab. rim	Patella/tibial tubercle	Femoral	Flex thigh, extend leg	Can avulse from AIIS (avulsion fracture)
Vastus lateralis	Gtr. trochanter, lat. linea aspera	Lateral patella/ tibia tubercle	Femoral	Extend leg	Oblique fibers can affect Q angle
Vastus intermedius	Proximal femoral shaft	Patella/tibia tubercle	Femoral	Extend leg	Covers articularis genu
Vastus medialis	Intertrochant. line, med. linea aspera	Medial patella/ tibia tubercle	Femoral	Extend leg	Weak in many patellofemoral disorders

Deep dissection

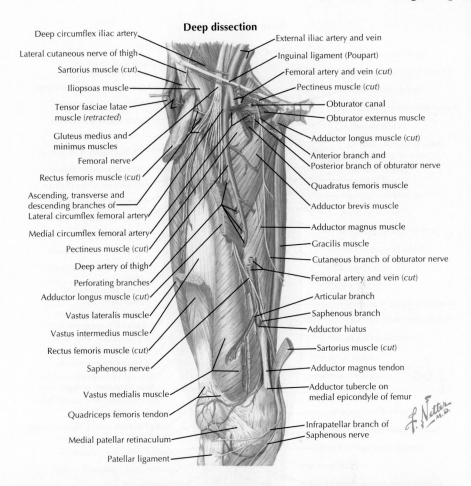

Deep circumflex iliac artery
Lateral cutaneous nerve of thigh
Sartorius muscle (*cut*)
Iliopsoas muscle
Tensor fasciae latae muscle (*retracted*)
Gluteus medius and minimus muscles
Femoral nerve
Rectus femoris muscle (*cut*)
Ascending, transverse and descending branches of Lateral circumflex femoral artery
Medial circumflex femoral artery
Pectineus muscle (*cut*)
Deep artery of thigh
Perforating branches
Adductor longus muscle (*cut*)
Vastus lateralis muscle
Vastus intermedius muscle
Rectus femoris muscle (*cut*)
Saphenous nerve
Vastus medialis muscle
Quadriceps femoris tendon
Medial patellar retinaculum
Patellar ligament

External iliac artery and vein
Inguinal ligament (Poupart)
Femoral artery and vein (*cut*)
Pectineus muscle (*cut*)
Obturator canal
Obturator externus muscle
Adductor longus muscle (*cut*)
Anterior branch and Posterior branch of obturator nerve
Quadratus femoris muscle
Adductor brevis muscle
Adductor magnus muscle
Gracilis muscle
Cutaneous branch of obturator nerve
Femoral artery and vein (*cut*)
Articular branch
Saphenous branch
Adductor hiatus
Sartorius muscle (*cut*)
Adductor magnus tendon
Adductor tubercle on medial epicondyle of femur
Infrapatellar branch of Saphenous nerve

MUSCLE	ORIGIN	INSERTION	NERVE	ACTION	COMMENT
MEDIAL					
Obturator externus	Ischiopubic rami, obturator memb	Piriformis fossa	Obturator	ER thigh	Insertion at start point of IM nail
Hip Adductors					
Adductor longus	Body of pubis (inferior)	Linea aspera (mid ⅓)	Obturator	Adducts thigh	Tendon can ossify
Adductor brevis	Body and inferior pubic ramus	Pectineal line, linea aspera	Obturator	Adducts thigh	Deep to pectineus
Adductor magnus	1. Pubic ramus 2. Ischial tub.	Linea aspera, add. tubercle	1. Obturator 2. Sciatic	Adducts & flex/ extend thigh	Muscle has two separate parts
Gracilis	Body and inferior pubic ramus	Prox. med. tibia (pes anserinus)	Obturator	Adduct thigh, flex/IR leg	Used in ligament reconstruction
Hip Flexors					
Pectineus	Pectineal line of pubis	Pectineal line of femur	Femoral	Flex and adducts thigh	Part of femoral triangle floor

Deep dissection

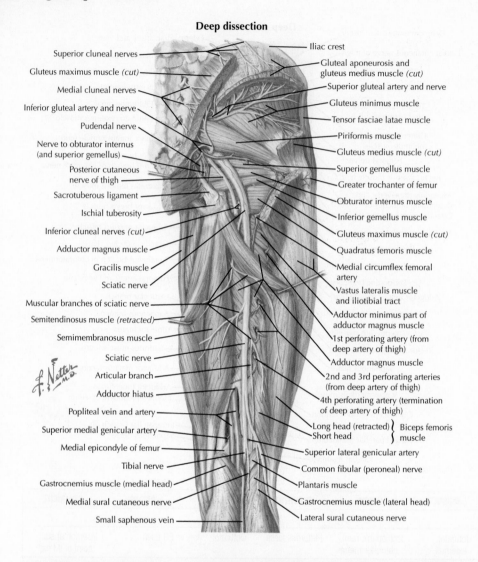

Superior cluneal nerves

Gluteus maximus muscle *(cut)*

Medial cluneal nerves

Inferior gluteal artery and nerve

Pudendal nerve

Nerve to obturator internus (and superior gemellus)

Posterior cutaneous nerve of thigh

Sacrotuberous ligament

Ischial tuberosity

Inferior cluneal nerves *(cut)*

Adductor magnus muscle

Gracilis muscle

Sciatic nerve

Muscular branches of sciatic nerve

Semitendinosus muscle *(retracted)*

Semimembranosus muscle

Sciatic nerve

Articular branch

Adductor hiatus

Popliteal vein and artery

Superior medial genicular artery

Medial epicondyle of femur

Tibial nerve

Gastrocnemius muscle (medial head)

Medial sural cutaneous nerve

Small saphenous vein

Iliac crest

Gluteal aponeurosis and gluteus medius muscle *(cut)*

Superior gluteal artery and nerve

Gluteus minimus muscle

Tensor fasciae latae muscle

Piriformis muscle

Gluteus medius muscle *(cut)*

Superior gemellus muscle

Greater trochanter of femur

Obturator internus muscle

Inferior gemellus muscle

Gluteus maximus muscle *(cut)*

Quadratus femoris muscle

Medial circumflex femoral artery

Vastus lateralis muscle and iliotibial tract

Adductor minimus part of adductor magnus muscle

1st perforating artery (from deep artery of thigh)

Adductor magnus muscle

2nd and 3rd perforating arteries (from deep artery of thigh)

4th perforating artery (termination of deep artery of thigh)

Long head (retracted) ⎫ Biceps femoris
Short head ⎭ muscle

Superior lateral genicular artery

Common fibular (peroneal) nerve

Plantaris muscle

Gastrocnemius muscle (lateral head)

Lateral sural cutaneous nerve

MUSCLE	ORIGIN	INSERTION	NERVE	ACTION	COMMENT
POSTERIOR: HAMSTRINGS					
Semitendinosus	Ischial tuberosity	Proximal medial tibia (pes anserinus)	Sciatic (tibial)	Extend thigh, flex leg	Tendon used in ligament reconstructions (ACL)
Semimembranosus	Ischial tuberosity	Posterior medial tibial condyle	Sciatic (tibial)	Extend thigh, flex leg	A border in medial approach
Biceps femoris: long head	Ischial tuberosity	Head of fibula	Sciatic (tibial)	Extend thigh, flex leg	Can avulse front origin (avulsion fx)
Biceps femoris: short head	Linea aspera, supracondylar line	Fibula, lateral tibia	Sciatic (peroneal)	Extend thigh, flex leg	Shares tendon insertion with long head

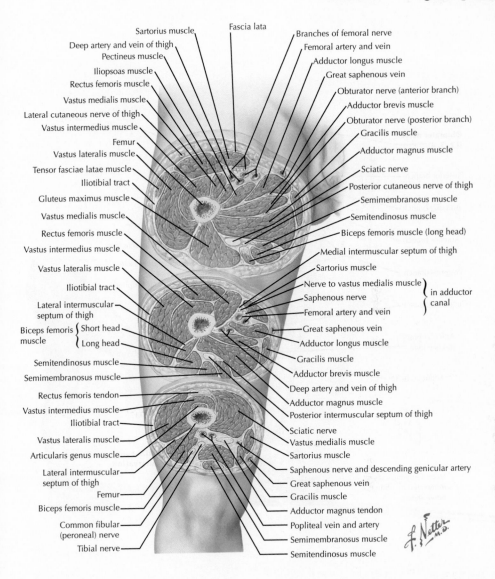

Sartorius muscle
Deep artery and vein of thigh
Pectineus muscle
Iliopsoas muscle
Rectus femoris muscle
Vastus medialis muscle
Lateral cutaneous nerve of thigh
Vastus intermedius muscle
Femur
Vastus lateralis muscle
Tensor fasciae latae muscle
Iliotibial tract
Gluteus maximus muscle
Vastus medialis muscle
Rectus femoris muscle
Vastus intermedius muscle
Vastus lateralis muscle
Iliotibial tract
Lateral intermuscular septum of thigh
Biceps femoris { Short head muscle { Long head
Semitendinosus muscle
Semimembranosus muscle
Rectus femoris tendon
Vastus intermedius muscle
Iliotibial tract
Vastus lateralis muscle
Articularis genus muscle
Lateral intermuscular septum of thigh
Femur
Biceps femoris muscle
Common fibular (peroneal) nerve
Tibial nerve

Fascia lata

Branches of femoral nerve
Femoral artery and vein
Adductor longus muscle
Great saphenous vein
Obturator nerve (anterior branch)
Adductor brevis muscle
Obturator nerve (posterior branch)
Gracilis muscle
Adductor magnus muscle
Sciatic nerve
Posterior cutaneous nerve of thigh
Semimembranosus muscle
Semitendinosus muscle
Biceps femoris muscle (long head)
Medial intermuscular septum of thigh
Sartorius muscle
Nerve to vastus medialis muscle }
Saphenous nerve } in adductor canal
Femoral artery and vein }
Great saphenous vein
Adductor longus muscle
Gracilis muscle
Adductor brevis muscle
Deep artery and vein of thigh
Adductor magnus muscle
Posterior intermuscular septum of thigh
Sciatic nerve
Vastus medialis muscle
Sartorius muscle
Saphenous nerve and descending genicular artery
Great saphenous vein
Gracilis muscle
Adductor magnus tendon
Popliteal vein and artery
Semimembranosus muscle
Semitendinosus muscle

STRUCTURE	RELATIONSHIP
COMPARTMENTS	
Anterior	Quadriceps: vastus lateralis, vastus intermedius, vastus medius, rectus femoris
Posterior	Biceps femoris (long head and short head), semitendinosus, semimembranosus, sciatic nerve
Medial	Adductor magnus, adductor longus, adductor brevis, gracilis, femoral artery and vein
FASCIOTOMIES	
Lateral incision	Release the anterior compartment and posterior compartment
Medial incision	Release the medial compartment

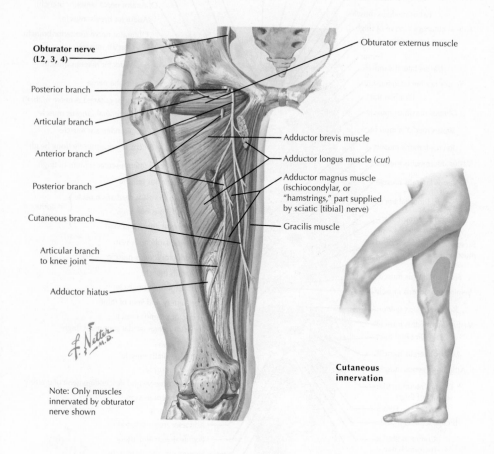

Obturator nerve
(L2, 3, 4)

Posterior branch

Articular branch

Anterior branch

Posterior branch

Cutaneous branch

Articular branch
to knee joint

Adductor hiatus

Note: Only muscles
innervated by obturator
nerve shown

Obturator externus muscle

Adductor brevis muscle

Adductor longus muscle (cut)

Adductor magnus muscle
(ischiocondylar, or
"hamstrings," part supplied
by sciatic [tibial] nerve)

Gracilis muscle

**Cutaneous
innervation**

LUMBAR PLEXUS
Anterior Division
Obturator (L2-4): exits via obturator canal, splits into anterior and posterior divisions. Can be injured by retractors placed behind the transverse acetabular ligament.
Sensory: Inferomedial thigh: via **cutaneous branch of obturator nerve**

Motor: Gracilis (anterior division)
           Adductor longus (anterior division)
           Adductor brevis (anterior/posterior divisions)
           Adductor magnus (posterior division)

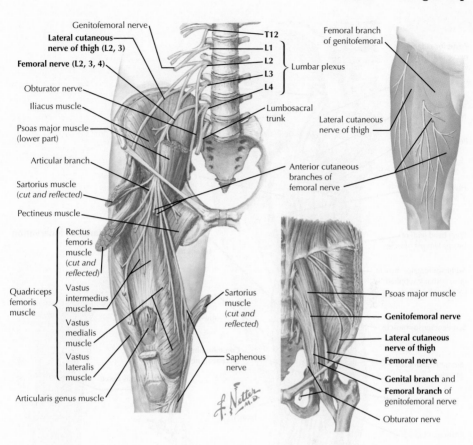

LUMBAR PLEXUS

Genitofemoral (L1-2): pierces psoas, lies on anteromedial surface of psoas and divides into two branches

Sensory: Femoral branch: proximal anterior thigh (over femoral triangle)
Genital branch: scrotum/labia
Motor: None (in thigh)

Posterior Division

Lateral femoral cutaneous (LFCN) (L2-3): crosses inferior to ASIS (can be compressed at or near ASIS)

Sensory: Lateral thigh
Motor: None

Femoral (L2-4): lies b/w psoas major & iliacus; branches in femoral triangle. Saphenous nerve runs under sartorius.

Sensory: Anteromedial thigh—via **anterior/intermediate cutaneous nerves**
Motor: Psoas
Pectineus
Sartorius
• Quadriceps
  ∘ Rectus femoris
  ∘ Vastus lateralis
  ∘ Vastus intermedialis
  ∘ Vastus medialis

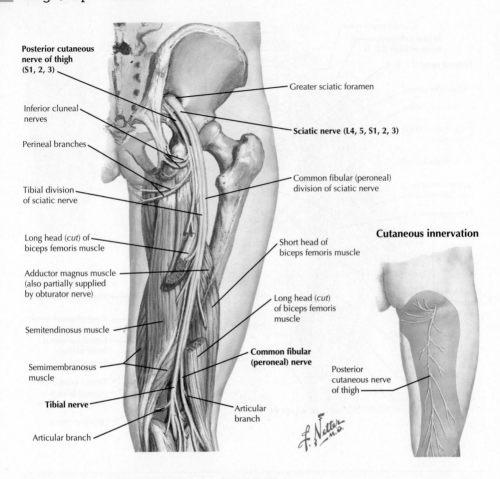

Posterior cutaneous nerve of thigh (S1, 2, 3)

Inferior cluneal nerves

Perineal branches

Tibial division of sciatic nerve

Long head (*cut*) of biceps femoris muscle

Adductor magnus muscle (also partially supplied by obturator nerve)

Semitendinosus muscle

Semimembranosus muscle

Tibial nerve

Articular branch

Greater sciatic foramen

Sciatic nerve (L4, 5, S1, 2, 3)

Common fibular (peroneal) division of sciatic nerve

Short head of biceps femoris muscle

Long head (*cut*) of biceps femoris muscle

Common fibular (peroneal) nerve

Articular branch

Cutaneous innervation

Posterior cutaneous nerve of thigh

SACRAL PLEXUS
Sciatic nerve: a single nerve with 2 distinct parts; it divides in the distal thigh into tibial & common peroneal nerves
Anterior Division
Tibial (L4-S3): descends (as sciatic) in posterior thigh deep to hamstrings and superficial to adductor magnus muscle
Sensory: None (in thigh) *Motor:* Biceps femoris (long head) Semitendinosus Semimembranosus
Posterior Division
Common peroneal (L4-S2): descends (as sciatic) in posterior thigh deep to hamstrings and superficial to adductor magnus
Sensory: None (in thigh) *Motor:* Biceps femoris (short head)
Posterior femoral cutaneous nerve (PFCN) (S1-3): through greater sciatic foramen, medial to sciatic nerve
Sensory: Posterior thigh *Motor:* None

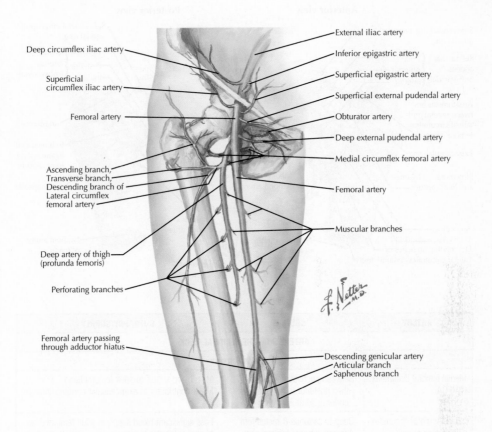

Deep circumflex iliac artery

Superficial circumflex iliac artery

Femoral artery

Ascending branch
Transverse branch
Descending branch of
Lateral circumflex
femoral artery

Deep artery of thigh
(profunda femoris)

Perforating branches

Femoral artery passing
through adductor hiatus

External iliac artery

Inferior epigastric artery

Superficial epigastric artery

Superficial external pudendal artery

Obturator artery

Deep external pudendal artery

Medial circumflex femoral artery

Femoral artery

Muscular branches

Descending genicular artery
Articular branch
Saphenous branch

ARTERY	BRANCHES	COMMENT
Obturator	Anterior/posterior branches	Runs through obturator foramen
FEMORAL ARTERY		
In femoral triangle, runs in adductor canal (under sartorius, b/w vastus medialis & adductor longus), then passes posterior through the adductor hiatus and becomes the popliteal artery posterior to the distal femur and knee.		
Femoral artery (superficial fem. [(SFA])	Superficial circumflex iliac Superficial epigastric Superficial and deep external pudendal Profunda femoris (deep artery) Descending genicular artery Articular branch Saphenous branch	Supplies superficial abdominal tissues Supplies superficial abdominal tissues Supplies subcutaneous tissues in pubic region and scrotum/labia majus Primary blood supply to thigh. See below Anastomosis at knee to supply knee
Profunda femoris (deep artery of thigh)	Medial femoral circumflex Lateral femoral circumflex Ascending branch Transverse branch Descending branch Perforators/muscular branch	Supplies femoral neck, under quad. femoris Supplies femoral neck Forms anastomosis at femoral neck To greater trochanter At risk in anteromedial approach to hip Supplies femoral shaft and thigh muscles

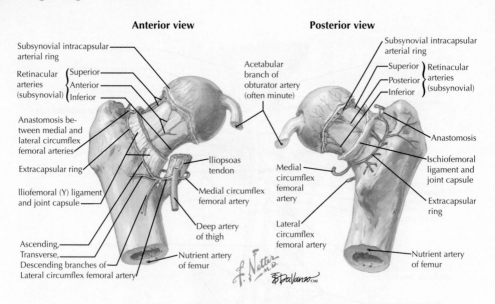

Anterior view · Posterior view

ARTERY	COURSE	COMMENT/SUPPLY
ARTERIES OF THE FEMORAL NECK		
Profunda Femoris		
Medial femoral circumflex (MFCA)	Between pectineus and psoas, then posterior to femoral neck under quadratus femoris	Main blood supply to adult femoral head Major contributor to extracapsular ring/anastomosis
Lateral femoral circumflex Ascending branch Transverse branch Descending branch	Deep to sartorius & rectus fem. Ascends anterior femoral neck Across proximal femur to GT Under rectus femoris	Less significant blood supply in adult femoral head Major contributor to extracapsular ring/anastomosis Gives partial supply to greater trochanter (GT) At risk in anterolateral approach to hip
1st Perforator	Ascending branch	Can contribute to extracapsular ring/anastomosis
Extracapsular ring—formed at the base of the femoral neck primarily from branches of MFCA and LFCA		
Lateral branches	From ring, laterally toward GT	Supply greater trochanter
Ascending cervical arteries Retinacular arteries	Along extracapsular femoral neck Along intracapsular femoral neck	Branch from the extracapsular ring Intracapsular continuation of cervical arteries Form a second intracapsular ring at base of head
Subsynovial intracapsular arterial ring—formed at the base of the femoral head		
Epiphyseal arteries Lateral epiphyseal art.	Enter bone at border of articular surface In posterosuperior neck	Will form intraosseous anastomoses Lat. epiphyseal supplies most of WB femoral head
Obturator Artery		
Artery of ligamentum teres Medial epiphyseal art.	Thru ligamentum teres to fovea Interosseous terminal branches	Minimal supply to the adult femoral head Anastomose with lateral epiphyseal arteries
Other Arteries		
Superior & inferior gluteal		Can contribute to extracapsular ring/anastomosis
Pediatric femoral head blood supply: 0-4yr MFCA, LFCA, and ligamentum teres artery; 4-8yr: mostly MFCA, minimal LFCA and ligamentum teres artery; >8yrs: MFCA is predominant		

**Lateral femoral
cutaneous nerve**

Entrapment of nerve
under inguinal ligament

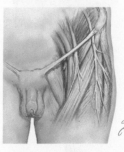

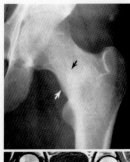

Arrows show the presence
of buttressing and sclerosis
in the femoral neck

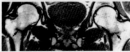

Coronal MRI reveals bilateral fatigue
fractures (arrows) in the femoral neck

Reprinted with permission from
Resnick D. Kransdorf M. Bone and Joint Imaging,
3rd edition, Elesevier, Philadelphia, 2005.

DESCRIPTION	Hx & PE	WORKUP/FINDINGS	TREATMENT
FEMOROACETABULAR IMPINGEMENT			

• Subtle abnormal hip morphology causes bony abutment. 2 types
  ○ *Cam:* femoral non-sphericity
  ○ *Pincer:* acetabulum overcoverage
• Causes early DJD
	Hx: Insidious onset, groin pain, worse with activity
	PE: Decreased ROM (esp. IR),+ impingement test (flex, add, IR hip)
		XR: AP/lateral of hip
		Cam: femoral neck "bump," +/− herniation pit, decreased offset
		Pincer: increased acetabular coverage
		MR: Labral tear, chondral injury
			1. NSAIDs, activity modification
			2. Surgical dislocation and neck and/or acetabular reshaping
			3. Osteotomy in selected cases
			4. THA if advanced DJD

FEMORAL NECK STRESS (FATIGUE) FRACTURE			
• Excessive loading of hip • 2 types: tension (superior neck), compression (inferior neck) • Common in military recruits	**Hx:** Increased activity with new onset of hip/groin pain **PE:** +/− pain with and/or diminished ROM	**XR:** AP, AP in IR, lateral **MR:** Best study for early detection of fracture **BS:** Shows fx subacutely	• Compression: limited weight-bearing • Tension: urgent percutaneous pinning (prevent displacement)
MERALGIA PARESTHETICA			
• Nerve trapped near ASIS • Due to activity (hip extension), clothing (e.g., belt), or repetitive compression	**Hx:** Pain/burning in lateral thigh **PE:** Decr. sensation on lateral thigh, + meralgia	**XR:** AP/lateral of hip: rule out other pathology	1. Remove compressive entity (e.g., belt, tight clothing, etc.) 2. Surgical release: rare
SNAPPING HIP (COXA SALTANS)			
Snapping in hip. 3 types 1. External: ITB over GT 2. Internal: psoas over femoral head or iliopectineal eminence 3. Intraarticular: usually loose body	**Hx:** Snapping at hip +/− pain **PE:** Palpate the tendon (ITB or psoas tendon) then flex & extend hip, feeling for snap. (external over GT; internal over LT)	**XR:** AP/lateral hip: rule out osseous abnormality (e.g., spur) and hip DJD **MR:** Loose body, labral tear **US/bursography:** Psoas tendon	External/Internal: 1. Activity modification, PT 2. Consider injection 3. Surgical release: very rare Intraarticular: LB removal
TROCHANTERIC BURSITIS			
• Inflammation of bursa over greater trochanter • F>M, middle age	**Hx:** Lateral hip pain, cannot sleep on affected side **PE:** Point tender at trochanter, pain w/adduction	**XR:** AP pelvis, AP/lateral of hip: rule out spur, OA, calcified tendons	1. NSAIDs, PT (ITB stretching) 2. Steroid injection 3. Surgical excision—rare

Osteoarthritis

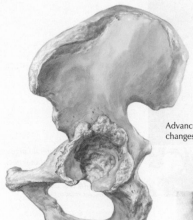

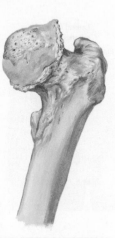

Advanced degenerative changes in acetabulum

Erosion of cartilage and deformity of femoral head

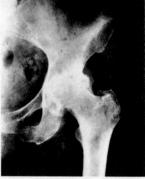

Radiograph of hip shows typical degeneration of cartilage and secondary bone changes with spurs at margins of acetabulum

DESCRIPTION	Hx & PE	WORKUP/FINDINGS	TREATMENT
OSTEOARTHRITIS			
• Loss or damage to articular cartilage • Etiology: Primary—idiopathic; Secondary—posttraumatic, infection, pediatric hip disease	**Hx:** Chronic hip or groin pain, increasing over time & with activity **PE:** Decreased ROM (first IR), + log roll, +/– flex contracture/antalgic gait	**XR:** AP pelvic/AP/lateral hip 1. Joint space narrowing 2. Osteophytes 3. Subchondral sclerosis 4. Bony cysts	1. NSAIDs/PT 2. Injection/activity modification, cane (in opposite hand) 3. Osteotomy (young) 4. Arthrodesis (young) 5. Total hip arthroplasty
OSTEONECROSIS (AVASCULAR NECROSIS/AVN)			
• Necrosis of femoral head due to vascular disruption • Assoc. w/trauma, steroid or EtOH use, inflammatory disorders. • M>F, 30-40's, 50% bilateral • Greater femoral head involvement, associated w/poor prognosis	**Hx:** Groin pain worse with activity **PE:** Limited ROM (esp IR & abd), antalgic gait **XR:** AP/lateral: stage-specific findings (see classification) **MRI:** Most sensitive study, shows early changes in femoral head **BS:** Replaced by MRI	**Classification:** Modified Ficat 0: Asymptomatic, nl XR, + MR 1: Symptomatic, nl XR, + MR 2: **XR:** sclerosis, no collapse 3: **XR:** + collapse (crescent sign) 4: Flat femoral head, nl acetabulum 5: Joint narrowing, early DJD 6: Advanced DJD incl. acetabulum	Stage: 0-1: Limited WB, observation 2: Core decompression 3: Consider vascularized fibula or femoral osteotomy 4-6: Total hip arthroplasty—appropriate for most patients. Hip fusion: in young laborers

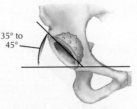

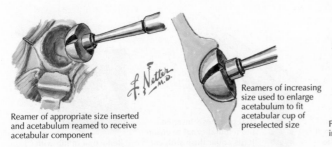

Reamer of appropriate size inserted
and acetabulum reamed to receive
acetabular component

Reamers of increasing
size used to enlarge
acetabulum to fit
acetabular cup of
preselected size

35° to
45°

Final position of cup 35° to 45° lateral
inclination and 15° anteversion

TOTAL HIP ARTHROPLASTY
General Information

- Goals: alleviate pain, maintain personal independence, allow performance of activities of daily living (ADLs).
- Common procedure with high satisfaction rates for primary procedure; revisions are also becoming more common.
- Advances in techniques and materials are improving implant survival; this procedure available to younger pts.

Materials

- **Cups** (acetabulum) **and stems** (femur). Usually made of titanium. Stainless steel or cobalt chrome stems may be too stiff (i.e., modulus mismatch) and cause stress shielding.
- **Bearing surfaces:** Acetabular liners and femoral head implants. Polyethylene (PE) liner and cobalt-chrome (Co-Cr) femoral head currently most common. Ceramic and metal also used.
  - UHMWPE (ultra high molecular weight PE): good surface, but high wear rates and debris lead to aseptic loosening. Direct compression molding is preferred manufacturing technique. Sterilization with irradiation in nonoxygen environment promotes cross-linking. Highly cross-linked PE has much better wear rates.
  - Co-Cr: "supermetal" alloy. Commonly used for femoral bearing surface with PE liner. Metal on metal implants available. Debris particles are much smaller, create less histocytic response. Carcinogenesis is a theoretic concern.
  - Ceramic (alumina): Excellent wear rates, but brittle (could fracture). Can be used with PE liner or ceramic cup.

Techniques

- **Two types of fixation:** 1. Cement, 2. Uncemented/biologic
  - **Cement:** Methylmethacrylate. Most often used in elderly patients. Provides immediate static fixation, no remodeling potential. Cement resists compression better than tension. As such, femoral implants do better than acetabular cups with this fixation. 3rd generation cementing techniques: pressurization, precoat stem, centralizer/restrictor, canal preparation, 2mm mantle
  - **Uncemented/biologic:** Used in younger patients (increasing popularity). Bone ongrowth or ingrowth—bone grows onto/into implant. Has remodeling potential, gives dynamic fixation. Not good a good choice in post-irradiated hip.
- Fixation is NOT immediate, needs initial fixation for stability: 2 techniques.
  - Press fit: Implant 1-2mm larger than bone. Bone hoop stresses provide initial fixation while bone on/ingrows.
  - Line to line: Implant and bone are same size. Screws used to provide initial fixation while bone on/ingrows.
- Optimal porous ongrowth pore size: 50-150 micrometers. Ongrowth surface area varies.
- Current gold standard implant: Uncemented (ingrowth) acetabular cup and cemented femoral steel. Trends are changing, and more uncemented femoral components and alternative bearing surfaces are being used more frequently.
- Head size affects stability (larger is more stable) and wear (large head = high volumetric wear). 28mm is optimal size.

Indications

- **Arthritis of hip**
  - Common etiologies: osteoarthritis, rheumatoid arthritis, osteonecrosis, prior pediatric hip disease
  - Clinical symptoms: groin/hip pain, worse with activity, gradually worsening over time, decreased functional capacity
  - Radiographic findings: appropriate radiographic evidence of hip arthritis should be present

Osteoarthritis	**Rheumatoid arthritis**
1. Joint space narrowing	1. Joint space narrowing
2. Sclerosis	2. Periarticular osteoporosis
3. Subchondral cysts	3. Joint erosions
4. Osteophyte formation	4. Ankylosis

  - Failed conservative treatment: NSAIDs, activity modification, weight loss, PT, cane (contralateral hand), injections
  - Other: Fractures (e.g., femoral neck with hip DJD), tumors, developmental disorders (e.g., DDH, etc)

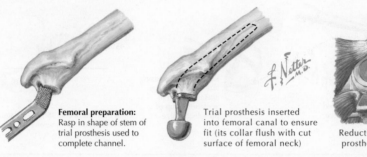

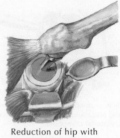

Femoral preparation:
Rasp in shape of stem of trial prosthesis used to complete channel.

Trial prosthesis inserted into femoral canal to ensure fit (its collar flush with cut surface of femoral neck)

Reduction of hip with prosthesis in place.

TOTAL HIP ARTHROPLASTY—CONTINUED
Contraindications
<ul><li>Absolute<ul><li>Neuropathic joint</li><li>Infection</li><li>Medically unstable patient (e.g., severe cardiopulmonary disease). Patient may not survive the procedure.</li></ul></li><li>Relative<ul><li>Young, active patients. These patients can wear out the prosthesis many times in their lives.</li></ul></li></ul>
Alternatives
<ul><li>Considerations: age, activity level, overall medical health</li><li>Osteotomy: femoral or pelvic; usually performed in younger patients</li><li>Arthrodesis/fusion: young laborers with isolated unilateral disease (i.e., normal spine, knee, ankle, contralateral hip)</li></ul>
Procedure
<ul><li>Approaches<ul><li>Posterior, lateral, and anterolateral approaches</li><li>Minimally invasive, one- and two-incision approaches are becoming more common.</li></ul></li><li>Steps<ul><li>Acetabulum: remove labrum & osteophytes, ream to a cortical rim, implant cup (35-45° coronal tilt, 15-30° anteversion)</li><li>Femur: dislocate head, cut neck, remove head, find and broach canal (lateralize as needed)—stem cannot be in varus, implant stem, trial head, & neck. Implant the appropriate head/neck and acetabular liner.</li></ul></li></ul>
Complications
<ul><li>Infection: Diagnose with labs and aspiration. Prevention is mainstay: perioperative antibiotics, meticulous prep/drape technique, etc. Acute/subacute: irrigation & debridement with PE exchange. Late: one- or two-stage revision.</li><li>Loosening: Patient often complains of "start up" pain. Radiolucent lines seen on plain radiographs. Most often caused by osteolysis. Osteolysis caused from macrophage response to submicron-sized wear particles (usually PE).</li><li>Dislocation: Can be caused from component (either femur or acetabulum) malalignment or soft tissue injury/dysfunction. Decreased in posterior approach when short external rotators are repaired during closure.</li><li>Neurovascular injury<ul><li>Sciatic nerve: peroneal division (resulting in foot drop) at risk from vigorous retraction in posterior approach</li><li>Femoral nerve: with vigorous retraction in anterolateral approach</li><li>Obturator vessels: under the transverse acetabular lig., injured with retractors or anteroinferior quadrant cup screw</li><li>External iliac vessels: at risk if cup screw placed in anterosuperior quadrant (posterosuperior quadrant is safe)</li><li>Medial femoral circumflex artery: under quadratus femoris, at risk in posterior approach if muscle is taken down</li></ul></li><li>Heterotopic ossification: Usually in predisposed patients. Can cause decreased ROM. One dose of XRT can prevent it.</li><li>Medical complications: Deep venous thrombosis (DVT) & pulmonary embolus (PE) known risk of THA. Prophylaxis must be initiated.</li><li>Periprosthetic fracture of femur<ul><li>Stable implant: ORIF (plates, cables, +/− bone graft).</li><li>Unstable implant: replace with longer stem that passes fx site.</li></ul></li></ul>

Development dysplasia of hip

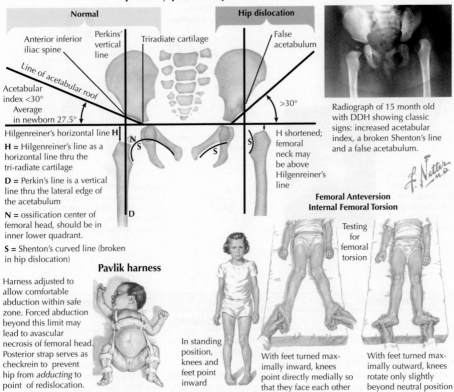

Normal

Anterior inferior iliac spine

Perkins' vertical line

Triradiate cartilage

Line of acetabular roof

Acetabular index <30°
Average in newborn 27.5°

Hilgenreiner's horizontal line **H**

H = Hilgenreiner's line as a horizontal line thru the tri-radiate cartilage

D = Perkin's line is a vertical line thru the lateral edge of the acetabulum

N = ossification center of femoral head, should be in inner lower quadrant.

S = Shenton's curved line (broken in hip dislocation)

Hip dislocation

False acetabulum

>30°

H shortened; femoral neck may be above Hilgenreiner's line

Radiograph of 15 month old with DDH showing classic signs: increased acetabular index, a broken Shenton's line and a false acetabulum.

Femoral Anteversion Internal Femoral Torsion

Testing for femoral torsion

Pavlik harness

Harness adjusted to allow comfortable abduction within safe zone. Forced abduction beyond this limit may lead to avascular necrosis of femoral head. Posterior strap serves as checkrein to prevent hip from *adducting* to point of redislocation.

In standing position, knees and feet point inward

With feet turned maximally inward, knees point directly medially so that they face each other

With feet turned maximally outward, knees rotate only slightly beyond neutral position

DESCRIPTION	EVALUATION	TREATMENT
DEVELOPMENTAL DYSPLASIA OF THE HIP (DDH)		
• Abnormal hip development resulting in dislocation, subluxation, or laxity of hip • Most from capsular laxity & positioning; irreducible teratologic form seen in congenital syndromes or neuromuscular diseases. • Risk factors: female, breech, first born, family hx, decreased uterine space conditions • Early diagnosis and treatment essential	**Hx:** Usually unnoticed by parents. +/− risk factors **PE:** Barlow (dislocation), + Ortolani (relocation), +/− Galeazzi test & decreased abduction **XR:** Useful after 6mo (femoral head begins to ossify). Look for position in acetabulum. Multiple radiographic lines help evaluate hip. **US:** Useful in neonate. Alpha angle >60 is nl.	**Obtain & maintain concentric reduction:** ○ 0-6mo: Pavlik harness ○ 6-24mo: Closed reduction, spica cast; open reduction if CR fails ○ 2-4yr: Open reduction with or without femoral osteotomy ○ >4yr: Acetabular osteotomy; teratologic hips need open treatment
COMPLICATIONS: Osteonecrosis of femoral head: can occur during reduction or from nonanatomic positioning postreduction.		
FEMORAL ANTEVERSION		
• Internal rotation of femur, femoral anteversion does not decrease properly • #1 cause of intoeing	**Hx:** Usually presents 3-6yr **PE:** Femur IR (IR>65°), patella points medial, intoeing gait	1. Most spontaneously resolve 2. Derotational osteotomy if it persists past age 10 (mostly cosmetic)

Slipped Capital Femoral Epiphysis

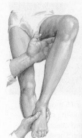

Best diagnostic sign is physical examination. With patient supine, as thigh is flexed it rolls into external rotation and abduction

Frog-leg radiograph, which demonstrates slipped epiphysis more clearly, always indicated when disorder is suspected

Slipped Capital Femoral Epiphysis: Operative Fixation

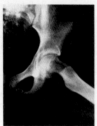

Threaded cannulated screw introduced over guide wire

Legg-Calve-Perthes Disease

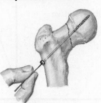

Young girl walking in Atlanta Scottish Rite Children's Hospital brace. Advantages of brace: allows child to walk without support, allows for further abduction by telescoping bar, and permits free knee and ankle motion

DESCRIPTION	EVALUATION	TREATMENT
LEGG-CALVE-PERTHES DISEASE		
• Idiopathic osteonecrosis of femoral head • Femoral head must revascularize, can take 2-5yr to complete • Prognosis good with onset <6yo & minimal lat. pillar involvement • Catterall & Herring classifications • Poor healing results in hip OA as adult	**Hx:** Boys (4:1), usually 4-8y.o. Limp with hip, thigh, or knee pain. No trauma. **PE:** Decr. ROM (esp. IR & abduction) **XR:** AP/lateral hip: sclerosis in early stages. "Crescent sign" sign of sub-chondral collapse/fx **MR:** Will show early necrosis when plain x-rays are still normal.	• Goals: 1. Relieve pain symptoms; 2. Maintain/obtain full ROM; 3. Contain femoral head • Traction, reduced weight-bearing • ROM: rest, traction, +/– therapy • Osteotomy: femoral or acetabular usually reserved for older patients
SLIPPED CAPITAL FEMORAL EPIPHYSIS (SCFE)		
• Displacement ("slip") of femoral epiphysis through the proximal physis • Classification: Stable: able to bear weight (WB); Unstable: unable to WB • Associated with obesity, renal & thyroid disease • Epiphysis is usually posterior to neck but remains in acetabulum.	**Hx:** 10-16y.o., obese, limp, hip or knee pain, +/– weight bear (WB) **PE:** Decr. ROM (esp. IR), hip ER with flexion, antalgic gait (if able to WB) **XR:** AP/lateral: BOTH hips, will show slip; Klein's line should intersect epiphysis. Graded on percent of epiphysis that slipped: Gr 1:<33%, Gr 2: 33-50%, Gr 3: >50%	• Percutaneous in situ screw fixation • One cannulated screw is gold stan-dard • Progressive slip may still occur • Forceful reduction NOT recom-mended • Prophylactic pinning of contralateral side is common and supported
COMPLICATIONS: Osteonecrosis (50% in unstable slips), chondrolysis, early osteoarthritis		
TRANSIENT SYNOVITIS		
• Aseptic hip effusion of unknown cause • May be caused by post viral syn-drome or overuse • Common cause of hip pain & limp • Diagnosis of exclusion, r/o septic hip	**Hx:** Ages 2-5y.o., M>F, insidious on-set limp **PE:** Decreased ROM (esp. abd), antal-gic gait **XR:** r/o other hip pathology **LABS:** CBC, ESR, blood culture **US:** Evaluate for effusion (if suspect septic hip)	• Aspirate hip under anesthesia with fluoroscopy if PE & labs indicate infection • Septic hip requires I&D and antibi-otics • Transient synovitis resolves: 2-10 days • Observation, rest, +/– NSAIDs

Anterior Approach to Hip

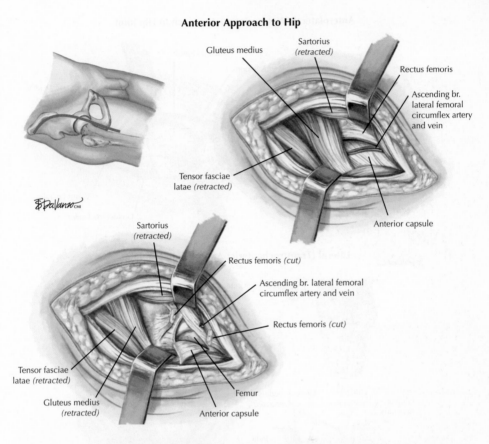

Illustration labels:

Gluteus medius
Sartorius *(retracted)*
Rectus femoris
Ascending br. lateral femoral circumflex artery and vein
Tensor fasciae latae *(retracted)*
Anterior capsule

Sartorius *(retracted)*
Rectus femoris *(cut)*
Ascending br. lateral femoral circumflex artery and vein
Rectus femoris *(cut)*
Tensor fasciae latae *(retracted)*
Gluteus medius *(retracted)*
Femur
Anterior capsule

USES	INTERNERVOUS PLANE	DANGERS	COMMENT
ANTERIOR (SMITH-PETERSON) APPROACH TO HIP			
Open reduction ○ Pediatric congenital hip dislocation ○ Adult anterior dislocations Irrigation & debridement Fractures: anterior femoral head (ORIF) Hemiarthroplasty Tumor excision	*Superficial* • Sartorius (femoral nerve) • Tensor fasciae latae (SGN) *Deep* • Rectus femoris (femoral n.) • Gluteus medius (SGN)	• Lateral femoral cutaneous n. • Femoral nerve • Ascending branch of lateral femoral circumflex artery	• Retract LFCN anteriorly • Ascending branch of LFCA must be ligated in approach • Take down both heads of rectus femoris to expose joint • Vigorous medial retraction can injure femoral nerve
MEDIAL (LUDLOFF) APPROACH TO HIP			
Pediatric hip dislocation Adductor or psoas release Irrigation & debridement	*Superficial:* Intermuscular plane • Adductor longus (obturator n.) • Gracilis (obturator n.) *Deep* • Adductor brevis (obturator n.) • Adductor magnus (obturator & sciatic n.)	• Obturator nerve (ant. division) • Medial femoral circumflex artery • Obturator nerve (post. division) • External pudendal artery (proximally)	• Used most in pediatric cases • Good access to transverse acetabular ligament & psoas tendon, which can block closed hip reduction. Poor access to acetabulum.

Anterolateral (Watson-Jones) Approach to Hip Joint

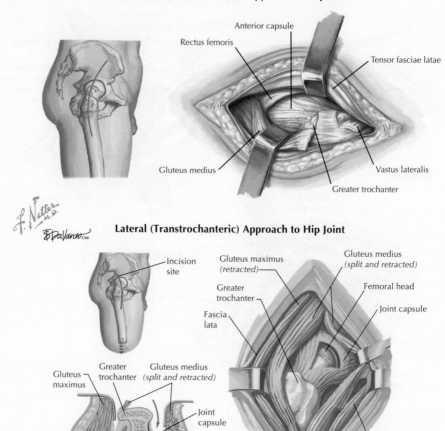

Anterior capsule

Rectus femoris

Tensor fasciae latae

Gluteus medius

Vastus lateralis

Greater trochanter

Lateral (Transtrochanteric) Approach to Hip Joint

Incision site

Gluteus maximus *(retracted)*

Gluteus medius *(split and retracted)*

Femoral head

Greater trochanter

Joint capsule

Fascia lata

Gluteus maximus

Greater trochanter

Gluteus medius *(split and retracted)*

Joint capsule

Femoral head

Acetabulum

Tensor fasciae latae

Vastus lateralis

USES	INTERNERVOUS PLANE	DANGERS	COMMENT
ANTEROLATERAL (WATSON-JONES) APPROACH TO HIP			
• Total hip arthroplasty • Hemiarthroplasty • ORIF of proximal femur fxs	Intermuscular plane • Tensor fasciae latae (SGN) • Gluteus medius (SGN)	• Descending branch of LFCA (under rectus femoris) • Femoral nerve	• Must detach abductors (either osteotomy or extensive release) • Vigorous medial retraction can injure femoral nerve
LATERAL (HARDINGE) APPROACH TO HIP			
• Total hip arthroplasty (not used for revisions)	• Split gluteus medius (superior gluteal n.) • Split vastus lateral n. distally (femoral n.)	• Superior gluteal artery • Femoral nerve • Femoral artery & vein • Superior gluteal nerve	• No osteotomy of greater trochanter required; less dislocation risk • Split gluteus medius ⅓ anterior, ⅔ posterior; release minimus

Posterior (Southern) Approach to Hip Joint

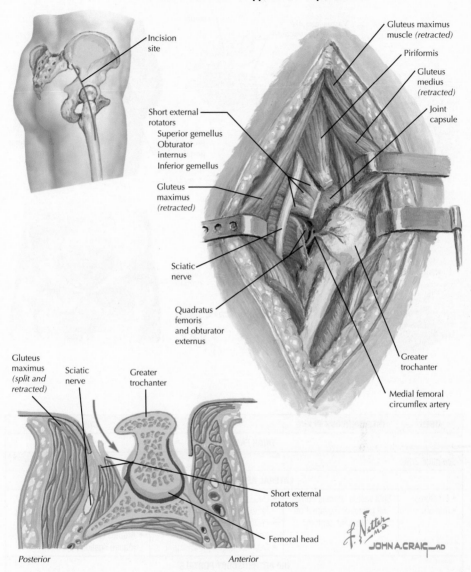

Incision site

Short external rotators
  Superior gemellus
  Obturator internus
  Inferior gemellus

Gluteus maximus *(retracted)*

Sciatic nerve

Quadratus femoris and obturator externus

Gluteus maximus muscle *(retracted)*

Piriformis

Gluteus medius *(retracted)*

Joint capsule

Greater trochanter

Medial femoral circumflex artery

Gluteus maximus *(split and retracted)*

Sciatic nerve

Greater trochanter

Short external rotators

Femoral head

Posterior

Anterior

JOHN A. CRAIG—AD

USES	INTERNERVOUS PLANE	DANGERS	COMMENT
POSTERIOR (MOORE/SOUTHERN) APPROACH TO HIP			
• Total hip arthroplasty • Hemiarthroplasty • Fractures/ORIF • Posterior hip dislocation	Split gluteus maximus (inferior gluteal n.)	• Sciatic nerve • Inferior gluteal artery • Medial femoral circum-flex artery (under quadratus femoris)	• Reflecting piriformis protects sciatic nerve • IGA injured in proximal extension • Repair short ERs to prevent dislocation

Lateral Approach to Thigh (Femur)

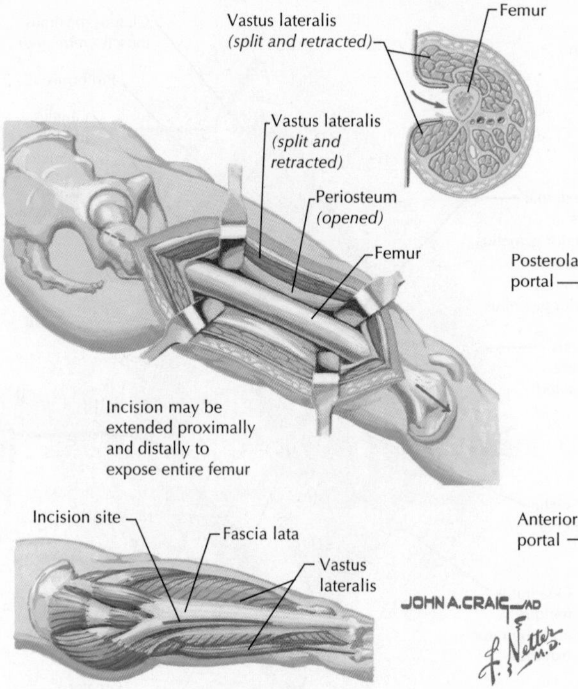

Hip Arthroscopy Portals

Vastus lateralis
(split and retracted)

Femur

Vastus lateralis
(split and retracted)

Periosteum
(opened)

Femur

Posterolateral portal

Anterolateral portal

Incision may be extended proximally and distally to expose entire femur

Incision site

Fascia lata

Vastus lateralis

Anterior portal

JOHN A. CRAIG—AD

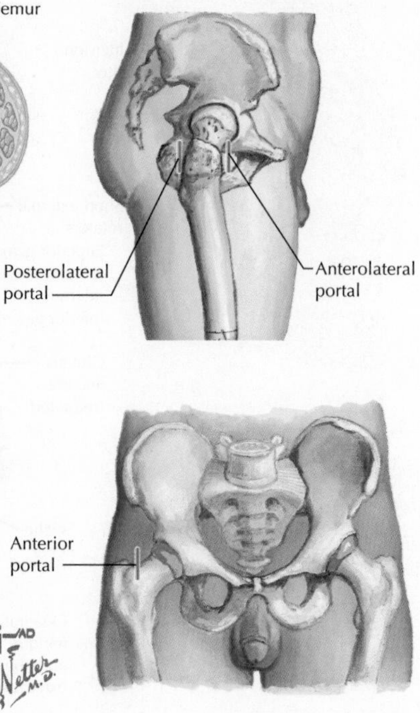

USES	INTERNERVOUS PLANE	DANGERS	COMMENT
THIGH FASCIOTOMIES			
See page 269.			
LATERAL APPROACH TO THIGH			
• Fractures • Tumors	Split vastus lateralis (femoral nerve) or elevate it off intermuscular septum	• Descending branch of lateral femoral circumflex artery • Perforates from profunda femoris • Superior lateral geniculate a.	• Incision can be large or small; made along line between greater trochanter and lateral condyle • Arteries (at left) encountered or require ligation
HIP ARTHROSCOPY PORTALS			
• Arthroscopy used for diagnosis, labral tears, loose body removal, synovectomy, irrigation, and debridement			
Anterior	Intersection of vertical line from ASIS and horizontal line from tip of GT	1. Lateral femoral cutaneous n. 2. Femoral nerve 3. Ascending branch of LFCA	Second portal. Angle 45° cephalad, 30° to midline. Pierce sartorius & rectus before capsule
Anterolateral	Anterior tip of greater trochanter (GT)	1. Superior gluteal nerve	Safest portal, establish 1st. Pierce gluteus medius & lateral capsule
Posterolateral	Posterior tip of greater trochanter (GT)	1. Sciatic nerve	Last portal. Pierce gluteus medius/minimus
• Long cannulae, arthroscope, instruments, and traction are needed for hip arthroscopy.			

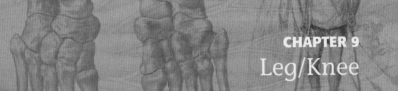

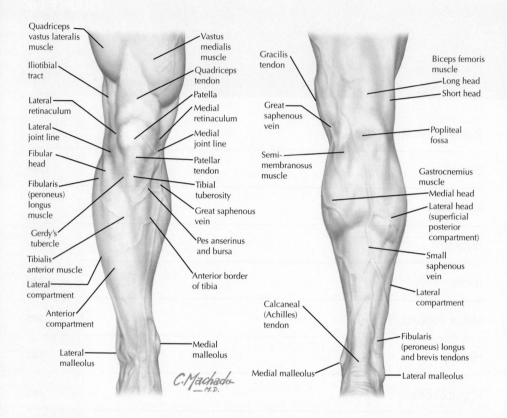

Labels (left figure):
- Quadriceps vastus lateralis muscle
- Iliotibial tract
- Lateral retinaculum
- Lateral joint line
- Fibular head
- Fibularis (peroneus) longus muscle
- Gerdy's tubercle
- Tibialis anterior muscle
- Lateral compartment
- Anterior compartment
- Lateral malleolus
- Vastus medialis muscle
- Quadriceps tendon
- Patella
- Medial retinaculum
- Medial joint line
- Patellar tendon
- Tibial tuberosity
- Great saphenous vein
- Pes anserinus and bursa
- Anterior border of tibia
- Medial malleolus

Labels (right figure):
- Gracilis tendon
- Great saphenous vein
- Semi-membranosus muscle
- Calcaneal (Achilles) tendon
- Medial malleolus
- Biceps femoris muscle
  - Long head
  - Short head
- Popliteal fossa
- Gastrocnemius muscle
  - Medial head
  - Lateral head (superficial posterior compartment)
- Small saphenous vein
- Lateral compartment
- Fibularis (peroneus) longus and brevis tendons
- Lateral malleolus

C.Machado —M.D.

STRUCTURE	CLINICAL APPLICATION
Iliotibial tract (band)	Tightness can cause lateral knee and/or thigh pain.
Quadriceps muscle	Atrophy can indicate an injury and/or contribute to knee pain.
Quadriceps tendon	Can rupture with eccentric loading. Defect is palpated here.
Patella	Tenderness can indicate fracture; swelling can be prepatellar bursitis.
Patellar tendon	Can rupture with eccentric loading. Defect is palpated here.
Patellar retinaculum	Patellar femoral ligaments palpated here. They can be injured in patellar dislocation. Plicae can also be palpated here.
Joint line	Tenderness here can indicate meniscal pathology.
Tibial tubercle	Tender in Osgood-Schlatter disease.
Pes anserinus & bursa	Insertion of medial hamstrings. Bursitis can develop. Site of hamstring tendon harvest.
Gerdy's tubercle	Insertion of the iliotibial tract (band).
Popliteal fossa	Popliteal artery pulse can be palpated here.
Muscle compartments	Will be firm or tense in compartment syndrome. Anterior most common.

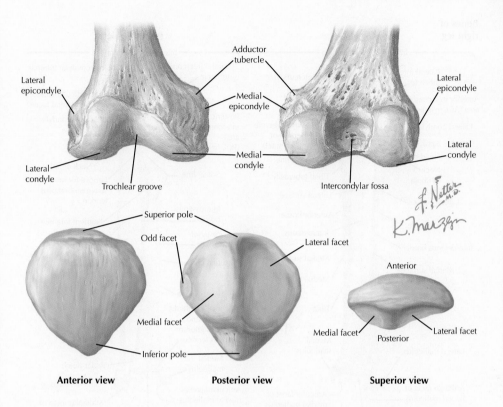

Anterior view   Posterior view   Superior view

CHARACTERISTICS	OSSIFY	FUSE	COMMENTS
DISTAL FEMUR			

• Distal femur—2 condyles
  ○ Medial: larger, more posterior
  ○ Lateral: more ant. & proximal
• Trochlear groove: a depression between the condyles anteriorly for patella articulation
• Intercondylar notch: between condyles, site of cruciate origins
	Secondary
	Distal Birth
	physis
		19yr	• Condyles: rounded posteriorly (for flexion) and flat anteriorly (for standing)
			  ○ Epicondyle: origin of collateral ligaments
			    ○ Epicondylar axis and/or post. condylar axis used to determine femur rotation (e.g., in TKA)
			• Sulcus terminale: groove in lateral condyle. Inferior to groove, it is weight-bearing portion of condyle.
			• Adductor tubercle: insertion of adductor magnus
			• Distal femoral physis: grows approx. 7mm/yr

PATELLA			

• Ovoid shaped, inf. & sup. poles
• Triangular in cross section
• 2 facets (larger lateral & medial) separated by a central ridge
  ○ Each facet is subdivided into superior, middle, inferior facets
  ○ Odd facet (7th sub-facet) is far medial on medial facet
	Primary 3yr
	(single center)
		11-13yr	• Largest sesamoid bone in body
			• Bipartite patella: failure of superolateral portion to fuse. It is often confused with a fracture.
			• Functions: 1. Enhances quadriceps pull (as fulcrum); 2. Protects knee; 3. Enhances knee lubrication
			• Contact point on patella moves proximally w/flexion
			• Odd facet articulates in deep flexion
			• Has thickest articular cartilage (up to 5mm)

Bones of right leg

Anterior view

Posterior view

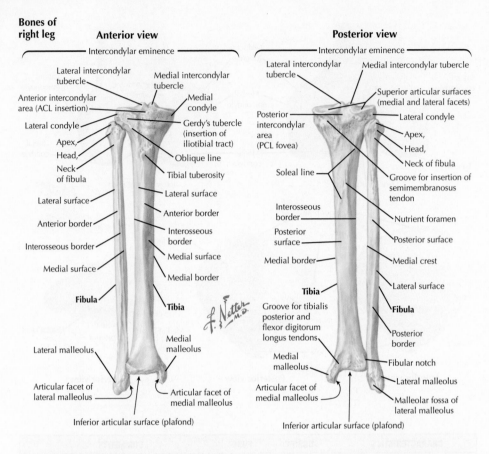

Intercondylar eminence

Lateral intercondylar tubercle

Medial intercondylar tubercle

Anterior intercondylar area (ACL insertion)

Medial condyle

Lateral condyle

Gerdy's tuberle (insertion of iliotibial tract)

Apex,

Head,

Neck of fibula

Oblique line

Tibial tuberosity

Lateral surface

Lateral surface

Anterior border

Anterior border

Interosseous border

Interosseous border

Medial surface

Medial surface

Medial border

Fibula

Tibia

Lateral malleolus

Medial malleolus

Articular facet of lateral malleolus

Articular facet of medial malleolus

Inferior articular surface (plafond)

Intercondylar eminence

Lateral intercondylar tubercle

Medial intercondylar tubercle

Superior articular surfaces (medial and lateral facets)

Lateral condyle

Posterior intercondylar area (PCL fovea)

Apex,

Head,

Neck of fibula

Soleal line

Groove for insertion of semimembranosus tendon

Interosseous border

Nutrient foramen

Posterior surface

Posterior surface

Medial border

Medial crest

Tibia

Lateral surface

Groove for tibialis posterior and flexor digitorum longus tendons

Fibula

Medial malleolus

Posterior border

Articular facet of medial malleolus

Fibular notch

Lateral malleolus

Malleolar fossa of lateral malleolus

Inferior articular surface (plafond)

CHARACTERISTICS	OSSIFY		FUSE	COMMENTS
TIBIA				
• Long bone characteristics	**Primary:** Shaft	7wk (fetal)	18 yr	• Lateral plateau fx more common
• Proximal end: plateau (canc.)				• Osgood-Schlatter: traction apophysitis at open tibial tubercle apophysis
◦ Medial plateau: concave				
◦ Lateral plateau: convex	**Secondary**		18-20yr	• Tubercle: patellar tendon insertion
◦ 7-10° posterior slope	1. Proximal epiphysis	9mo		• IM nail insertion point proximal to tibial tubercle
• Tubercle: 3cm below joint line	2. Distal epiphysis	1yr		
• Eminence: medial & lateral tubercles (spines)	3. Tibial tuberosity			• Tibial spine avulsion fx of ACL (peds)
• Shaft: triangular cross section				• Gerdy's tubercle on proximal tibia: insertion site of iliotibial tract (band)
• Distal end: pilon (cancellous)				• Fibularis incisura: lat. groove for fibula
◦ Articular surface: plafond				• Plafond is roof and medial malleolus is medial wall of ankle mortise
◦ Distal tip: medial malleolus				
FIBULA				
• Long bone characteristics	**Primary:** Shaft	7wk (fetal)	20yr	• LCL & biceps femoris insert on head
• Proximal end: head				• Neck has groove for peroneal nerve
◦ Neck				• Nerve can be injured in fibula fx
• Shaft: long, cylindrical	**Secondary**		18-22yr	• Shaft used for vascularized BG
• Distal end: lateral malleolus	1. Proximal epiphysis	1-3yr		• Lat. mal. is lat. wall of ankle mortise
	2. Distal epiphysis	4yr		

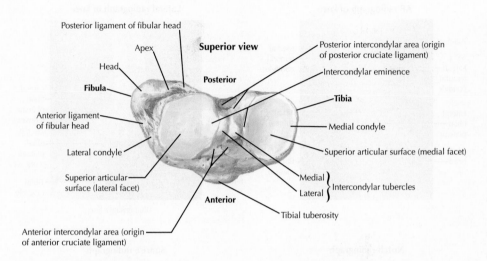

Posterior ligament of fibular head

Apex **Superior view** Posterior intercondylar area (origin of posterior cruciate ligament)

Head

Posterior Intercondylar eminence

Fibula

Tibia

Anterior ligament of fibular head

Medial condyle

Lateral condyle

Superior articular surface (medial facet)

Superior articular surface (lateral facet)

Medial ⎫
Lateral ⎬ Intercondylar tubercles
      ⎭

Anterior

Tibial tuberosity

Anterior intercondylar area (origin of anterior cruciate ligament)

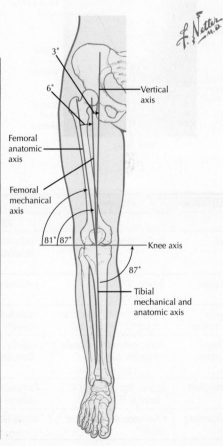

LOWER EXTREMITY ALIGNMENT	
Definitions	
Anatomic axis of femur	Line drawn along the axis of the femur
Anatomic axis of tibia	Line drawn along the axis of the tibia
Mechanical axis of femur	Line drawn between center of femoral head and intercondylar notch
Mechanical axis of tibia	Line drawn between center of knee and center of ankle mortise
Knee axis	Line drawn along inferior aspect of both femoral condyles
Vertical axis	Vertical line, perpendicular to the ground
Lateral distal femoral angle	Angle formed between knee axis and femoral axis laterally
Medial tibial angle	Angle formed between knee axis and tibial axis
Relationships	
Knee axis	Parallel to the ground and perpendicular to vertical axis
Mechanical axis of femur	Average of 6° from anatomic axis Approximately 3° from vertical axis
Mechanical axis of tibia	Normally same as anatomic axis of tibia unless tibia has a deformity
Lateral distal femoral angle	81° from femoral anatomic axis 87° from femoral mechanical axis
Medial proximal tibial angle	87° from tibial mechanical axis

3°

6°

Vertical axis

Femoral anatomic axis

Femoral mechanical axis

81° 87°

Knee axis

87°

Tibial mechanical and anatomic axis

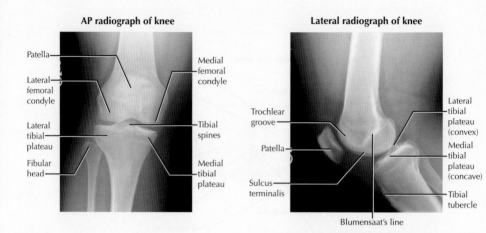

AP radiograph of knee

Patella

Lateral femoral condyle

Lateral tibial plateau

Fibular head

Medial femoral condyle

Tibial spines

Medial tibial plateau

Lateral radiograph of knee

Trochlear groove

Patella

Sulcus terminalis

Blumensaat's line

Lateral tibial plateau (convex)

Medial tibial plateau (concave)

Tibial tubercle

Notch radiograph

Lateral femoral condyle

Lateral tibial plateau

Intercondylar notch

Medial femoral condyle

Medial tibial plateau

Tibial spines

Sunrise radiograph

Lateral patellar facet

Lateral femoral condyle

Trochlear groove

Medial femoral condyle

Medial patellar facet

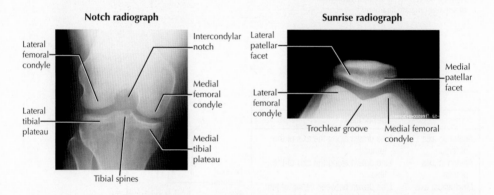

RADIOGRAPH	TECHNIQUE	FINDINGS	CLINICAL APPLICATION
KNEE			
AP	Supine; beam at 90°	Medial/lateral compartments; varus/valgus deformity	Femoral condyle, tibial plateau/ spine, patella fx, OCD, osteo- arthritis (weight-bearing)
Lateral	Supine; 30° flexion	Patellofemoral compartment	Fractures, quadriceps/patellar tendon rupture
Axial/ sunrise	Prone; knee 115° flex; beam at patella 15° cephalad	Patellofemoral compartment (patellar articular facets)	Patellofemoral arthritis, mal- alignment or patellar tilt
Tunnel/ notch	Prone; knee 45° flex; beam is caudal at knee joint	Posterior femoral condyles, inter- condylar notch, tibial eminence	Osteochondral fx/defect, femo- ral condyle or tibial eminence fx, DJD/osteoarthritis
Merchant	Supine; legs of table at 45°; beam at PF joint	Patellofemoral compartment (patellar articular facets)	Articular surface lesions, DJD, tilt or malalignment
Rosenberg	PA (weight-bearing); knees at 45°	Medial/lateral compartments	Osteoarthritis of WB portion of posterior condyles

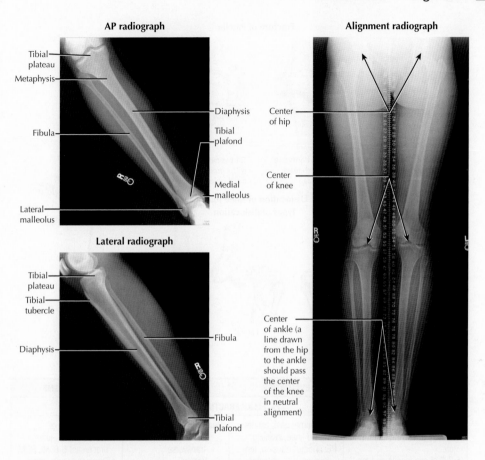

AP radiograph

Tibial plateau
Metaphysis
Fibula
Lateral malleolus
Diaphysis
Tibial plafond
Medial malleolus

Alignment radiograph

Center of hip
Center of knee
Center of ankle (a line drawn from the hip to the ankle should pass the center of the knee in neutral alignment)

Lateral radiograph

Tibial plateau
Tibial tubercle
Diaphysis
Fibula
Tibial plafond

RADIOGRAPH	TECHNIQUE	FINDINGS	CLINICAL APPLICATION
LEG			
AP tibia	Supine; beam at mid tibia	Tibia and surrounding soft tissues	Fractures, deformity, infection, etc
Lateral tibia	Supine; beam laterally mid-tibia	Tibia and surrounding soft tissues	Fractures, deformity, infection, etc
See Foot & Ankle chapter to see views of the ankle.			
OTHER STUDIES			
Alignment films	Bilateral full length hip to ankle, WB	Full lower extremity alignment	Determine malalignment/deformity
Scanogram	Entire bilateral LE with ruler	Measure length of bones	Used for leg length discrepancy
CT	Axial, coronal, & sagittal views	Articular congruity, fracture fragments	Intraarticular condyle, plateau, pilon fxs
MRI	Sequence protocols vary	Soft tissues: ligaments, meniscus, articular cartilage, bone marrow	Ligament ruptures, meniscal tears, OCD, stress fxs, tumor, infection
Bone scan	Radioisotope	All bones evaluated	Stress fxs, infection, tumor

Fracture of Patella

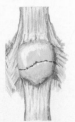

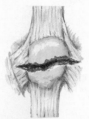

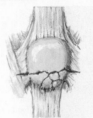

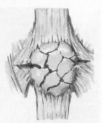

Nondisplaced trans-verse fracture with intact retinacula

Displaced transverse fracture with tears in retinacula

Transverse fracture with comminution of distal pole

Severely comminuted fracture

Dislocation of Knee Joint
Types of dislocation

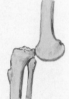

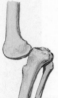

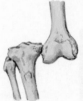

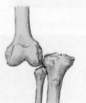

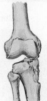

Anterior   Posterior   Lateral   Medial   Rotational

DESCRIPTION	EVALUATION	CLASSIFICATION	TREATMENT
PATELLAR FRACTURE			

• Mechanism: direct & indirect: e.g., fall, dashboard, etc.
• Pull of quadriceps and tendons displace most fxs
• If intact, retinaculum resists displacement of fragments
• Do not confuse with bipartite patella (unfused superolateral corner)
	Hx: Trauma, pain, cannot extend knee, swelling
	PE: "Dome" effusion, tenderness, +/– palpable defect, inability to extend knee
	XR: Knee trauma series
	CT: Not usually needed, will show fx fragments
		Descriptive/location:
		  ○ Nondisplaced
		  ○ Transverse
		  ○ Vertical
		  ○ Stellate
		  ○ Inferior/superior pole
		  ○ Comminuted
			• Nondisplaced or comminuted—knee brace/cast 6-8 wk, ROM
			• Displaced (>2-3mm): ORIF (e.g., tension bands) to restore articular surface
			• Severely comminuted: may require full or partial patellectomy

COMPLICATIONS: Osteoarthritis and/or pain, decreased motion and/or strength, osteonecrosis, refracture			
KNEE DISLOCATION			

• Rare: ortho. emergency
• Usually high-energy injury
• Multiple ligaments & other soft tissue are disrupted
• High incidence of associated fx & neurovascular injury
• Many spontaneously reduce; must keep index of suspicion for injury
• Close follow-up is important for good result
	Hx: Trauma, pain, inability to bear weight
	PE: Large effusion, soft tissue swelling, deformity, pain, +/– distal pulses/peroneal nerve function
	XR: AP/lateral
	AGRAM: Evaluate for arterial injury
	MR: Ligament injury, meniscus, articular cartilage injury
		By position:
		  ○ Anterior
		  ○ Posterior
		  ○ Lateral
		  ○ Medial
		  ○ Rotatory: anteromedial or anterolateral
			• Early reduction essential; postreduction neurologic exam and x-rays
			• Immobilize (cast) 6-8wk (if ligaments not torn)
			• Surgery if irreducible or vascular injury (revascularize within 6 hr + fasciotomy).
			• Early vs. delayed ligament repair/reconstruction

COMPLICATIONS: Neurovascular: popliteal artery, peroneal nerve injury, knee stiffness (#1), chronic instability			

Tibial Plateau Fracture

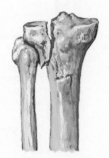

I. Split fracture of lateral tibial plateau

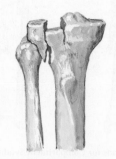

II. Split fracture of lateral condyle plus depression of tibial plateau

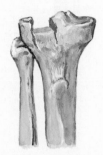

III. Depression of lateral tibial plateau without split fracture

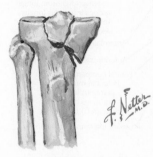

IV. Comminuted split fracture of medial tibial plateau and tibial spine

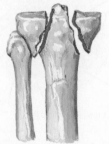

V. Bicondylar fracture involving both tibial plateaus with widening

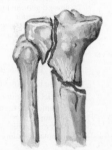

VI. Fracture of lateral tibial plateau with separation of metaphyseal-diaphyseal junction

DESCRIPTION	EVALUATION	CLASSIFICATION	TREATMENT
TIBIAL PLATEAU FRACTURE			
• Mechanism: axial load AND varus/valgus stress • Restoration of articular surface/congruity is important • Metaphyseal injury: bone will compress, leading to functional bone loss; may need bone graft • Lateral fracture more common than medial • Associated meniscal (50%) and ligament (MCL>ACL) tears	**Hx:** Trauma, pain, swelling, inability to bear weight **PE:** Effusion, tenderness; do thorough neurovascular exam. **XR:** Knee trauma series **CT:** To better define fx lines & comminution. Needed for preop planning. **AGRAM:** If decreased pulses. Consider in all type IV fxs	**Schatzker (6 types):** I: Lateral plateau split fx II: Lat. split/depression fx III: Lat. plateau depression IV: Medial plat. split fx V: Bicondylar plateau fx VI: Fx w/metaphyseal-diaphyseal separation Types IV-VI usually result from high-energy trauma	• Consider joint aspiration • Nondisplaced (<3mm step off,<5mm gapping): knee brace/cast 6-8wk, NWB 6-12wk • Displaced: ORIF +/− bone graft (plates & screws). Early ROM but NWB 12wk • Avoid both medial & lateral periosteal stripping (incr. nonunion rate) • Repair torn ligaments/menisci
COMPLICATIONS: compartment syndrome, posttraumatic osteoarthritis, persistent knee pain, popliteal artery injury			

Fracture of Shaft of Tibia

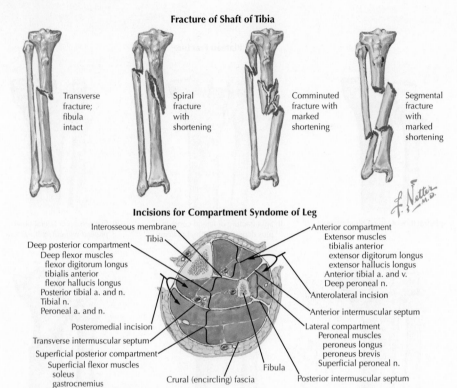

Transverse fracture; fibula intact

Spiral fracture with shortening

Comminuted fracture with marked shortening

Segmental fracture with marked shortening

Incisions for Compartment Syndome of Leg

Interosseous membrane
Tibia
Deep posterior compartment
Deep flexor muscles
flexor digitorum longus
tibialis anterior
flexor hallucis longus
Posterior tibial a. and n.
Tibial n.
Peroneal a. and n.
Posteromedial incision
Transverse intermuscular septum
Superficial posterior compartment
Superficial flexor muscles
soleus
gastrocnemius
plantaris tendon
Crural (encircling) fascia
Fibula

Anterior compartment
Extensor muscles
tibialis anterior
extensor digitorum longus
extensor hallucis longus
Anterior tibial a. and v.
Deep peroneal n.
Anterolateral incision
Anterior intermuscular septum
Lateral compartment
Peroneal muscles
peroneus longus
peroneus brevis
Superficial peroneal n.
Posterior intermuscular septum

DESCRIPTION	EVALUATION	CLASSIFICATION	TREATMENT
TIBIA SHAFT FRACTURE			
• Common long bone fx • Usually high-E trauma • Condition of surrounding soft tissues is critically important to success of outcome • Compartment syndrome: consider in ALL fxs • Subcutaneous position of tibia predisposes it to open fractures • May lead to amputation	**Hx:** Trauma, pain, swelling, inability to bear weight **PE:** Swelling, deformity, +/− firm/tense compartments **XR:** AP & lateral of tib./fib. (also knee & ankle series) **CT:** Not usually needed **AGRAM:** If decreased pulses	**Descriptive:** Location Displaced/comminuted Type: transverse, spiral oblique Rotation/angulation	• Nondisplaced: long leg cast 8wk (best for pediatrics, seldom used in adults) • Displaced/unstable: reamed, locked IM nail • Open fractures: thorough I&D is critical. External fixation is useful for these fractures. • Fasciotomies for compartment syndrome
COMPLICATIONS: compartment syndrome, nonunion & malunion, knee pain (from IM nail), ankle and/or knee stiffness			
COMPARTMENT SYNDROME			
• Incr. pressure in closed space/compartment • Compartments (4): have rigid fibroosseous borders • Mechanism: trauma (fracture, crush) vascular injury, burn	**Hx:** Trauma, pain **PE:** 5 P's: pain (w/passive stretch), paresthesia, pallor, pulseless, paralysis Firm/tense compartments	**XR:** Evaluate for fractures **Angiogram:** If needed to evaluate for vascular inj. **Compartment Pressures:** 1. Absolute: >30-40mmHg 2. ΔP: <30mmHg of diastolic blood pressure	• Usually a clinical diagnosis • Emergent fasciotomy (usually two incisions)

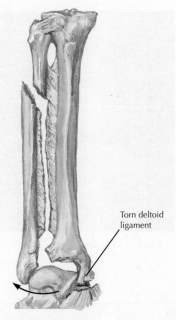

Torn deltoid ligament

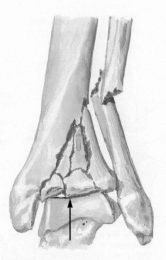

Pilon fracture
Usual cause is vertical loading of ankle joint, eg, falling from height and landing on heel (usually with ankle dorsiflexed). Fracture and compression of articular surface of tibia plus separation of malleoli and fracture of fibula

Maisonneuve fracture
Complete disruption of tibiofibular syndesmosis with diastasis caused by external rotation of talus and transmission of force to proximal fibula, resulting in high fracture of fibula. Interosseous membrane torn longitudinally. Radiograph shows repair with long transverse screw (these fractures easily missed on radiographs)

DESCRIPTION	EVALUATION	CLASSIFICATION	TREATMENT
MAISONNEUVE FRACTURE			

• Complete syndesmosis disruption with diastasis & proximal fibula fx
• Variant of ankle fracture & deltoid ligament rupture
• Unstable fracture
	Hx: Trauma, ankle pain, +/− knee pain
	PE: Ankle pain, swelling, proximal fibula tenderness
	XR: Leg and ankle series. May need stress views of ankle to see instability
		Descriptive:
		Location
		Type: Spiral
		     Oblique
		     Comminuted
			Reduce and stabilize syndesmosis (e.g., with a screw); immobilize while healing

COMPLICATIONS: ankle instability, ankle arthritis			
PILON (DISTAL TIBIA) FRACTURE			
• Intraarticular: through distal articular/WB surface • Soft tissue swelling leads to complications with early open treatment • Restoration of articular surface congruity is essential • Healing is often slow	**Hx:** Trauma, cannot bear weight, pain, swelling **PE:** Effusion, tenderness; do good neurovascular exam **XR:** AP/lateral (obliques) **CT:** Needed to better define fx and preop plan	**Ruedi/Allgower** (3 types): I: Non or minimally displaced II: Displaced: articular surface incongruous III: Comminuted articular surface	• Nondisplaced: cast & NWB for 6-12wk • Displaced/comminuted: early external fixation and delayed (14 days) ORIF; (plates & screws +/− bone grafting)
COMPLICATIONS: posttraumatic DJD, (almost 100% in comminuted fxs), stiffness, malunion, wound complications			

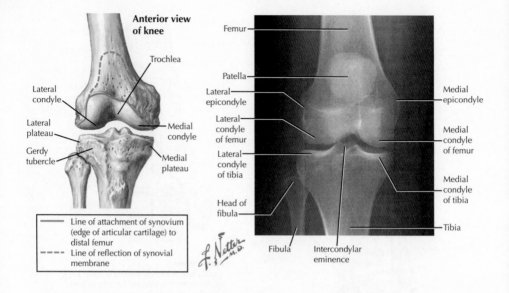

Anterior view of knee

Trochlea

Lateral condyle

Lateral plateau

Gerdy tubercle

Medial condyle

Medial plateau

——— Line of attachment of synovium (edge of articular cartilage) to distal femur

– – – Line of reflection of synovial membrane

Femur

Patella

Lateral epicondyle

Lateral condyle of femur

Lateral condyle of tibia

Head of fibula

Medial epicondyle

Medial condyle of femur

Medial condyle of tibia

Tibia

Fibula   Intercondylar eminence

KNEE
Structure

- Comprises 3 separate articulations
  - Medial & lateral femorotibial joints (2)—condyloid (hinge) joints. Femoral condyles articulate with corresponding tibial plateaus.
  - Patellofemoral joint (1)—sellar (gliding) joint. Patella articulates with femoral trochlear groove.
- 3 compartments in the knee: medial, lateral, patellofemoral
- Capsule surrounds entire joint (all three articulations/compartments) and extends proximally into the suprapatellar pouch.
  - The capsule has a synovial lining that also covers the cruciate ligaments (making them intraarticular but extrasynovial)
- Articular (hyaline) cartilage (type II collagen) covers the femoral condyles, tibial plateaus, trochlear groove, and patellar facets.
- Menisci are interposed in the medial & lateral femorotibial joints to: 1.protect the articular cartilage, 2. give support to the knee.
- Knee axis (line drawn between weight-bearing portion of medial & lateral femoral condyles) is parallel to the ground.
  - Mechanical axis of the femur is 3° valgus to the vertical axis, allowing the larger MFC to align with the LFC parallel to the ground.
  - Mechanical axis of the tibia is 3° varus to the vertical axis (87° to knee axis).

Kinematics

- Inherently unstable joint. Bony morphology adds little stability. Stability primarily provided by surrounding static and dynamic stabilizers. (Dynamic stabilizers may compensate when static stabilizers are injured [e.g., complete or partial ACL rupture].)
  - Medial: Static—superficial and deep medial collateral ligaments (MCL), posterior oblique ligament (POL).
    Dynamic—semimembranosus, vastus medialis, medial gastrocnemius, PES tendons
  - Lateral: Static—lateral collateral ligament (LCL), iliotibial band (ITB), arcuate ligament.
    Dynamic—popliteus, biceps femoris, lateral gastrocnemius
- Not a simple hinge joint. The knee has 6 degrees of motion:
  - Extension/flexion, IR/ER, varus/valgus, anterior/posterior translation, medial/lateral translation, compression/distraction
- Flexion & extension are the primary motions in the knee.
  - Flexion is a combination of both "rolling" and "sliding" of the femur on the tibia in varying ratios depending on the degree of flexion.
  - Rolling: equal translation of tibiofemoral contact point & joint axis. Rolling predominates in early flexion.
  - Gliding: translation of tibiofemoral contact point without moving the joint axis. Increased gliding is needed for deep flexion.
  - The cruciate ligaments control the roll/glide function. The PCL alone can maintain this function (e.g., PCL retaining TKA).
  - Normal motion: Extension/flexion: −5 to 140°. 115° needed to get out of a chair; 130° needed for fast running.
- IR/ER: about 10° total through arc of motion. Tibia IRs in swing, and ERs in stance via "screw home mechanism."
  - Screw home mechanism: larger MFC ERs tibia in full extension, tightening cruciates and stabilizing the knee in stance.
  - Popliteus IRs the tibia to "unlock" the knee, loosen the cruciates, which allows the knee to initiate flexion.
- Other motions: Medial/lateral translation: minimal in normal knees
  - Anterior/posterior translation: dependent on tissue laxity, usually within 2mm of contralateral side in normal knees
  - Varus/valgus: approximately 5mm of gapping laterally or medially when stressed in normal knees

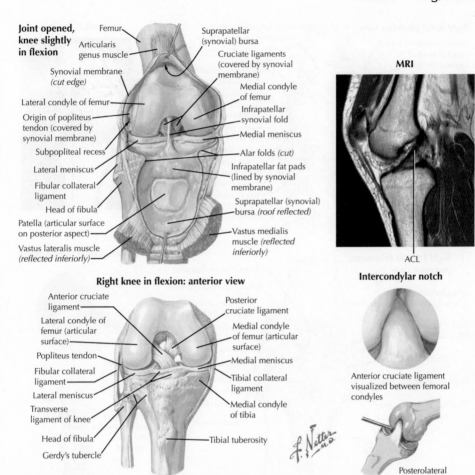

Joint opened, knee slightly in flexion

- Femur
- Articularis genus muscle
- Synovial membrane *(cut edge)*
- Lateral condyle of femur
- Origin of popliteus tendon (covered by synovial membrane)
- Subpopliteal recess
- Lateral meniscus
- Fibular collateral ligament
- Head of fibula
- Patella (articular surface on posterior aspect)
- Vastus lateralis muscle *(reflected inferiorly)*

- Suprapatellar (synovial) bursa
- Cruciate ligaments (covered by synovial membrane)
- Medial condyle of femur
- Infrapatellar synovial fold
- Medial meniscus
- Alar folds *(cut)*
- Infrapatellar fat pads (lined by synovial membrane)
- Suprapatellar (synovial) bursa *(roof reflected)*
- Vastus medialis muscle *(reflected inferiorly)*

MRI

ACL

Right knee in flexion: anterior view

- Anterior cruciate ligament
- Lateral condyle of femur (articular surface)
- Popliteus tendon
- Fibular collateral ligament
- Lateral meniscus
- Transverse ligament of knee
- Head of fibula
- Gerdy's tubercle

- Posterior cruciate ligament
- Medial condyle of femur (articular surface)
- Medial meniscus
- Tibial collateral ligament
- Medial condyle of tibia
- Tibial tuberosity

Intercondylar notch

Anterior cruciate ligament visualized between femoral condyles

Posterolateral

LIGAMENTS	ATTACHMENTS	FUNCTION/COMMENT
KNEE		
Femorotibial Joint—Anterior Structures		
Anterior cruciate ligament (ACL) Anteromedial bundle Posterolateral bundle	Posteromedial aspect of lateral femoral condyle to anterior tibial eminence	Primary restraint to anterior tibial translation; secondary restraint to varus (in extension) & IR Tight in knee flexion, lax in extension Tight in knee extension, lax in flexion
Transverse meniscal ligament	Connects both anterior horns of menisci to tibia	Stabilizes menisci; can be torn/injured
Other Structures		
Ligamentum mucosum (anterior plica)	Distal femoral articulation to anterior tibial plateau	Synovial remnant. Covers anterior notch (ACL); may need to be debrided for full visualization
Infrapatellar fat pad	Posterior to patellar tendon, anterior to intercondylar notch	Cushions patellar tendon. Can become fibrotic or impinged on, causing knee pain (Hoffa syndrome)
See Patellofemoral Joint for other anterior structures		

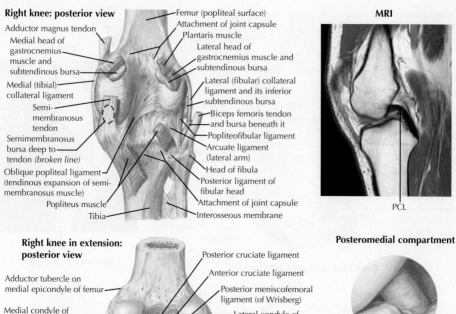

Right knee: posterior view

- Femur (popliteal surface)
- Attachment of joint capsule
- Adductor magnus tendon
- Plantaris muscle
- Medial head of gastrocnemius muscle and subtendinous bursa
- Lateral head of gastrocnemius muscle and subtendinous bursa
- Medial (tibial) collateral ligament
- Lateral (fibular) collateral ligament and its inferior subtendinous bursa
- Semi-membranosus tendon
- Biceps femoris tendon and bursa beneath it
- Semimembranosus bursa deep to tendon (broken line)
- Popliteofibular ligament
- Arcuate ligament (lateral arm)
- Oblique popliteal ligament (tendinous expansion of semimembranosus muscle)
- Head of fibula
- Posterior ligament of fibular head
- Popliteus muscle
- Attachment of joint capsule
- Tibia
- Interosseous membrane

MRI

PCL

Right knee in extension: posterior view

- Posterior cruciate ligament
- Adductor tubercle on medial epicondyle of femur
- Anterior cruciate ligament
- Posterior meniscofemoral ligament (of Wrisberg)
- Medial condyle of femur (articular surface)
- Lateral condyle of femur (articular surface)
- Medial meniscus
- Popliteus tendon
- Tibial collateral ligament
- Fibular collateral ligament
- Medial condyle of tibia
- Lateral meniscus
- Head of fibula

F. Netter M.D.

Posteromedial compartment

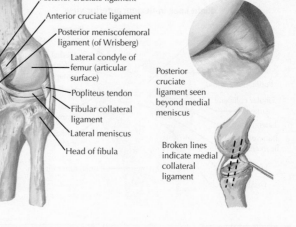

Posterior cruciate ligament seen beyond medial meniscus

Broken lines indicate medial collateral ligament

LIGAMENTS	ATTACHMENTS	COMMENTS
KNEE		
Femorotibial Joint—Posterior Structures		
Posterior cruciate ligament (PCL)	Lateral aspect (in notch) of medial femoral condyle to post. proximal tibia (below joint line)	Primary restraint to posterior tibial translation Secondary restraint to varus, valgus, and ER
Anterolateral bundle	Ant. origin on condyle, lat. on tibia	Tight in knee flexion, lax in extension
Posteromedial bundle	Post. origin on condyle, med. on tibia	Tight in knee extension, lax in flexion
Meniscofemoral ligaments	Posterior lateral meniscus to MFC and/or PCL, either:	Variably present. Rarely are both present
Ligament of Humphrey	Anterior to PCL	Contributes to PCL function & stabilizes meniscus
Ligament of Wrisberg	Posterior to PCL	Contributes to PCL function & stabilizes meniscus
Oblique popliteal ligament (OPL)	Origin on semimembranosus insertion on posterior tibia; inserts on posterior LFC & capsule	Tightens posterior capsule when semimembranosus contracts; considered part of "posteromedial" corner

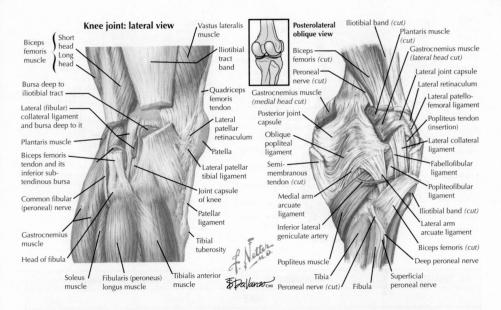

Knee joint: lateral view — Posterolateral oblique view

LIGAMENTS	ATTACHMENTS	FUNCTION/COMMENT
KNEE		
Femorotibial Joint—Lateral and Posterolateral Structures		
First Layer—Superficial		
Iliotibial band (tract) (ITB)	3 insertions: 1.Gerdy's tubercle, 2. patella and patellar tendon, 3. supracondylar tubercle	Stabilizes lateral knee—"accessory anterolateral ligament." Post. in flexion (ERs tibia), ant. in extension
Biceps femoris	2 heads insert on fibular head, lateral to LCL	Lateral stabilizer, also externally rotates tibia
Second Layer—Middle		
Lateral patellofemoral ligament Lateral patellar retinaculum	Lateral femur to lateral edge of patella Vastus fascia to tibia & patella	May need release if tightened and causing patella tilt and abnormal lateral articular cartilage wear
Third Layer—Deep		
SUPERFICIAL LAMINA		
Lateral collateral lig. (LCL)	Lateral epicondyle to medial fibular head	Primary restraint to varus stress, also resists ER
Fabellofibular ligament	Fibula head to fabella, usually with arcuate lig.	Variably present, also called "short collateral"
DEEP LAMINA		
Popliteus muscle and tendon	Inserts anterior and distal to LCL origin	Resists tibia ER, varus, and posterior translation
Popliteofibular ligament (PFL)	Popliteus musculotendinous jxn to fibula head	Primary static restraint to external rotation (ER)
Capsule	Femur to tibia. Extends 15mm below joint line	Reinforced by other structures; resists varus & ER
Arcuate ligament	Lateral arm: fibular head to posterior femur Medial arm: post-lat femur, blends with OPL	Variably present, Y-shaped: two arms. Lateral arm covers popliteus supporting posterolateral knee
Other		
Lateral meniscus	To lateral plateau via coronary ligaments	Gives concavity to the convex lateral plateau
Lateral head of gastrocnemius	Origin is on posterior lateral condyle	Adds dynamic support to posterolateral knee

- The inferior lateral geniculate artery passes between the superficial and deep lamina of the third layer of the posterolateral corner.
- The LCL, popliteus, and popliteofibular ligament are the most consistent structures and are the focus of surgical reconstruction.
- Most of the posterolateral structures act as stabilizers to varus & ER forces. They also are secondary stabilizers to posterior translation.
- Arcuate "complex" refers to posterolateral stabilizing structures including: LCL, arcuate ligament, popliteus, & lateral gastrocnemius.

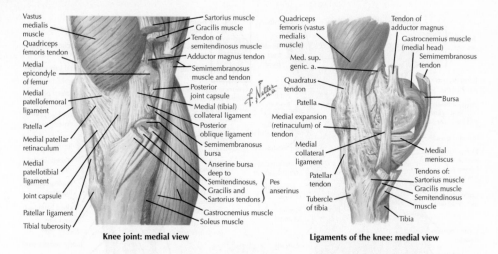

Knee joint: medial view

Ligaments of the knee: medial view

LIGAMENTS	ATTACHMENTS	FUNCTION/COMMENT
	KNEE	
	Femorotibial Joint—Medial Structures	
	First Layer—Superficial	
Sartorius	Becomes fascial layer at insertion at Pes	Covers other tendons at Pes insertion
Fascia	Deep fascia from thigh continues to knee	Blends with retinaculum (ant.) & capsule (post.)
	Second Layer—Middle	
Superficial medial collateral (MCL)	Medial epicondyle to tibia (deep to Pes) Broad insertion is 5-7cm below joint line	Primary restraint to valgus force (esp. at 30°) Secondary stabilizer to anterior translation & IR
Posterior oblique ligament (POL)	Adductor tubercle (post. to MCL) to posterior tibia, PH of med. meniscus, & capsule	Static stabilizer against valgus. Lax in flexion but tightens dynamically due to semimembr.
Medial patellofemoral ligament (MPFL)	Medial patella to medial femoral epicondyle	Primary static stabilizer against patella lateralization; may need repair/reconstruction after dx
Medial patellar retinaculum	Continuous w/vastus fascia to tibia & patella	Can also be injured in lateral patellar subluxation
Semimembranosus	Inserts posteromedial on tibia	Gives posteromedial support
	Third Layer—Deep	
Deep medial collateral (MCL) Meniscofemoral fibers Meniscotibial fibers	Inserts on medial meniscus & tibia plateau 2 sets of fibers: Femur to meniscus Tibia to meniscus	Stabilizes meniscus. Also known as medial capsular ligament or middle ⅓ capsular ligament
Capsule	Femur to tibia, extends 15mm below joint	Reinforced by other posteromedial structures
	Other	
Medial meniscus	Attached firmly to medial tibial plateau via coronary ligaments	Posterior horn is secondary stabilizer to anterior translation. Becomes 1° in ACL
Medial head of gastrocnemius	Origin on the posteromedial femur	Provides some minor additional dynamic support

- Gracilis and semitendinosus tendons are between layers 1 and 2 and act as secondary dynamic medial stabilizers.
- The POL is a confluence of layers 2 and 3 tissues that are indistinct in the posteromedial aspect of the knee.

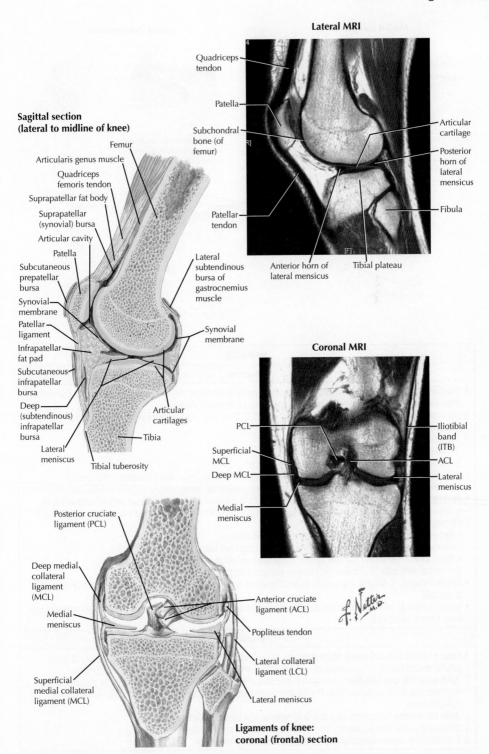

Lateral MRI

Quadriceps tendon

Patella

Subchondral bone (of femur)

Patellar tendon

Anterior horn of lateral mensicus

Tibial plateau

Articular cartilage

Posterior horn of lateral mensicus

Fibula

Sagittal section (lateral to midline of knee)

Femur

Articularis genus muscle

Quadriceps femoris tendon

Suprapatellar fat body

Suprapatellar (synovial) bursa

Articular cavity

Patella

Subcutaneous prepatellar bursa

Synovial membrane

Patellar ligament

Infrapatellar fat pad

Subcutaneous infrapatellar bursa

Deep (subtendinous) infrapatellar bursa

Lateral meniscus

Tibial tuberosity

Lateral subtendinous bursa of gastrocnemius muscle

Synovial membrane

Articular cartilages

Tibia

Coronal MRI

PCL

Superficial MCL

Deep MCL

Medial meniscus

Iliotibial band (ITB)

ACL

Lateral meniscus

Posterior cruciate ligament (PCL)

Deep medial collateral ligament (MCL)

Medial meniscus

Superficial medial collateral ligament (MCL)

Anterior cruciate ligament (ACL)

Popliteus tendon

Lateral collateral ligament (LCL)

Lateral meniscus

Ligaments of knee: coronal (frontal) section

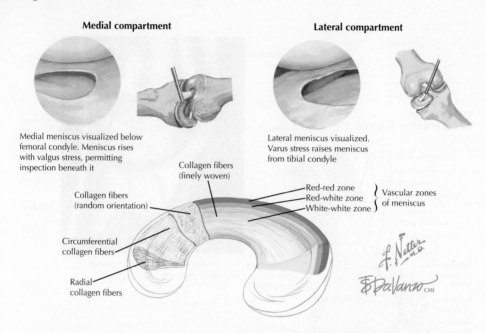

Medial compartment

Medial meniscus visualized below femoral condyle. Meniscus rises with valgus stress, permitting inspection beneath it

Lateral compartment

Lateral meniscus visualized. Varus stress raises meniscus from tibial condyle

Collagen fibers (finely woven)

Collagen fibers (random orientation)

Circumferential collagen fibers

Radial collagen fibers

Red-red zone
Red-white zone
White-white zone

} Vascular zones of meniscus

MENISCUS
Structure

- Fibrocartilage discs interposed in femorotibial joints between femoral condyles and tibial plateaus. Have a triangular cross section—thickest at the periphery, then tapering to a thin central edge.
- Histologically made up of collagen (mostly type 1, also 2, 3, 5, 6), cells (fibrochondrocytes), water, proteoglycans, glycoproteins, elastin
- 3 layers seen microscopically:
  1. Superficial layer: woven collagen fiber pattern
  2. Surface layer: randomly oriented collagen fiber pattern
  3. Middle (deepest) layer: circumferential (longitudinal) oriented fibers. These fibers dissipate hoop stresses. Radial fibers. These fibers acts as "ties" to hold the circumferential fibers.
- Vascular supply from superior and inferior medial and lateral geniculate arteries. They form perimeniscal plexus in synovium/capsule. Peripheral portion (10-30% medially, 10-25% laterally) is vascular via vessels from the perimeniscal plexus. 3 zones:
  ○ Red zone: 3mm from capsular junction (most tears will heal)
  ○ Red/white zone: 3-5mm from capsular junction (some tears will heal)
  ○ White zone: >5mm from capsular junction (most tears will not heal)
  The central, avascular ⅔ of the menisci receive nutrition from the synovial fluid
- Medial meniscus: C-shaped, less mobile, firmly attached to tibia (via coronary ligaments) and capsule (via deep MCL) at midbody
- Lateral meniscus: "circular", more mobile, loose peripheral attachments, no attachment at popliteal hiatus (where popliteus tendon enters joint)

Function

1. **Load transmission and shock absorption:** the menisci absorb 50% (in extension) or 85% (in flexion) of forces across femorotibial joint. The transmission of this load to the menisci helps protect the articular cartilage
2. **Joint congruity and stability:** the menisci create congruity between the curved condyles and flat plateaus, which increases stability. The menisci (esp. PHMM) also act as secondary stabilizers to translation (esp. in the ligament-deficient knee)
3. **Joint lubrication:** the menisci help distribute synovial fluid across the articular surfaces.
4. Joint nutrition: the menisci absorb, then release synovial fluid nutrients for the cartilage.
5. Proprioception: nerve endings provide sensory feedback for joint position.

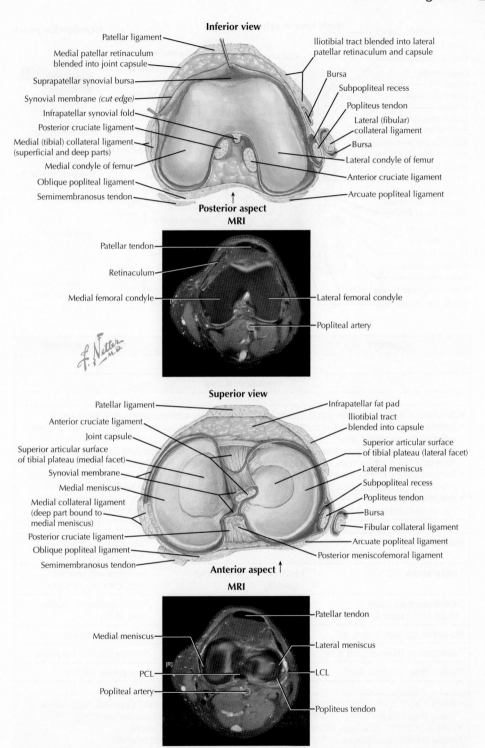

Inferior view

Patellar ligament

Medial patellar retinaculum blended into joint capsule

Suprapatellar synovial bursa

Synovial membrane *(cut edge)*

Infrapatellar synovial fold

Posterior cruciate ligament

Medial (tibial) collateral ligament (superficial and deep parts)

Medial condyle of femur

Oblique popliteal ligament

Semimembranosus tendon

Iliotibial tract blended into lateral patellar retinaculum and capsule

Bursa

Subpopliteal recess

Popliteus tendon

Lateral (fibular) collateral ligament

Bursa

Lateral condyle of femur

Anterior cruciate ligament

Arcuate popliteal ligament

Posterior aspect

MRI

Patellar tendon

Retinaculum

Medial femoral condyle

Lateral femoral condyle

Popliteal artery

Superior view

Patellar ligament

Anterior cruciate ligament

Joint capsule

Superior articular surface of tibial plateau (medial facet)

Synovial membrane

Medial meniscus

Medial collateral ligament (deep part bound to medial meniscus)

Posterior cruciate ligament

Oblique popliteal ligament

Semimembranosus tendon

Infrapatellar fat pad

Iliotibial tract blended into capsule

Superior articular surface of tibial plateau (lateral facet)

Lateral meniscus

Subpopliteal recess

Popliteus tendon

Bursa

Fibular collateral ligament

Arcuate popliteal ligament

Posterior meniscofemoral ligament

Anterior aspect

MRI

Medial meniscus

PCL

Popliteal artery

Patellar tendon

Lateral meniscus

LCL

Popliteus tendon

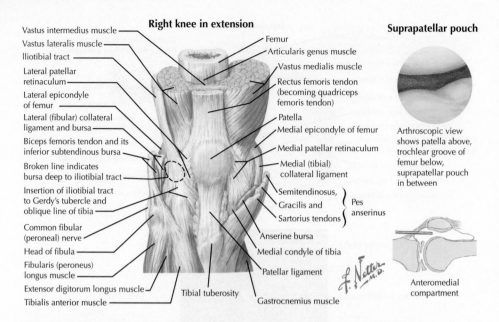

Right knee in extension

Vastus intermedius muscle
Vastus lateralis muscle
Iliotibial tract
Lateral patellar retinaculum
Lateral epicondyle of femur
Lateral (fibular) collateral ligament and bursa
Biceps femoris tendon and its inferior subtendinous bursa
Broken line indicates bursa deep to iliotibial tract
Insertion of iliotibial tract to Gerdy's tubercle and oblique line of tibia
Common fibular (peroneal) nerve
Head of fibula
Fibularis (peroneus) longus muscle
Extensor digitorum longus muscle
Tibialis anterior muscle

Femur
Articularis genus muscle
Vastus medialis muscle
Rectus femoris tendon (becoming quadriceps femoris tendon)
Patella
Medial epicondyle of femur
Medial patellar retinaculum
Medial (tibial) collateral ligament
Semitendinosus, Gracilis and Sartorius tendons } Pes anserinus
Anserine bursa
Medial condyle of tibia
Patellar ligament
Tibial tuberosity
Gastrocnemius muscle

Suprapatellar pouch

Arthroscopic view shows patella above, trochlear groove of femur below, suprapatellar pouch in between

Anteromedial compartment

LIGAMENTS	ATTACHMENTS	FUNCTION/COMMENT
KNEE		
Patellofemoral Joint		
Function		
• Composed of quadriceps tendon, patella, patellar tendon (ligament), and additional patella-stabilizing ligaments.		
• Extensor mechanism (of the knee) is primary role of this joint. The patella increases the moment arm from joint axis, increasing the mechanical advantage and quadriceps pull in extension.		
• Stability of the patella in the trochlear groove results from both bony morphology and static and dynamic stabilizers. Hypoplastic LFC or patellar ridge, a flat trochlea, or increased "Q" angle can all predispose the patella to dislocation.		
• The patella begins to engage the trochlea at 20° of flexion and is fully engaged by 40°. The articulation point moves proximally with increased flexion. The odd facet (far medial) of the patella articulates in full flexion.		
• Joint reaction forces can be very high in this joint: 3× body weight with stairs, 7× body weight with deep bending. The articular cartilage is up to 5mm (thickest in the body) to accommodate for these high forces.		
Structure		
Quadriceps tendon	Quadriceps to superior pole of patella	Can rupture with eccentric contraction (usu. >40y.o.)
Patellar tendon (ligament)	Inferior pole of patella to tibial tuberosity	Can rupture with eccentric contraction (usu. >40y.o.)
Patellofemoral ligaments Medial (MPFL), lateral (LPFL)	Femoral epicondyles to medial/lateral patella	Primary stabilizers of patella (esp. MPFL)
Patellotibial ligaments (med. & lat.)	Tibial plateaus to medial/lateral patella	Minor patellar stabilizer
Patellomeniscal ligaments (med. & lat.)	Patella to periphery of menisci	Secondary stabilizers of patella
Patellar retinaculum (med. & lat.)	Inserts on both the femur and tibia	Minor patellar stabilizer
Other		
• Patella position can evaluated on lateral radiograph (30° flexion) with Insall ratio (patella [diagonal] length/patellar tendon length). Normal ratio is 1.0 (0.8 to 1.2). >1.2 indicates patella baja, <0.8 indicates patella alta.		
• Dynamic stabilizers: quadriceps, adductor magnus, ITB, and vastus medialis and lateralis		
• Medial patellofemoral ligament (MPFL): primary restraint to lateral dislocation (most common)		

Patellofemoral Joint

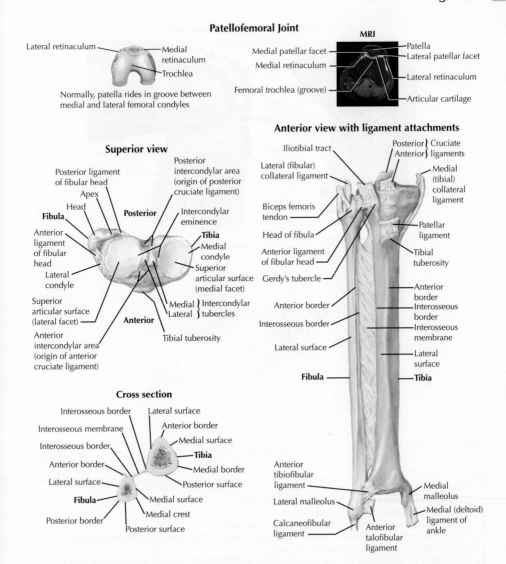

Lateral retinaculum — Medial retinaculum — Trochlea

Normally, patella rides in groove between medial and lateral femoral condyles

MRI

Medial patellar facet — Medial retinaculum — Femoral trochlea (groove) — Patella — Lateral patellar facet — Lateral retinaculum — Articular cartilage

Superior view

Posterior ligament of fibular head — Apex — Head — **Fibula** — Anterior ligament of fibular head — Lateral condyle — Superior articular surface (lateral facet) — Anterior intercondylar area (origin of anterior cruciate ligament)

Posterior

Posterior intercondylar area (origin of posterior cruciate ligament) — Intercondylar eminence — **Tibia** — Medial condyle — Superior articular surface (medial facet) — Medial } Intercondylar Lateral } tubercles — Tibial tuberosity

Anterior

Anterior view with ligament attachments

Iliotibial tract — Lateral (fibular) collateral ligament — Biceps femoris tendon — Head of fibula — Anterior ligament of fibular head — Gerdy's tubercle — Anterior border — Interosseous border — Lateral surface — **Fibula**

Posterior } Cruciate Anterior } ligaments — Medial (tibial) collateral ligament — Patellar ligament — Tibial tuberosity — Anterior border — Interosseous border — Interosseous membrane — Lateral surface — **Tibia**

Cross section

Interosseous border — Interosseous membrane — Interosseous border — Anterior border — Lateral surface — **Fibula** — Posterior border

Lateral surface — Anterior border — Medial surface — **Tibia** — Medial border — Posterior surface — Medial surface — Medial crest — Posterior surface

Anterior tibiofibular ligament — Lateral malleolus — Calcaneofibular ligament — Anterior talofibular ligament — Medial malleolus — Medial (deltoid) ligament of ankle

LIGAMENTS	ATTACHMENTS	FUNCTION/COMMENT
PROXIMAL TIBIOFIBULAR JOINT		
Anterior tibiofibular ligament	Fibular head to anterior lateral tibia	Broader and stronger than posterior ligament
Posterior tibiofibular ligament	Fibular head to posterior lateral tibia	Weaker than anterior ligament
Other		
Interosseous membrane	Lateral tibia to medial fibula	Stout fibrous membrane separates anterior & posterior compartments. Is disrupted in Maisonneuve fracture

- This joint has minimal motion. Dislocation or disruption of this joint indicates high-energy trauma to the knee region.
- For distal tibiofibular joint, please see Chapter 10, Foot/Ankle.

Technique for injection of knee joint

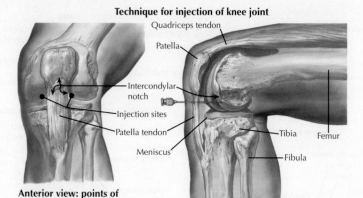

Quadriceps tendon
Patella
Intercondylar notch
Injection sites
Patella tendon
Meniscus
Tibia
Femur
Fibula

Anterior view: points of needle insertion indicated

Lateral view: needle in place

Knee arthrocentesis

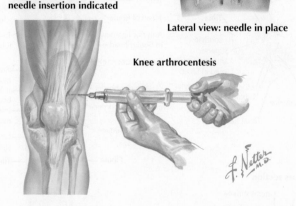

STEPS
INJECTION
1. Ask patient about allergies.
2. Place patient in seated position with knee flexed and hanging.
3. Prep skin (iodine/soap) over the anterior knee.
4. Prepare syringe with local/steroid mixture on 21/22 gauge needle.
5. Palpate the "soft spot" between the border of the patellar tendon, the tibial plateau, and the femoral condyle.
6. May locally anesthetize the skin over the "soft spot."
7. Horizontally insert the needle into the "soft spot," aiming approximately 30° to the midline toward the intercondylar notch. If the needle hits the condyle, redirect it more centrally into the notch.
8. Gently aspirate to confirm that you are not in a vessel.
9. Inject solution into knee. The fluid should flow easily.
10. Withdraw needle and dress the injection site.
ASPIRATION/ARTHROCENTESIS
1. Ask patient about allergies.
2. Place patient supine with the knee fully extended.
3. Palpate the borders of the patella and femoral condyle.
4. Prep skin (iodine/antiseptic soap) over this area.
5. Insert needle, usually 21 or 18 gauge (for thick fluid), horizontally into suprapatellar pouch at level of superior pole of the patella.
6. Aspirate fluid into syringe (may use multiple syringes if needed).
7. Gently compress knee to "milk" fluid to the pouch for aspiration.
8. Withdraw needle and dress the injection site.

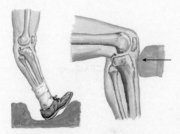
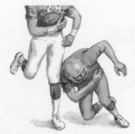
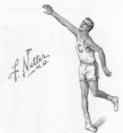

PCL Injury
Usual causes include hyperextension injury, as occurs from stepping into hole, and direct blow to flexed knee

Sprains
Usual cause is forceful impact on posterolateral aspect of knee with foot anchored, producing valgus stress on knee joint

ACL Injury
Usual cause is twisting of hyperextended knee, as in landing after basketball jump shot

QUESTION	ANSWER	CLINICAL APPLICATION
1. Age	Young	Trauma: ligamentous or meniscal injury, fracture
	Middle aged, elderly	Arthritis
2. Pain		
a. Onset	Acute	Trauma: fx, dislocation, soft tissue (ligament/meniscus) injury, septic bursitis/arthritis
b. Location	Chronic	Arthritis, infection, tendinitis/bursitis, overuse, tumor
	Anterior	Quadriceps or patellar tear or tendinitis, prepatellar bursitis, patellofemoral dysfunction
	Posterior	Meniscus tear (posterior horn), Baker's cyst, PCL injury
	Lateral	Meniscus tear (joint line), collateral lig. injury, arthritis, ITB syndrome
		Meniscus tear (joint line), collateral ligament injury, arthritis, pes bursitis
	Medial	Tumor, infection
c. Occurrence	Night pain	Etiology of pain likely from joint
	With activity	
3. Stiffness	Without locking	Arthritis, effusion (trauma, infection)
	With locking/catching	Loose body, meniscal tear (esp. bucket handle), arthritis, synovial plica
4. Swelling	Intraarticular	Infection, trauma (OCD, meniscal tear, ACL/PCL injury, fracture)
	Extraarticular	Collateral ligament injury, bursitis, contusion, sprain
	Acute (post injury)	Acute (hours): ACL injury; subacute (day): meniscus injury, OCD
	Acute (without injury)	Infection: prepatellar bursitis, septic joint
5. Instability	Giving away/collapse	Cruciate or collateral ligament injury/extensor mechanism injury
	Giving away & pain	Patellar subluxation/dislocation, pathologic plica, OCD
6. Trauma	Mechanism: valgus	MCL injury (+/– terrible triad: MCL, ACL, medial meniscus injuries)
	Varus force	LCL or posterolateral corner injury
	Flexion/posterior	PCL injury (e.g., dashboard injury)
	Twisting	Noncontact: ACL injury; Contact: multiple ligaments
	Popping noise	Cruciate ligament injury (esp. ACL), osteochondral fx, meniscal tear
	None	Degenerative and overuse etiology
7. Activity	Agility/cutting sports	Cruciate (ACL #1) or collateral ligament
	Running, cycling etc.	Patellofemoral etiology
	Squatting	Meniscus tear
	Walking	Distance able to ambulate equates with severity of arthritic disease
8. Neurologic sx	Numbness, tingling	Neurologic disease, trauma (consider L-spine etiology)
9. Systemic	Fevers, chills	Infection, septic joint, tumor
10. Hx of arthritides	Multiple joints involved	Rheumatoid arthritis, gout, etc

Quadriceps atrophy

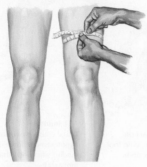

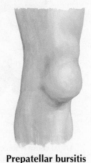

Prepatellar bursitis
(housemaid's knee)

JOHN A.CRAIG—MD

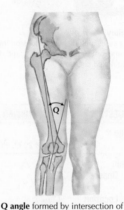

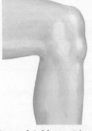

Line of
incision

Cellulitis and
induration

Osgood-Schlatter Disease
Clinical appearance. Prominence over tibial
tuberosity partly due to soft-tissue swelling
and partly to avulsed fragments

Incision and drainage
often necessary

Q angle formed by intersection of
lines from anterior superior iliac spine
and from tibial tuberosity through mid-
point of patella. Large Q angle pre-
disposes to patellar subluxation.

EXAM	TECHNIQUE/FINDINGS	CLINICAL APPLICATION/DDX
	INSPECTION	
Gait	Varus thrust	Can indicate LCL or posterolateral corner injury/insufficiency
	Patella tracking	Maltracking can lead to patellofemoral symptoms
	Flexed knee gait	From tight Achilles tendon or hamstrings, can lead to patellofemoral symptoms
Anterior	Knee alignment	Normal knee alignment is clinically neutral (6° valgus radiographically). Evaluate while weight-bearing. Variations can be developmental or post-traumatic.
	Genu valgum (knock knee)	Can predispose to lateral compartment DJD, patella instability/maltracking
	Genu varum (bow leg)	Can predispose to medial compartment DJD, ligamentous incompetency
	Q angle	Angle from ASIS to mid-patella to tibial tubercle. Nl: male ≤10°, female ≤15°; increased angle predisposes to patellar subluxation, patellofemoral symptoms
	Swelling	Prepatellar: prepatellar bursitis (inflammatory or septic); intraarticular effusion: arthritis, infection, trauma (hemarthrosis): intraarticular fracture, meniscal tear, ligament rupture
	Enlarged tibial tubercle	May be result of Osgood-Schlatter disease (esp. in adolescents)
Posterior	Mass	Baker's cyst
Lateral	Knee alignment	Evaluated while weight-bearing
	Recurvatum	Possible PCL injury
	Patella position	Best evaluated radiographically with Insall ratio (see Joints, Patellofemoral)
	High-riding patella	Patella alta: can predispose to patella instability
	Low-riding patella	Patella baja: usually posttraumatic or postsurgical (possible arthrofibrosis)
Musculature	Quadriceps	Atrophy can result from injury, postoperative, or neurologic conditions
	Vastus medialis	VMO atrophy may contribute to patellofemoral symptoms

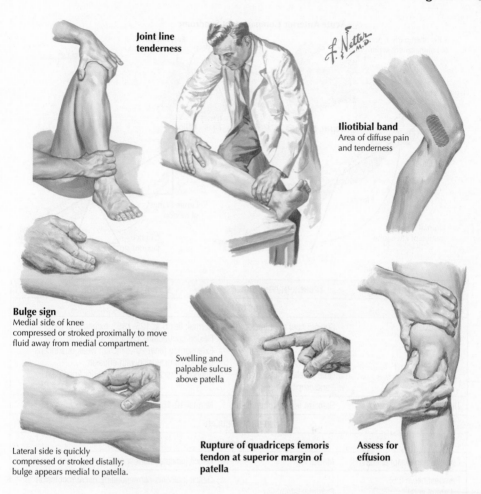

Joint line tenderness

Iliotibial band
Area of diffuse pain and tenderness

Bulge sign
Medial side of knee compressed or stroked proximally to move fluid away from medial compartment.

Lateral side is quickly compressed or stroked distally; bulge appears medial to patella.

Swelling and palpable sulcus above patella

Rupture of quadriceps femoris tendon at superior margin of patella

Assess for effusion

EXAM	TECHNIQUE/FINDINGS	CLINICAL APPLICATION/DDX
PALPATION		
Bony structures	Patella	Tenderness at distal pole: tendinitis (jumper's knee)
	Tibial tubercle	Tenderness with Osgood-Schlatter disease
Soft tissues	Quadriceps tendon	Defect: tendon rupture; tenderness: tendinitis
	Patellar tendon	Defect: tendon rupture; tenderness (esp. at insertion): tendinitis (jumper's knee)
	Compress suprapatellar pouch	Ballotable patella (effusion): arthritis, trauma, infection
	Prepatellar bursa	Edematous/tender bursae indicate correlating bursitis
	Pes anserine bursa	Tenderness indicates bursitis
	Retinaculum/plica	Thickened, tender plica is pathologic
	Medial joint line and MCL	Tenderness: medial meniscus tear or MCL injury
	Lateral joint line and LCL	Tenderness: lateral meniscus tear or LCL injury
	Iliotibial band/LFC (anterolateral knee)	Pain or tightness is pathologic
	Popliteal fossa	Mass consistent with Baker's cyst, popliteal aneurysm
	Compartments of leg (anterior, posterior, lateral)	Firm or tense compartment: compartment syndrome

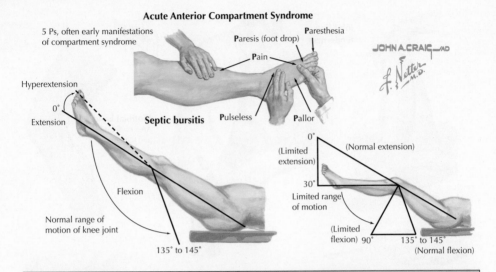

Acute Anterior Compartment Syndrome

5 Ps, often early manifestations of compartment syndrome

Paresthesia

Paresis (foot drop)

Pain

JOHN A.CRAIG—MD

Hyperextension

0°

Extension

Septic bursitis

Pulseless

Pallor

Flexion

Normal range of motion of knee joint

135° to 145°

0°
(Limited extension)

(Normal extension)

30°
Limited range of motion

(Limited flexion) 90°

135° to 145°
(Normal flexion)

EXAM	TECHNIQUE/FINDINGS	CLINICAL APPLICATION/DDX
RANGE OF MOTION		
Flexion/extension	Supine: heel to buttocks, then straight	Normal: flex 0 to 125-135°, extend 0 to 5-15° Flexion contracture: common in OA/DJD Extensor lag (final 20° difficult): weak quadriceps Decreased extension with effusion
	Note patellar tracking, pain, and crepitus	Abnormal tracking leads to anterior knee pain
Tibial IR & ER	Stabilize femur, rotate tibia	Normal 10-15° IR/ER
NEUROVASCULAR		
Sensory		
Femoral nerve/saphenous (L4)	Medial leg	Deficit indicates corresponding nerve/root lesion

Peroneal nerve (L5)
  Lateral sural
  Superficial branch
	
	Proximal lateral leg
	Distal lateral leg
		Deficit indicates corresponding nerve/root lesion

Tibial nerve (S1) Medial sural	 Proximal posterolateral leg	Deficit indicates corresponding nerve/root lesion
Sural nerve	Distal posterolateral leg	Deficit indicates corresponding nerve/root lesion
Motor		
Femoral nerve (L2-4)	Knee extension	Weakness = Quadriceps or nerve/root lesion
Sciatic: Tibial (L4-S3) Peroneal (L4-S3)	Knee flexion Knee flexion	Weakness = Biceps (LH) or nerve/root lesion Weakness = Biceps (SH) or nerve/root lesion
Tibial nerve (S1)	Foot plantarflexion	Weakness = TP, FHL, FDL, or nerve/root lesion
Peroneal (deep) n. (L4) Peroneal (superficial) n. (L5)	Foot dorsiflexion Hallux dorsiflexion	Weakness = TA or nerve/root lesion Weakness = EHL or nerve/root lesion
Other		
Reflex (L4)	Patellar	Hypoactive/absence indicates L4 radiculopathy Hyperactive may indicate UMN/myelopathic condition
Pulse	Popliteal	Diminished pulse can result from trauma

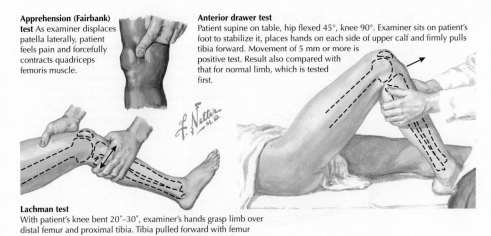

Apprehension (Fairbank) test As examiner displaces patella laterally, patient feels pain and forcefully contracts quadriceps femoris muscle.

Anterior drawer test
Patient supine on table, hip flexed 45°, knee 90°. Examiner sits on patient's foot to stabilize it, places hands on each side of upper calf and firmly pulls tibia forward. Movement of 5 mm or more is positive test. Result also compared with that for normal limb, which is tested first.

Lachman test
With patient's knee bent 20°–30°, examiner's hands grasp limb over distal femur and proximal tibia. Tibia pulled forward with femur stabilized. Movement of 5 mm or more than that in normal limb indicates rupture of anterior cruciate ligament.

EXAM	TECHNIQUE	CLINICAL APPLICATION/DDX
SPECIAL TESTS		
Patellofemoral Joint		
Patella displacement	Translate patella medially & laterally	Divide patella into 4 quadrants. Patella should translate 2 quadrants in both directions. Decreased mobility indicates a tight retinaculum.
Patella apprehension	Relax knee, push patella laterally	Pain/apprehension of subluxation: patellar instability or medial retinaculum/MPFL injury
J sign	Actively extend knee from flexed position	Lateral displacement of patella in full extension: maltracking
Patella compression/grind	Extend knee, fire quads, compress patella	Pain: chondromalacia, OCD, PF arthritis/DJD of patella
Meniscus		
Joint line tenderness	Palpate both joint lines	Most sensitive exam for meniscal tear when tender (see page 309)
McMurray	Flex/varus/ER knee, then extend Flex/valgus/IR knee, then extend	Pop or pain suggests medial, meniscal tear Pop or pain suggests lateral, meniscal tear
Apley's compression	Prone, knee 90°, compress & rotate	Pain or pop indicates meniscal tear
Anterior Cruciate Ligament		
Lachman	Flex knee 20-30°, anterior force on tibia	Laxity indicates ACL injury. Most sensitive exam for ACL rupture. Grade 1: 0-5mm, 2: 6-10mm, 3: >10mm; A: good, B: no endpoint
Anterior drawer	Flex knee 90°, anterior force on tibia	Laxity/anterior translation: ACL injury
Pivot shift	Supine, extend knee, IR, valgus force on proximal tibia, then flex knee	Clunk with knee flexion indicates ACL injury. (If ACL is deficient, the tibia starts subluxated and reduces with flexion, causing the clunk.)

Pivot shift test for anterolateral knee instability

Patient supine and relaxed. Examiner lifts heel of foot to flex hip 45° keeping knee fully extended; grasps knee with other hand, placing thumb beneath head of fibula. Examiner applies strong internal rotation to tibia and fibula at both knee and ankle while lifting proximal fibula. Knee permitted to flex about 20°; examiner then pushes medially with proximal hand and pulls with distal hand to produce a valgus force at knee

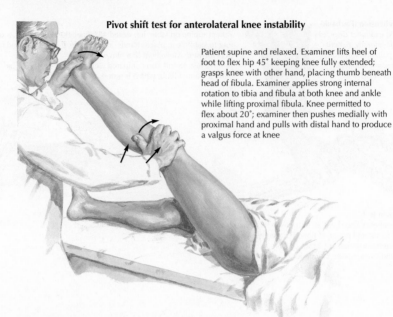

As internal rotation, valgus force, and forward displacement of lateral tibial condyle maintained, knee passively flexed. If anterior subluxation of tibia (anterolateral instability) present, sudden visible, audible, and palpable reduction occurs at about 20°–40° flexion. Test positive if anterior cruciate ligament ruptured, especially if lateral capsular ligament also torn

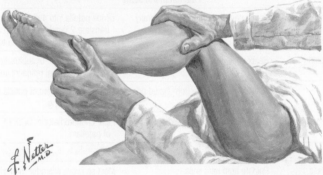

Posterior drawer test

Posterior sag sign

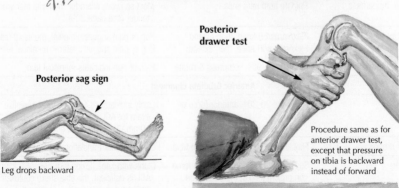

Leg drops backward

Procedure same as for anterior drawer test, except that pressure on tibia is backward instead of forward

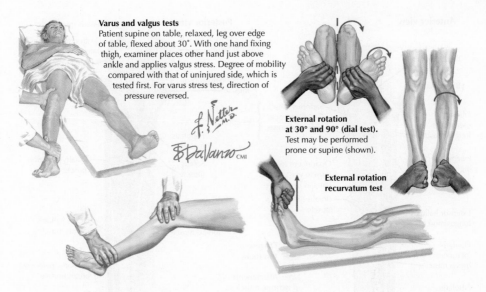

Varus and valgus tests
Patient supine on table, relaxed, leg over edge of table, flexed about 30°. With one hand fixing thigh, examiner places other hand just above ankle and applies valgus stress. Degree of mobility compared with that of uninjured side, which is tested first. For varus stress test, direction of pressure reversed.

External rotation at 30° and 90° (dial test). Test may be performed prone or supine (shown).

External rotation recurvatum test

EXAM	TECHNIQUE	CLINICAL APPLICATION/DDX
SPECIAL TESTS		
Posterior Cruciate Ligament		
Posterior drawer	Flex knee 90°, posterior force on tibia	Posterior translation: PCL injury
Posterior sag	Supine, hip 45°, knee 90°, view laterally	Posterior translation of tibia (by gravity) on femur indicates PCL injury
Quadriceps active	Supine, knee 90°, fire quadriceps	Posteriorly subluxated tibia translates anteriorly if PCL is deficient
Reverse pivot shift	Supine, flex knee 45°, ER, valgus force on proximal tibia, then extend knee	Clunk with knee extension indicates PCL injury. (If PCL is deficient, the tibia is subluxated posteriorly, then reduces w/extension, causing the clunk.)
Collateral Ligaments		
Valgus stress	Lateral force to knee at 30°, then 0°	Laxity at 30°—MCL injury; 0°—MCL and cruciate ligament injury
Varus stress	Medial force to knee at 30°, then 0°	Laxity at 30°— LCL injury; 0°—LCL and cruciate ligament injury
Other		
Prone ER at 30° & 90° (Dial)	Prone, ER both knees at 90°, then 30° (can be done supine)	Increased ER at 30°: posterolateral corner (PLC) injury; at 90° PLC & PCL injuries
ER recurvatum	Supine, legs straight, raise legs by toes	Recurvatum, varus, and IR of knee indicates PLC (+/– PCL) injury
Slocum	Knee 90°, IR tibia 30°, anterior force / Knee 90°, ER tibia 30°, anterior force	Displacement: anterior & lateral injury (ACL & PLC)) / Displacement: anterior & medial inj. (ACL, MCL, POL)
Posterior lateral drawer	Knee 90°, ER tibia 15°, posterior force	Laxity indicates posterolateral corner and/or PCL injury
Posterior medial drawer	Knee 90°, IR tibia 30°, posterior force	Laxity indicates PCL and medial ligament (MCL, POL) injury

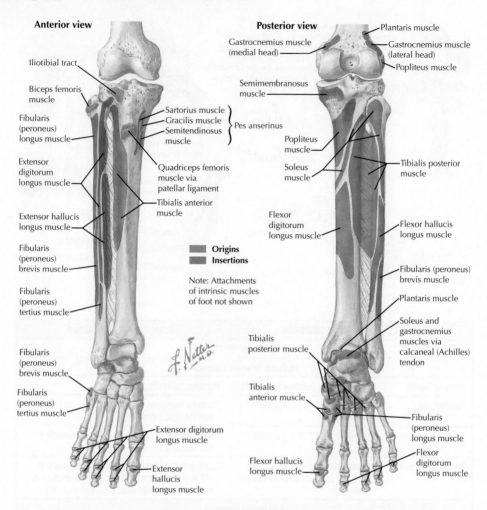

Anterior view

- Iliotibial tract
- Biceps femoris muscle
- Fibularis (peroneus) longus muscle
- Extensor digitorum longus muscle
- Extensor hallucis longus muscle
- Fibularis (peroneus) brevis muscle
- Fibularis (peroneus) tertius muscle
- Sartorius muscle
- Gracilis muscle
- Semitendinosus muscle } Pes anserinus
- Quadriceps femoris muscle via patellar ligament
- Tibialis anterior muscle

- Fibularis (peroneus) brevis muscle
- Fibularis (peroneus) tertius muscle
- Extensor digitorum longus muscle
- Extensor hallucis longus muscle

Posterior view

- Plantaris muscle
- Gastrocnemius muscle (medial head)
- Semimembranosus muscle
- Popliteus muscle
- Soleus muscle
- Flexor digitorum longus muscle
- Gastrocnemius muscle (lateral head)
- Popliteus muscle
- Tibialis posterior muscle
- Flexor hallucis longus muscle
- Fibularis (peroneus) brevis muscle
- Plantaris muscle
- Soleus and gastrocnemius muscles via calcaneal (Achilles) tendon

- Tibialis posterior muscle
- Tibialis anterior muscle
- Flexor hallucis longus muscle
- Fibularis (peroneus) longus muscle
- Flexor digitorum longus muscle

■ Origins
■ Insertions

Note: Attachments of intrinsic muscles of foot not shown

LATERAL FEMORAL CONDYLE	MEDIAL FEMORAL CONDYLE	FIBULAR HEAD	PROXIMAL TIBIA
ORIGINS			
Lateral gastrocnemius Plantaris Popliteus (ant. & inf. to LCL) **Ligaments:** Lateral collateral lig. (LCL)	Medial gastrocnemius	Soleus	Tibialis anterior (Gerdy's tub.) Extensor digitorum longus
INSERTIONS			

	Adductor magnus (ad-
	ductor tub.)
	Ligaments:
	  Medial collateral
	  lig. (MCL)
		Biceps femoris
		Ligaments:
		  Lateral collateral lig. (LCL)
		  Popliteofibular ligament
		  Arcuate ligament
		  Fabellofibular ligament
			Quadriceps (tibial tubercle)
			Iliotibial band (Gerdy's tub.)
			Pes tendons (sar, grac, semi)
			Semimembranosus (postmed.)
			Popliteus (posteriorly)
			Ligaments:
			  Medial collateral lig. (MCL)

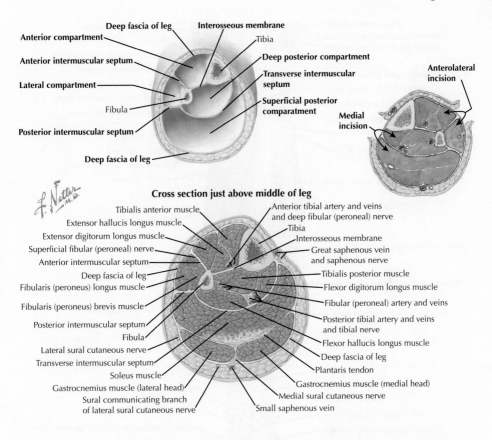

Cross section just above middle of leg

COMPARTMENT	MUSCLES	NEUROVASCULAR STRUCTURE
COMPARTMENTS (4)	
Anterior	Tibialis anterior (TA) Extensor hallucis longus (EHL) Extensor digitorum longus (EDL) Peroneus tertius	Deep peroneal nerve Anterior tibial artery and vein
Lateral	Peroneus longus Peroneus brevis	Superficial peroneal nerve
Superficial posterior	Gastrocnemius Soleus Plantaris	None
Deep posterior	Posterior tibialis (PT) Flexor hallucis longus (FHL) Flexor digitorum longus (FDL) Popliteus	Tibial nerve Posterior tibial artery and vein Peroneal artery and vein
FASCIOTOMIES	
Anterolateral	Centered over the intermuscular septum between the anterior and lateral compartments
Medial	Centered over the posterior tibial border/septum between the superficial and deep posterior compartments

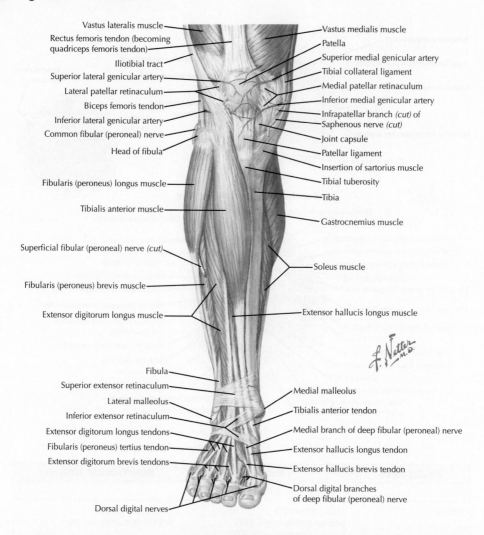

MUSCLE	ORIGIN	INSERTION	NERVE	ACTION	COMMENT
ANTERIOR COMPARTMENT					
Tibialis anterior (TA)	Proximal lateral tibia, (Gerdy's tubercle)	Med. cuneiform, plantar 1st metatarsal base	Deep peroneal	Dorsiflex, invert foot	Test L4 motor function
Extensor hallucis longus (EHL)	Medial fibula, interosseous membrane	Base of distal phalanx of great toe	Deep peroneal	Dorsiflex, extend great toe	Test L5 motor function
Extensor digitorum longus (EDL)	Lateral tibia condyle & proximal fibula	Base of middle & distal phalanges (4 toes)	Deep peroneal	Dorsiflex, extend lateral 4 toes	Single tendon divides into four tendons
Peroneus tertius	Distal fibula, interosseous membrane	Base of 5th metatarsal	Deep peroneal	Dorsiflex, evert foot (weak)	Often adjoined to the EDL

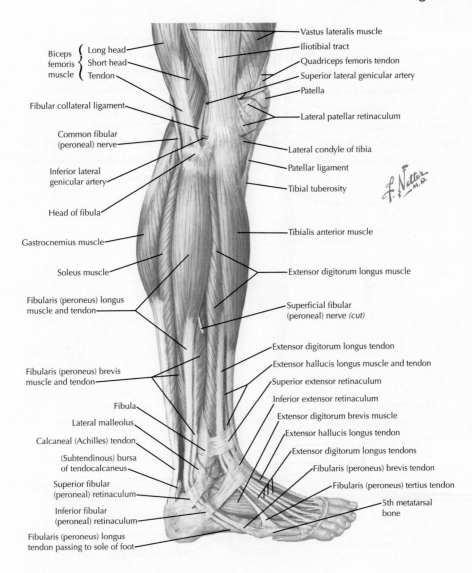

Biceps femoris muscle
- Long head
- Short head
- Tendon

Fibular collateral ligament

Common fibular (peroneal) nerve

Inferior lateral genicular artery

Head of fibula

Gastrocnemius muscle

Soleus muscle

Fibularis (peroneus) longus muscle and tendon

Fibularis (peroneus) brevis muscle and tendon

Fibula

Lateral malleolus

Calcaneal (Achilles) tendon

(Subtendinous) bursa of tendocalcaneus

Superior fibular (peroneal) retinaculum

Inferior fibular (peroneal) retinaculum

Fibularis (peroneus) longus tendon passing to sole of foot

Vastus lateralis muscle

Iliotibial tract

Quadriceps femoris tendon

Superior lateral genicular artery

Patella

Lateral patellar retinaculum

Lateral condyle of tibia

Patellar ligament

Tibial tuberosity

Tibialis anterior muscle

Extensor digitorum longus muscle

Superficial fibular (peroneal) nerve *(cut)*

Extensor digitorum longus tendon

Extensor hallucis longus muscle and tendon

Superior extensor retinaculum

Inferior extensor retinaculum

Extensor digitorum brevis muscle

Extensor hallucis longus tendon

Extensor digitorum longus tendons

Fibularis (peroneus) brevis tendon

Fibularis (peroneus) tertius tendon

5th metatarsal bone

MUSCLE	ORIGIN	INSERTION	NERVE	ACTION	COMMENT
LATERAL COMPARTMENT					
Peroneus longus	Proximal lateral fibula	Plantar medial cuneiform, 1st metatarsal base	Superficial peroneal	Plantar flex foot (1st ray)	Test S1 motor function; runs under the foot
Peroneus brevis	Distal lateral fibula	Base of 5th metatarsal	Superficial peroneal	Evert foot	Can cause avulsion fx at base of 5th MT; has most distal muscle belly

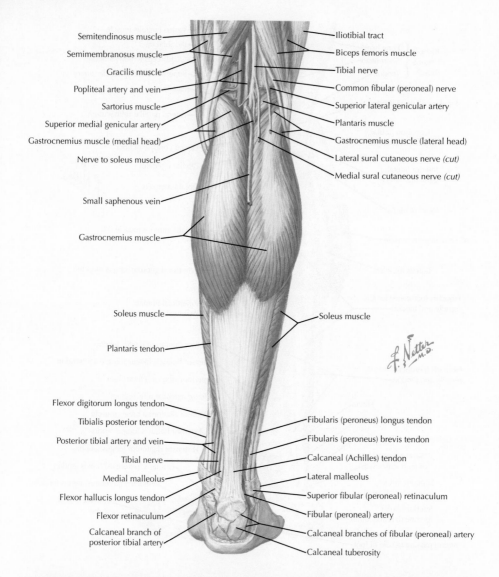

Semitendinosus muscle
Semimembranosus muscle
Gracilis muscle
Popliteal artery and vein
Sartorius muscle
Superior medial genicular artery
Gastrocnemius muscle (medial head)
Nerve to soleus muscle
Small saphenous vein
Gastrocnemius muscle
Soleus muscle
Plantaris tendon
Flexor digitorum longus tendon
Tibialis posterior tendon
Posterior tibial artery and vein
Tibial nerve
Medial malleolus
Flexor hallucis longus tendon
Flexor retinaculum
Calcaneal branch of posterior tibial artery

Iliotibial tract
Biceps femoris muscle
Tibial nerve
Common fibular (peroneal) nerve
Superior lateral genicular artery
Plantaris muscle
Gastrocnemius muscle (lateral head)
Lateral sural cutaneous nerve *(cut)*
Medial sural cutaneous nerve *(cut)*
Soleus muscle
Fibularis (peroneus) longus tendon
Fibularis (peroneus) brevis tendon
Calcaneal (Achilles) tendon
Lateral malleolus
Superior fibular (peroneal) retinaculum
Fibular (peroneal) artery
Calcaneal branches of fibular (peroneal) artery
Calcaneal tuberosity

MUSCLE	ORIGIN	INSERTION	NERVE	ACTION	COMMENT
SUPERFICIAL POSTERIOR COMPARTMENT					
Gastrocnemius	Lateral and medial femoral condyles	Calcaneus (via Achilles tendon)	Tibial	Plantar flex foot	Test S1 motor function; two heads, fabella is in tendon of lateral head
Soleus	Posterior fibular head/soleal line of tibia	Calcaneus (via Achilles tendon)	Tibial	Plantar flex foot	Fuses to gastrocnemius at Achilles tendon
Plantaris	Lateral femoral supracondylar line	Calcaneus	Tibial	Plantar flex foot (weak)	Long tendon can be harvested for tendon reconstruction

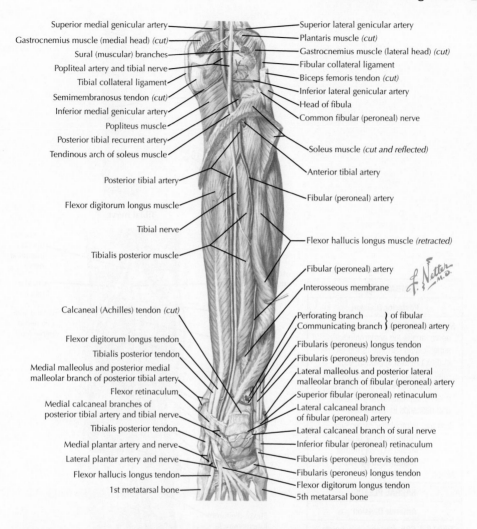

MUSCLE	ORIGIN	INSERTION	NERVE	ACTION	COMMENT
DEEP POSTERIOR COMPARTMENT					
Popliteus	Lateral femoral condyle (anterior and distal to LCL)	Proximal posterior tibia	Tibial	IR tibia/knee (during "swing" phase)	Origin is intraarticular; primary restraint to ER of knee
Flexor hallucis longus (FHL)	Posterior fibula	Base of distal phalanx of great toe	Tibial	Plantar flex great toe	Test S1 motor function
Flexor digitorum longus (FDL)	Posterior tibia	Bases of distal phalanges of 4 toes	Tibial	Plantar flex lateral 4 toes	At ankle, tendon is just anterior to tibial artery
Tibialis posterior (TP)	Posterior tibia, fibula, interosseous membrane	Plantar navicular cuneiforms, MT bases	Tibial	Plantar flex and invert foot (in "heel off" phase)	Tendon rupture/degen. can cause acquired flat foot

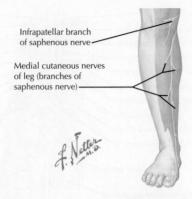

Tibial nerve

LUMBAR PLEXUS

Posterior Division

***Saphenous* (L2-4):** Branch of femoral nerve, enters leg posteromedially, superficial to sartorial fascia (at risk in direct medial approach, e.g., MMR). It then gives off infrapatellar branch (at risk in anteromedial & midline approaches, e.g., ACLR), and descends in medial leg.

Sensory: Infrapatellar region: via
         infrapatellar branch
         Medial leg: via **medial**
         cutaneous nerves
Motor: None (in leg)

SACRAL PLEXUS

Anterior Division

***Tibial* (L4-S3):** descends b/w heads of gastrocnemius into leg, posterior to posterior tibialis muscle (in deep posterior compartment) to ankle just posterior to medial malleolus b/w FDL and FHL tendons.

Sensory: Proximal posterolateral leg:
         via **medial sural nerve**
Motor: • Super. post. compartment
         ∘ Plantaris
         ∘ Gastrocnemius
         ∘ Soleus: via **n. to soleus**
        • Deep post. compartment
         ∘ Popliteus: via **n. to**
           popliteus
         ∘ Posterior tibialis (PT)
         ∘ Flexor digitorum longus
         ∘ Flexor hallucis longus

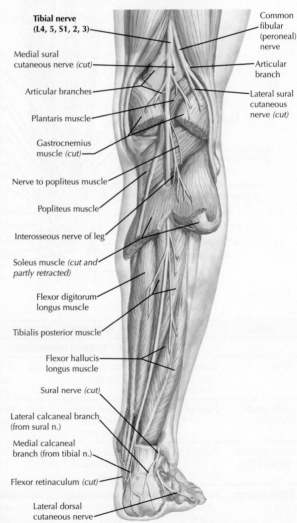

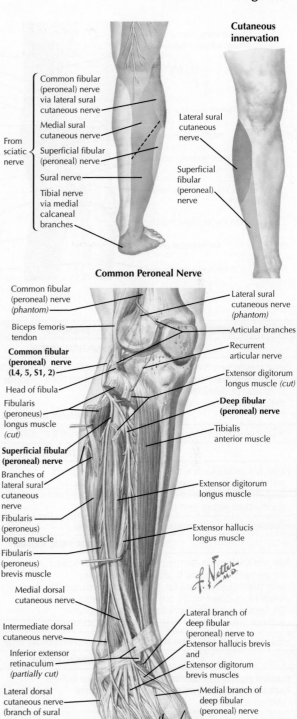

Cutaneous innervation

From sciatic nerve:
- Common fibular (peroneal) nerve via lateral sural cutaneous nerve
- Medial sural cutaneous nerve
- Superficial fibular (peroneal) nerve
- Sural nerve
- Tibial nerve via medial calcaneal branches

Lateral sural cutaneous nerve

Superficial fibular (peroneal) nerve

Common Peroneal Nerve

Common fibular (peroneal) nerve *(phantom)*

Biceps femoris tendon

Common fibular (peroneal) nerve (L4, 5, S1, 2)

Head of fibula

Fibularis (peroneus) longus muscle *(cut)*

Superficial fibular (peroneal) nerve

Branches of lateral sural cutaneous nerve

Fibularis (peroneus) longus muscle

Fibularis (peroneus) brevis muscle

Medial dorsal cutaneous nerve

Intermediate dorsal cutaneous nerve

Inferior extensor retinaculum *(partially cut)*

Lateral dorsal cutaneous nerve *(branch of sural nerve)*

Dorsal digital nerves

Lateral sural cutaneous nerve *(phantom)*

Articular branches

Recurrent articular nerve

Extensor digitorum longus muscle *(cut)*

Deep fibular (peroneal) nerve

Tibialis anterior muscle

Extensor digitorum longus muscle

Extensor hallucis longus muscle

Lateral branch of deep fibular (peroneal) nerve to Extensor hallucis brevis and Extensor digitorum brevis muscles

Medial branch of deep fibular (peroneal) nerve

SACRAL PLEXUS
Posterior Division

Common peroneal (L4-S2): divides from sciatic nerve in distal posterior thigh, runs posteroinferior to biceps femoris, around fibular neck (can be compressed or injured), then divides into 2 branches.

Sensory: Proximal lateral leg: via **lateral sural nerve**

Motor: None (before dividing)

Deep peroneal: runs in anterior compartment of leg with anterior tibial artery, posterior to tibialis anterior on interosseous membrane.

Sensory: None (in leg)

Motor: • Anterior compartment
- ○ Tibialis anterior (TA)
- ○ Extensor hallucis longus
- ○ Ext. digitorum longus
- ○ Peroneus tertius

Superficial peroneal: Runs in lateral compartment of leg, crosses anteriorly 12cm above lateral malleolus (injured in lateral ankle approach, e.g., ankle ORIF) to dorsal foot, then divides into 2 branches.

Sensory: Anterolateral leg

Motor: • Lateral compartment
- ○ Peroneus longus (PL)
- ○ Peroneus brevis (PB)

Other

Sural: Formed from **medial sural** cutaneous (tibial nerve) & **lateral sural** cutaneous (peroneal nerve), runs subcutaneously in posterolateral leg, crosses Achilles tendon 10cm above insertion, then to lateral heel.

Sensory: Posterolateral distal leg

Motor: None

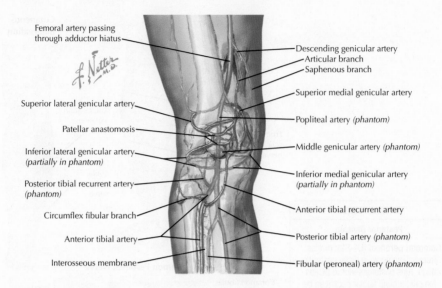

Femoral artery passing through adductor hiatus

Descending genicular artery
Articular branch
Saphenous branch

Superior medial genicular artery

Superior lateral genicular artery

Popliteal artery *(phantom)*

Patellar anastomosis

Middle genicular artery *(phantom)*

Inferior lateral genicular artery *(partially in phantom)*

Inferior medial genicular artery *(partially in phantom)*

Posterior tibial recurrent artery *(phantom)*

Anterior tibial recurrent artery

Circumflex fibular branch

Anterior tibial artery

Posterior tibial artery *(phantom)*

Interosseous membrane

Fibular (peroneal) artery *(phantom)*

COURSE	BRANCHES	COMMENT/SUPPLY
POPLITEAL ARTERY		
Begins at adductor hiatus and runs through the popliteal fossa, posterior to PCL (can be injured here), then divides at the popliteus muscle	Superior medial and lateral geniculate Inferior medial and lateral geniculate Middle geniculate **Anterior** and **posterior** tibial arteries	SLGA at risk in lateral release ILGA separates lateral knee layer 3 ligaments/structures Supplies ACL, PCL, and synovium Terminal branches of popliteal artery
• All four geniculate arteries anastomose around the knee and the patella.		
ANTERIOR TIBIAL ARTERY		
Passes b/w the two heads of the posterior tibialis into the anterior compartment and lies on interosseous membrane w/deep *peroneal* n.	Anterior tibial recurrent Circumflex fibular Anterior medial and lateral malleolar Dorsalis pedis	Supplies and anastomoses at knee Supplies fibular head and lateral knee Supplies anterior portion of malleoli Terminal branch in foot
• Supplies muscles of the anterior compartment of the leg		
POSTERIOR TIBIAL ARTERY		
Runs with *tibial* nerve in deep posterior compartment, posterior to posterior tibialis muscle to the ankle, where it lies between the FDL and FHL tendons posterior to the medial malleolus (pulse is palpable here).	Posterior tibial recurrent **Peroneal** artery Perforating muscular branches Posterior medial malleolar *Medial calcaneal* *Medial and lateral plantar*	Supplies and anastomoses at knee Supplies lateral compartment To muscles of post. compartments Supplies posterior medial malleolus Supplies medial calcaneus/heel Terminal branches in the foot
• Supplies muscles of the superficial and deep posterior compartments of the leg		
PERONEAL ARTERY		
Branches from posterior tibial artery, runs between PT & FHL muscles in posterior compartment	Posterior lateral malleolar *Lateral calcaneal*	Supplies posterior lateral malleolus Supplies lateral calcaneus/heel
• Supplies muscles of the lateral compartment of the leg		
• See muscle pages 315-319 for additional pictures of the arteries		

Joint Pathology in Osteoarthritis

Progressive stages in joint pathology

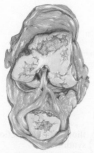
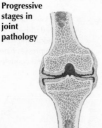
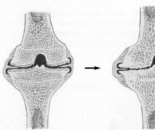

Knee joint opened anteriorly reveals large erosion of articular cartilages of femur and patella with cartilaginous excrescences at intercondylar notch

Early degenerative changes with surface fraying of articular cartilages

Further erosion of cartilages, pitting, and cleft formation. Hypertrophic changes of bone at joint margins

Cartilages almost completely destroyed and joint space narrowed. Subchondral bone irregular and eburnated; spur formation at margins. Fibrosis of joint capsule

Joint Pathology in Rheumatoid Arthritis

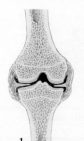
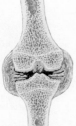
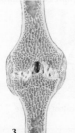
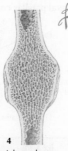

1   2   3   4

Progressive stages in joint pathology.1. Acute inflammation of synovial membrane (synovitis) and beginning proliferative changes. 2. Progression of inflammation with pannus formation; beginning destruction of cartilage and mild osteoporosis. 3. Subsidence of inflammation; fibrous ankylosis. 4. Bony ankylosis; advanced osteoporosis

Knee joint opened anteriorly, patella reflected downward. Thickened synovial membrane inflamed; polypoid outgrowths and numerous villi (pannus) extend over rough articular cartilages of femur and patella

DESCRIPTION	Hx & PE	WORKUP/FINDINGS	TREATMENT
ARTHRITIS			
Osteoarthritis			

• Primary/idiopathic or secondary (e.g., posttraumatic)
• Loss/deterioration of articular cartilage
• Can affect 1 (medial #1) or all 3 compartments in knee
	Hx: Older, decreasing activity level. Pain w/ weight-bearing and activities
	PE: Effusion, joint line tenderness, +/− contracture or deformity (varus #1)
		XR
		1. Arthritis series
		  ◦ Joint space narrowing
		  ◦ Osteophytes
		  ◦ Subchondral sclerosis
		  ◦ Subchondral cysts
		2. Alignment views
			1. NSAIDs, activity modification
			2. Physical therapy, brace, cane
			3. Glucocorticosteroid injections
			4. Unicompartmental
			  ◦ HTO
			  ◦ Unicompartment arthroplasty
			5. Tricompartmental: Total knee arthroplasty (TKA)

Inflammatory			

• Multiple types: rheumatoid, gout, seronegative (e.g., Reiter's)
• In RA, synovitis/pannus formation destroys cartilage & eventually whole joint.
	Hx: Usually younger pts. Pain, often multiple joints
	PE: Effusion, +/− warmth, decr. ROM & deformity
		XR: Arthritis series: joint narrowing, joint erosions, ankylosis, joint destruction
		LABS: CBC, RF, ANA, CRP, crystals, culture
			1. Early: manage medically
			2. Late
			  ◦ Nonop: like osteoarthritis
			  ◦ Synovectomy
			  ◦ Total knee arthroplasty

Patellofemoral stress syndrome

With knee extended, patella lies above and between femoral condyles in contact with suprapatellar fat pad

As knee flexes, tension in quadriceps femoris tendon and patellar tendon compresses patella against femoral condyles

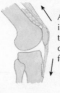

Chondromalacia

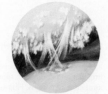
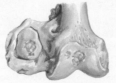

Iliotibial tract friction syndrome
As knee flexes and extends, iliotibial tract glides back and forth over lateral femoral epicondyle, causing friction

Arthroscopic view shows fragmented patellar cartilage

Chondromalacia of patella with "kissing" lesion on femoral condyle

Lateral patellar compression syndrome

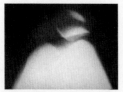
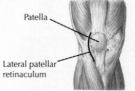
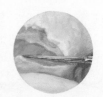

Patella

Lateral patellar retinaculum

Preoperative x-ray showing lateral tilt of patella.

Line indicates extent of release

Arthroscopic view of transcutaneous release of lateral retinaculum

DESCRIPTION	Hx & PE	WORKUP/FINDINGS	TREATMENT
ANTERIOR KNEE PAIN			
Patellofemoral Syndrome			
• Pain in patellofemoral joint • Contributing factors: overuse, subtle instability or malalignment, quadriceps weakness • Chondromalacia may be present, but not necessarily	**Hx:** Young female and athletes. Pain w/activities (esp. running, stairs) and prolonged sitting **PE:** +patella compression, +/− incr. Q angle and/or J-sign	**XR:** 4 views: AP & notch: eval. for OCD, OA Lateral: OA & Insall ratio Sunrise: subluxation or tilt, OA, OCD	• NSAIDs, activity modification • Physical therapy: ROM, quad. strengthening, hamstring stretching, +/− foot orthoses • Patella realignment (if malalignment is present)
Chondromalacia Patellae			
• Softening or wear of the articular cartilage of the patella • Term often misused to imply any anterior knee pain	**Hx:** Usually younger pts.; pain, often multiple jts. **PE:** Effusion, decr. ROM & deformity	**XR:** 4 view: evaluate like PFS (see above)	• NSAIDs, activity modification • Physical therapy • Arthroscopic debridement/chondroplasty may help
Lateral Patellar Compression Syndrome			
• Overloading of lateral facet during flexion • Due to tight lateral structures (esp. lateral retinaculum)	**Hx:** Usually younger pts.; anterior knee pain **PE:** PF pain, decreased mobility/patella glide	**XR:** 3 or 4 views Sunrise/merchant: evaluate for lateral patella tilt	• PT: stretch lateral tissues, quad. strengthening +/− taping or centralizing brace • Arthroscopic lateral release
Iliotibial Band Syndrome			
• ITB rubs on lateral femoral condyle • Common w/runners/cyclists	**Hx:** Pain w/activity **PE:** Lateral femoral condyle; TTP (knee at 30°)	**XR:** AP/lateral: normal, r/o tumor	• NSAIDs, activity modification, stretching (ITB) • Partial excision (rare)

Synovial plica

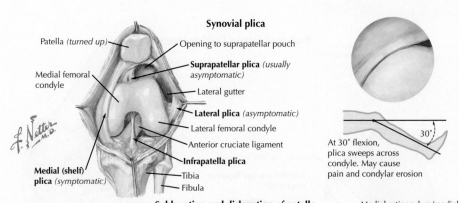

Patella *(turned up)*
Opening to suprapatellar pouch
Suprapatellar plica *(usually asymptomatic)*
Medial femoral condyle
Lateral gutter
Lateral plica *(asymptomatic)*
Lateral femoral condyle
Anterior cruciate ligament
Infrapatella plica
Medial (shelf) plica *(symptomatic)*
Tibia
Fibula

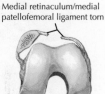

At 30° flexion, plica sweeps across condyle. May cause pain and condylar erosion

Subluxation and dislocation of patella

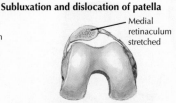

Lateral retinaculum
Medial retinaculum

Medial retinaculum stretched

Medial retinaculum/medial patellofemoral ligament torn

Skyline view. Normally, patella rides in groove between medial and lateral femoral condyles

In subluxation, patella deviates laterally; can be due to weakness of vastus medialis muscle, tightness of lateral retinaculum, and high Q angle

In dislocation, patella displaced completely out of intercondylar groove

DESCRIPTION	Hx & PE	WORKUP/FINDINGS	TREATMENT
ANTERIOR KNEE PAIN			
Patellar Instability			
• Subluxation or dislocation of patella (lateral #1) • Associated w/anatomic variants • MPFL is key structure	**Hx:** Pain & patella instability **PE:** + patellar apprehension, +/− increased Q angle, genu valgum, femoral anteversion	**XR:** 3 or 4 views: eval. for fx and patella position (lateral and/or patella alta) **MR:** eval. MPFL if acute	• Acute: MPFL repair • Recurrent/chronic: physical therapy, brace; patellar realignment surgery
Patellar Tendinitis			
• Seen in jumpers (e.g., basketball/volleyball players) • Microtears at tendon insertion at distal pole	**Hx:** Sports, anterior knee pain (worse with activity) **PE:** Patellar inferior pole TTP	**XR:** AP/lateral: normal **MR:** Increased signal at insertion (inferior pole) or intrasubstance	• NSAIDs, stretch and strengthen quadriceps and hamstrings • Surgical debridement (rare)
Plica			
• Fold in synovium (embryonic remnant) becomes thickened or inflamed • Medial plica #1	**Hx:** Anteromedial pain, +/− popping/catching **PE:** Tender, palpable plica, +/− snap with flexion	**XR:** Knee series. Eval. for other pain sources **MR:** Of questionable value	• Ice, NSAIDs • Activity modification • Arthroscopic debridement (if symptoms persist)
Prepatellar Bursitis			
• Etiology: trauma or overuse (e.g., prolonged kneeling) • "Housemaid's knee" • Inflammatory or septic	**Hx:** Knee pain & swelling **PE:** Egg-shaped swelling on anterior patella, TTP, +/− signs of infection	**XR:** Knee series: usu. normal **LAB:** CBC, ESR, +/− aspirate: gram stain & cell count	• Inflammatory: ice, NSAIDs, knee pads, rest, +/− aspiration; bursectomy if persistent • Septic: bursectomy, abx

Rupture of Anterior Cruciate Ligament

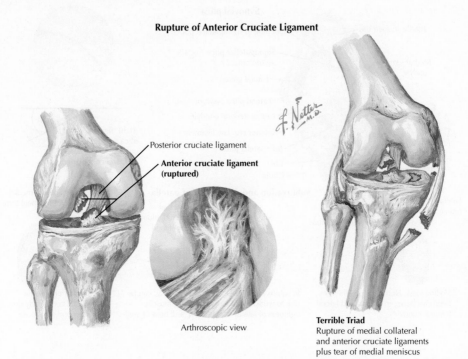

Posterior cruciate ligament

Anterior cruciate ligament (ruptured)

Arthroscopic view

Terrible Triad
Rupture of medial collateral and anterior cruciate ligaments plus tear of medial meniscus

DESCRIPTION	Hx & PE	WORKUP/FINDINGS	TREATMENT
LIGAMENT INJURIES			
Anterior Cruciate			
• Mechanism: twisting injury, often noncontact pivoting • Associated with other injuries: meniscal tears, collateral ligament (all 3 = terrible triad) • Common in female athletes	**Hx:** Twisting injury, "pop," swelling, inability to continue playing **PE:** Effusion (hemarthrosis) + Lachman (most sensitive), + anterior drawer, + pivot shift	**XR:** Knee series (Segond fx is pathognomic for ACL) **MR:** Absent/detached ACL, +/− bone bruise (middle LFC–posterior lateral tibia plateau) **Arthrocentesis:** Hemarthrosis	Based on functional stability ○ Stable/low demand pt: activity modification, PT, brace ○ Unstable/athletes/active pt: surgical reconstruction (grafts: BTB, hamstring, allograft)
COMPLICATIONS: arthrofibrosis, failure/recurrence (1. technical error, 2. missed ligamentous injury, 3. recurrent trauma)			
Posterolateral Corner			
• Mechanism: direct blow or hyperextension/varus injury • LCL, popliteus, popliteofibular ligament are injured. These are focus of surgical reconstruction. • Can be associated w/PCL injury	**Hx:** Trauma, pain, instability **PE:** +/− effusion, + prone ER test at 30°, +/− posterolateral drawer & ER recurvatum tests	**XR:** Knee series. Avulsions can occur (fibular head). Alignment: eval. for varus **MR:** To evaluate all ligaments and other soft tissues	• Nonoperative: low grade (grades 1& 2 injury): brace & physical therapy • Surgical repair: acute grade 3 • Surgical reconstruction: chronic or combined injury, HTO if varus

Rupture of posterior cruciate ligament

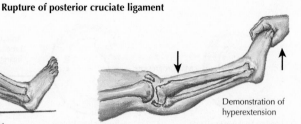

Demonstration of hyperextension

Posterior sag sign. Leg drops backward

Collateral ligament injury

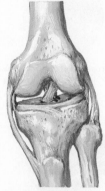

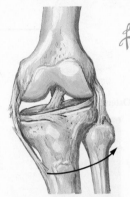

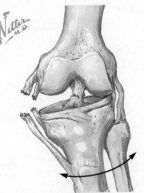

1st-degree sprain. Localized joint pain and tenderness but no joint laxity

2nd-degree sprain. Detectable joint laxity with good end point plus localized pain and tenderness

3rd-degree sprain. Complete disruption of ligaments and gross joint instability

DESCRIPTION	Hx & PE	WORKUP/FINDINGS	TREATMENT
LIGAMENT INJURIES			
Posterior Cruciate			
• Mechanism: anterior force on tibia (e.g., dashboard injury) or sports (hyperextension) • Associated with collateral and/or PL corner injuries	**Hx:** Trauma (dashboard) or sports injury, pain **PE:** +/− effusion, + posterior drawer, quadriceps active test, & posterior sag	**XR:** Knee series. Look for avulsion fracture. **MR:** Confirms diagnosis. Evaluates meniscus and articular cartilage.	• Nonoperative: isolated (esp. grades 1& 2 injury): brace & PT • Surgical reconstruction: failed nonop treatment, combined injury, some isolated grade 3's
Medial Collateral			
• Mechanism: valgus force • Common in football • Usually injured at femoral origin (medial epicondyle)	**Hx:** Trauma, pain, instability **PE:** Tenderness at medial epicondyle along tendon. Pain/laxity w/valgus stress	**XR:** Knee series. Medial epicondyle avulsion can occur (calcified = Pelligrini-Steida). **MR:** Confirms diagnosis	• Hinged knee brace • Physical therapy: ROM and strengthening • Surgery: uncommon
Lateral Collateral			
• Mechanism: varus force • Isolated injuries are rare, usually combined with posterolateral corner (PLC)	**Hx:** Trauma, pain, instability **PE:** Lateral tenderness. Pain/laxity w/varus stress	**XR:** Knee series. Fibular head avulsions can occur. **MR:** Confirms diagnosis	• Isolated injury: hinged brace • Combined injury: surgical repair or reconstruction

Tears of meniscus

Longitudinal (vertical) tear

May progress to

Bucket handle tear

Anterior cruciate ligament

Femoral condyle

Bucket handle

Arthroscopic view of bucket handle tear shows handle displaced into intercondylar fossa

Radial tear

May progress to

Parrot beak tear

Arthroscopic view of parrot beak tear with fibrillation of meniscal margin

Osteochondral defect

Fragment of cartilage and bone

Stage 2 lesion

Tunnel view radiographs of small OCD lesion involving medial femoral condyle

Arthroscopic view of knee with osteochondral defect

DESCRIPTION	Hx & PE	WORKUP/FINDINGS	TREATMENT
INTRAARTICULAR CONDITIONS			
Meniscus Tear			
• Acute: young, twisting injury • Degenerative: older +/– OA • Multiple tear patterns • Associated w/other injuries (ACL rupture, OCD, etc) • Medial>lateral 3:1 (posterior horn most common)	**Hx:** Pain & swelling esp. with flexion activities, +/– catching or locking (e.g., bucket handle tear) **PE:** Effusion, joint line tenderness, + McMurray/Apley tests	**XR:** Knee series: usually normal. Early OA often seen in pts w/degenerative tears **MR:** Very sensitive for tears. "Double PCL" sign for displaced bucket handle tears	• Small/minimally symptomatic: treat conservatively • Peripheral tears (red zone): repair (heal best w/ACL reconstruction) • Central tears (white zone): partial meniscectomy
Osteochondral Defect			

• Spectrum: purely chondral to osteochondral lesions
• Traumatic or degenerative
• Osteochondritis dissecans is separate but similar entity
	Hx: Often young/active pts. Pain (usually w/WB), +/– popping, catching
	PE: Inconsistent: +/– effusion, bony tenderness
		XR: Knee series: 4 views (need 45° PA & notch views), consider alignment series
		MR: Good modality for purely chondral lesions
			Displaced OCD: internal fixation
			Chondral:
			  ○ Debridement
			  ○ Microfracture
			  ○ Osteochondral transfer
			  ○ Chondrocyte implantation

Quadriceps tendon rupture

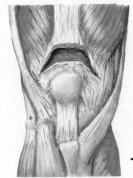

Rupture of quadriceps femoris tendon at superior margin of patella

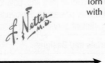

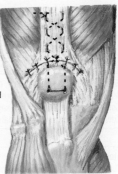

Torn retinaculum closed with interrupted sutures

Patellar tendon rupture

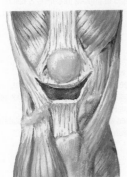

Rupture of patellar ligament at inferior margin of patella

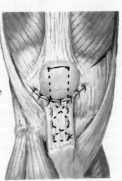

Ruptured patellar ligament repaired with nonabsorbable sutures through drill holes in patella; torn edges of retinaculum approximated with interrupted sutures

DESCRIPTION	Hx & PE	WORKUP/FINDINGS	TREATMENT
OTHER			
Quadriceps Tendon Rupture			
• Mechanism: eccentric contraction or indirect trauma • Patients usually >40y.o. • Usually at musculotendinous junction	**Hx:** Older, fall/trauma **PE:** Effusion, palpable defect above patella. Inability to do or maintain straight leg raise	**XR:** Knee series. Look for patella baja **MR:** Will show tendon tear. Usually not needed. May be helpful in partial tears.	• Acute: primary surgical repair • Chronic: surgical reconstruction (tendon lengthening or allograft procedure)
Patellar Tendon Rupture			
• Mechanism: direct or indirect (eccentric load) trauma • Patients usually <40y.o. • Associated with underlying tendon and/or metabolic disorder	**Hx:** Younger pts, trauma, pain, loss of knee extension **PE:** Effusion, palpable defect in tendon. Cannot do straight leg raise	**XR:** Knee series. Look for patella alta **MR:** Will show tendon tear. Usually *not* needed. May be helpful in partial tears.	• Acute: primary surgical repair • Chronic: surgical reconstruction (tendon lengthening or allograft procedure)
Tumor			
#1 in adolescents: osteosarcoma; #1 in adults: chondrosarcoma; #1 benign (young adults): giant cell tumor			

TOTAL KNEE ARTHROPLASTY
General Information
• Goals: 1. Clinical: alleviate pain, maintain personal independence, allow performance of activities of daily living (ADLs) & recreation; 2. Surgical: restore mechanical alignment, restore joint line, balance soft tissues (e.g., collateral ligs.) • Common procedure with high satisfaction rates for primary procedure. Revisions are also becoming more common. Advances in techniques and materials are improving implant survival; this procedure now available to younger pts.
Materials and Designs

Materials
• Femur component: cobalt-chrome commonly used for femoral-bearing surface with titanium stem
• Tibia component/tray: does not articulate with femoral component. Often made of titanium.
• Tibial tray insert: articulates with femoral component; made of polyethylene (UHMWPE, ultra high molecular weight PE)
   ∘ Polyethylene (PE) wears well but does produce microscopic particles that may lead to implant loosening & failure.
   ∘ Polyethylene should be at least 8mm thick, cross-linked for better wear, & sterilized in inert (non-O_2) environment.
   ∘ Congruent design (not flat) improves wear rate and rollback (increased knee flexion).
   ∘ Direct compression molding is preferred manufacturing technique.
• Cement: methylmethacrylate
Prosthetic Designs
• Unconstrained: 2 types. These are most common for primary surgical procedures with minimal deformity.
   ∘ Posterior cruciate (PCL) retaining ("CR"): preserves femoral rollback for incr. knee flexion but has incr. PE wear.
   ∘ Posterior cruciate (PCL) substituting ("posterior stabilized") ("PS"): provides mechanical rollback, but may dislocate. Indicated for patellectomy, inflammatory arthritis, incompetent PCL (e.g., previous PCL rupture, etc).
• Constrained (non-"hinged"): Used for moderate ligament (MCL/LCL) deficiency. Uses a central post to provide stability.
• Constrained ("hinged"): Used for global ligament deficiency. Has high wear and failure rates.
• Other: Mobile-bearing designs are available.
Fixation
• Cement. Most common.
• Biologic. Bone ingrowth techniques. Theoretically have longer life, but have higher failure rates.

Indications

• Arthritis of knee
   ∘ Common etiologies: osteoarthritis (idiopathic, posttraumatic), rheumatoid arthritis, osteonecrosis
   ∘ Clinical symptoms: knee pain, worse with activity, gradually worsening over time, decreased ambulatory capacity.
   ∘ Radiographic findings: appropriate radiographic evidence of knee arthritis

OSTEOARTHRITIS	RHEUMATOID ARTHRITIS
1. Joint space narrowing	1. Joint space narrowing
2. Sclerosis	2. Periarticular osteoporosis
3. Subchondral cysts	3. Joint erosions
4. Osteophyte formation	4. Ankylosis

• Failed conservative treatment: NSAIDs, activity modification, weight loss, physical therapy, orthosis (e.g., medial off-loader brace), ambulatory aid (e.g., cane in contralateral hand), injections (corticosteroid, viscosupplementation)
Contraindications
• **Absolute:** Neuropathic joint, infection, extensor mechanism dysfunction, medically unstable patient (e.g., severe cardiopulmonary disease). Patient may not survive the procedure. • **Relative:** Young, active patients. These patients can wear out the prostheses many times in their lives.
Alternatives

• Considerations: age, activity level, overall medical health
• Osteotomy: relatively young patients with unicompartmental disease
   ∘ Valgus knee/lateral compartment DJD: distal femoral varus–producing osteotomy
   ∘ Varus knee/medial compartment DJD: proximal tibia valgus–producing osteotomy
• Unicompartmental arthroplasty: unicompartmental disease
• Arthrodesis/fusion: young laborers with isolated unilateral disease (e.g., normal spine, hip, ankle)

All components
in place

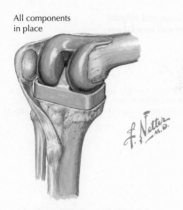

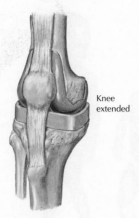

Knee
extended

TOTAL KNEE ARTHROPLASTY
Procedure

Approaches
- Midline incision with medial parapatellar arthrotomy is most common.
- Minimally invasive incisions are also being used. Special equipment is often needed for the smaller incisions.

Steps
- Bone cuts
  - Cut femur and tibia perpendicular to mechanical axis. Can use intramedullary (femur/tibia) or extramedullary (tibia) reference; this will restore the mechanical alignment
  - Bone removed from femur and tibia should be equal to that replaced by the implants to maintain/restore joint line.
- Implants—trial implants are first inserted to test adequacy of the bone cuts
  - Implants should be best fit possible to native bone
  - Femur placed in 3° of external rotation to accommodate a perpendicular bone cut of the proximal tibia (typically in 3° of varus)
  - Femoral axis determined in 3 ways: 1. epicondylar axis, 2. posterior condylar axis, 3. AP axis—perpendicular to trochlea
- Balancing
  - Sagittal plane: goal is to make flexion & extension gaps equal. May need to cut more bone or add implant augments.
  - Coronal plane: soft tissues are of primary concern. Rule is to release the concave side of the deformity.
  - Varus deformity: release medial side: 1. deep MCL, 2. postmed capsule/semimemb insertion, 3.superficial MCL
  - Valgus deformity: release lateral side: 1. lateral capsule, 2a. ITB (tight in ext.), 2b. popliteus (tight in flexion), 3. LCL
  - Polyethylene trial: the knee should be stable and well balanced with the trial polyethylene in place.
- Final implantation of components

Complications

- Patellofemoral complications are most common: patella maltracking, patellofemoral pain, patellar fracture.
- Arthrofibrosis: may respond early (<6 wk) to manipulation under anesthesia.
- Extensor mechanism failure: patellar tendon rupture or avulsion (difficult to repair/reconstruct); patellar fracture
- Infection: diagnose with labs and aspiration. Prevention is mainstay: perioperative antibiotics, meticulous prep/drape technique, etc. Treatment: acute/subacute: irrigation & debridement with PE exchange. Late: 1- or 2-stage revision
- Loosening: more common with biologic fixation. Also caused by microscopic particles from polyethylene wear
- Neurovascular injury
  - Peroneal nerve: esp. after mechanical axis correction of a valgus knee (nerve is stretched)
  - Superolateral geniculate artery: should be identified and cauterized
- Medical complications: Deep venous thrombosis (DVT) and pulmonary embolus (PE) are known risks of TKA. Prophylaxis must be initiated.
- Periprosthetic fracture
  - Femur: stable implant—nail or fixed angle device; unstable implant—replace with longer stem that passes fx site

Genu varum and valgum (bow leg and knock-knee)

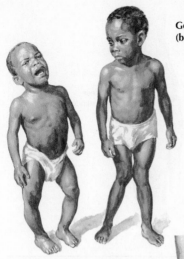

Two brothers, younger (left) with bowleg, older (right) with knock-knee. In both children, limbs eventually became normally aligned without corrective treatment

Infantile tibia vara (Blount's disease)

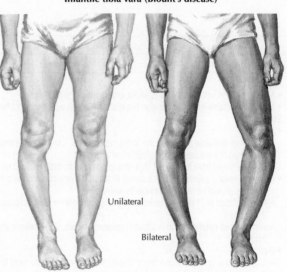

Unilateral

Bilateral

DESCRIPTION	EVALUATION	TREATMENT
GENU VARUM		

• Normal (physiologic): ages 0-2
• Pathologic: Blount's disease:
  2 types
  ◦ Infantile: <3y.o., obesity, early
    walking
  ◦ Adolescent: insidious onset
    >8y.o.
	Hx: Parents notice a deformity
	PE: Unilateral or bilateral genu varum
	XR: Tibia metadiaphyseal angle
	  (TMDA): <9° is normal, >16° is
	  pathologic/Blount's
		• Physiologic: observation
		• Infantile: <3y.o.: brace; >3y.o.:
		  osteotomy
		• Adolescent: hemiepiphysiodesis
		  (open physis) or osteotomy (closed
		  physis)

GENU VALGUM		

• Normal (physiologic): ages 2-5
• Pathologic: skeletal tumors
  ◦ Metabolic: renal osteodystrophy
  ◦ Other: trauma, infection
	Hx: Parents notice a deformity
	PE: Unilateral or bilateral genu valgum
	XR: Alignment x-rays: valgus is 6° in
	  normal adults
		• Physiologic: observation
		• Pathologic: hemiepiphysiodesis
		  or osteotomy

Posteromedial bowing of tibia

Posteromedial bowing.
Convexity of bow in distal third of tibia and fibula directed posteriorly and medially. Spontaneous correction usually obviates need for realignment osteotomy, but leg-length discrepancy often persistent.

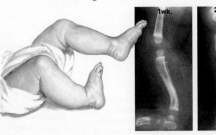

1 wk.   2 yrs.

Anterolateral bowing of tibia and congenital pseudarthrosis

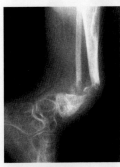

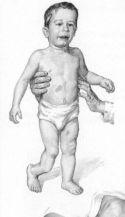

Congenital pseudoarthrosis of the tibia.
Angulation of right leg. Café au lait spots on thigh and abdomen suggest relationship to neurofibromatosis.

Anterolateral bowing.
In infancy it may be difficult to predict if anterolateral bowing will correct spontaneously or if bone will progress to fracture and congenital pseudarthrosis. Progression to pseudarthrosis is more likely if the medullary canal is narrow and has sclerotic changes.

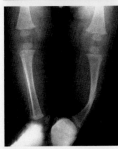

Anterolateral bowing. Medullary canal present but narrow with sclerotic changes; cyst apparent. Prone to spontaneous fracture and pseudarthrosis

DESCRIPTION	EVALUATION	TREATMENT
TIBIA BOWING		
Posteromedial Bowing		
• Congenital convexity of tibia • Idiopathic, unilateral • Deformity corrects but a leg length discrepancy usually results	**Hx:** Deformity present at birth **PE:** Foot appears dorsiflexed (calcaneovalgus), leg is bowed **XR:** Bowing of tibia and fibula	• Bowing resolves with growth • Resultant leg length discrepancy ○ Mild: shoe lift ○ Severe: hemiepiphysiodesis
Anterolateral Bowing/Congenital Tibia Pseudarthrosis		
• Bowing of tibia, unknown etiology • Associated with neurofibromatosis • Anterolateral bowing can lead to pseudarthrosis	**Hx/PE:** Leg deformity & disability. Bowed leg, +/– signs of neurofibromatosis (e.g., café au lait spots) **XR:** Reveals bowing or pseudarthrosis	• Young/bowing tibia: full contact brace • Pseudarthrosis: tibial nail/external fixation & bone graft • Amputation: if surgical treatment fails

Osgood-Schlatter disease

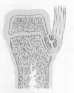

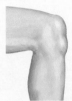

Normal insertion of patellar ligament to ossifying tibial tuberosity

In Osgood-Schlatter lesion, superficial portion of tuberosity pulled away, forming separate bone fragments

In Osgood-Schlatter condition, the apophysis of the tibial tuberosity is prominent and has irregular ossification. Fragmentation and separate ossicles may develop

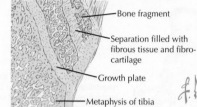

Bone fragment

Separation filled with fibrous tissue and fibro-cartilage

Growth plate

Metaphysis of tibia

High-power magnification of involved area

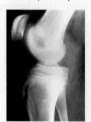

Radiograph shows separation of superficial portion of tibial tuberosity

Tibial torsion

Evaluating patient for internal tibial torsion. Child seated with knees flexed 90°, heels against flat, vertical surface. Patellae point directly forward, indicating that femurs are in neutral position, but feet point inward, indicating internal tibial torsion

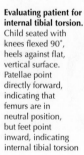

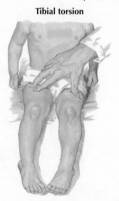

DESCRIPTION	EVALUATION	TREATMENT
OSGOOD-SCHLATTER DISEASE		
• Traction apophysitis/osteochondrosis of the tibial tubercle (2° ossification site) • Repetitive stress to extensor mechanism (e.g., in athletics [most common])	**Hx:** Adolescent w/knee pain, worse after activity **PE:** Tibial tubercle swollen & tender to palpation **XR:** Shows ossification center at tibial tubercle +/− heterotopic ossification	Symptoms resolve w/apophysis closure (during adolescence) • Activity modification/restriction • Cast/brace if symptoms severe • Excision of unfused ossicle
TIBIAL TORSION		
• Congenital internal rotation of tibia • Assoc. w/decreased intrauterine space & other "packaging problems" • Most common cause of intoeing gait	**Hx:** 1-2y.o., frequent tripping, "pigeon toed" **PE:** Intoeing gait, negative foot to thigh angle, medial foot progression angle, transmalleolar axis IR/medial with thigh/patella pointed forward	• Will spontaneously resolve • Orthoses of no proven benefit • Supramalleolar osteotomy if deformity persists into late childhood

Anteromedial Approach to Knee Joint

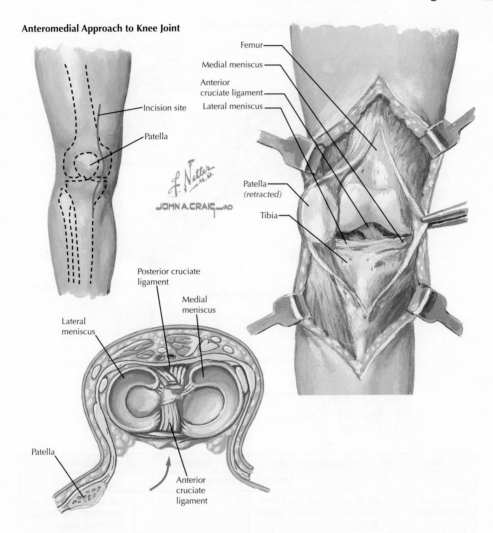

USES	INTERNERVOUS PLANE	DANGERS	COMMENT
KNEE: MEDIAL PARAPATELLAR APPROACH			
• Ligament reconstruction • Total knee arthroplasty • Meniscectomy	• No planes: capsule is under skin	• Infrapatellar branch of saphenous nerve	• Most commonly used approach • Most/best exposure • Neuroma may develop from cut nerve
LEG/TIBIA: POSTEROLATERAL APPROACH (HARMON)			
• Fractures • Nonunions	• Gastrocnemius/soleus/FHL (tibial) • Peroneus longus/brevis (superficial peroneal)	• Lesser saphenous vein • Posterior tibial artery	• A technically difficult approach • Bone grafting of nonunion
FASCIOTOMY			
See pages 294 and 315			

Posterolateral approach to tibia

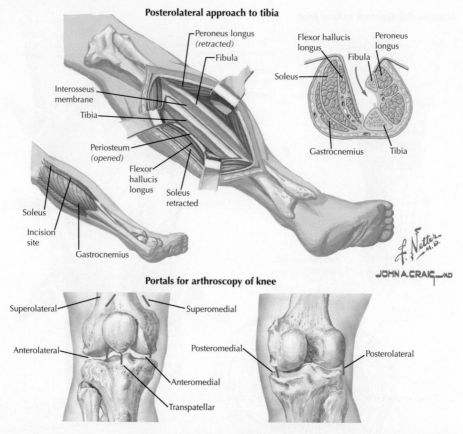

Portals for arthroscopy of knee

USES	INTERNERVOUS PLANE	DANGERS	COMMENT
ARTHROSCOPY PORTALS			
Anteromedial (inferomedial)	Just above joint line, 1cm inferior to patella; 1cm medial to patellar tendon	Anterior horn of medial meniscus	Most common portal to use instruments; also helpful for viewing lateral compartment
Anterolateral (inferolateral)	Just above joint line, 1cm inferior to patella; 1cm lateral to patellar tendon	Anterior horn of lateral meniscus	Most common portal for the arthroscope
Superolateral/ superomedial	2.5cm above joint line, lateral or medial to quadriceps tendon		Used to view patellofemoral articulation, patella tracking, also inflow/outflow
Posteromedial	Flex knee to 90°, 1cm above joint line, posterior to MCL	Saphenous nerve	Used to view PCL, posterior horns of menisci, retrieve loose bodies
Posterolateral	Flex knee, 1cm above joint line, posterior to LCL	Peroneal nerve	Used to view PCL, posterior horns of menisci, retrieve loose bodies
Transpatellar	1cm below inferior pole of patella in midline	Patellar tendon	Central joints and notch viewing

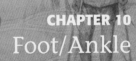

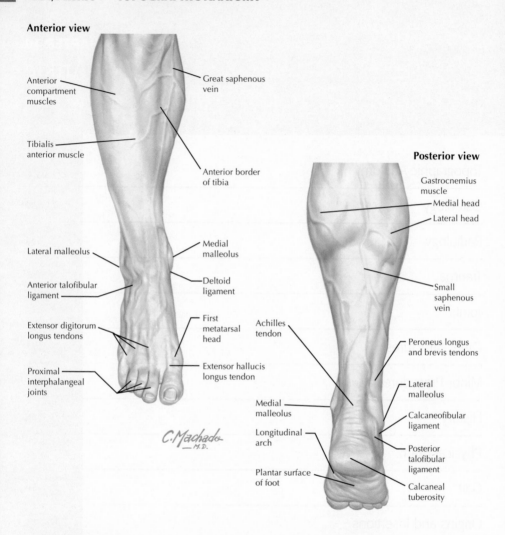

Anterior view

Anterior compartment muscles

Great saphenous vein

Tibialis anterior muscle

Anterior border of tibia

Lateral malleolus

Medial malleolus

Anterior talofibular ligament

Deltoid ligament

Extensor digitorum longus tendons

First metatarsal head

Proximal interphalangeal joints

Extensor hallucis longus tendon

C.Machado
_ M.D.

Posterior view

Gastrocnemius muscle

Medial head

Lateral head

Small saphenous vein

Achilles tendon

Peroneus longus and brevis tendons

Medial malleolus

Lateral malleolus

Longitudinal arch

Calcaneofibular ligament

Posterior talofibular ligament

Plantar surface of foot

Calcaneal tuberosity

STRUCTURE	CLINICAL APPLICATION
Anterior compartment muscles	Peroneal nerve injury results in weakness and foot drop.
Gastrocnemius muscle	Muscle tears/strains commonly occur at musculotendinous junction.
Achilles tendon	Loss of contour and/or defect occurs when tendon is ruptured.
Valgus heel	Best seen posteriorly; heel should be in a valgus position.
Medial and lateral malleoli	Swelling indicates ankle injury: fracture or sprain.
Longitudinal arch of foot	Loss of arch indicates pes planus: congenital or acquired.
Plantar foot	Site of many ulcers; site of pain in plantar fasciitis.
1st metatarsal head	Head is prominent and painful in hallux valgus/bunion.
1st metatarsophalangeal joint	Common site for gout. Joint will be red and swollen.
Proximal interphalangeal joints	Hammertoes cause these joints to be prominent dorsally.

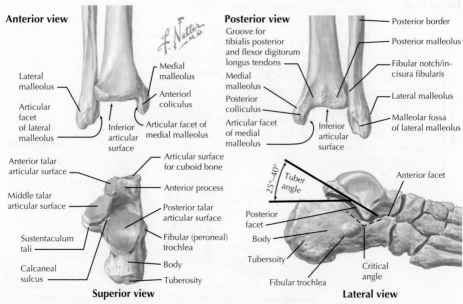

Anterior view

- Lateral malleolus
- Articular facet of lateral malleolus
- Medial malleolus
- Anteriorl coliculus
- Inferior articular surface
- Articular facet of medial malleolus

Posterior view

- Groove for tibialis posterior and flexor digitorum longus tendons
- Medial malleolus
- Posterior colliculus
- Articular facet of medial malleolus
- Inferior articular surface
- Posterior border
- Posterior malleolus
- Fibular notch/in-cisura fibularis
- Lateral malleolus
- Malleolar fossa of lateral malleolus

Superior view

- Anterior talar articular surface
- Middle talar articular surface
- Sustentaculum tali
- Calcaneal sulcus
- Articular surface for cuboid bone
- Anterior process
- Posterior talar articular surface
- Fibular (peroneal) trochlea
- Body
- Tuberosity

Lateral view

- 25°–40° Tuber angle
- Anterior facet
- Posterior facet
- Body
- Tuberosity
- Fibular trochlea
- Critical angle

CHARACTERISTICS	OSSIFY		FUSE	COMMENTS
DISTAL FIBULA				
Lateral malleolus	Distal physis	4yr	18-20yr	• ATFL, CFL, & PTFL all insert on lateral malleolus • Small avulsion fractures commonly occur here
DISTAL TIBIA				
Plafond: weight-bearing portion of distal tibia	Distal physis	1yr	18-20yr	• Concave and congruent with talar body/dome • Unique adolescent ankle fractures result from phased closure of distal tibia physis
Lateral distal tibia ∘ Anterior tubercle ∘ Posterior tubercle				• Incisura: lat. groove for fibula b/w 2 tubercles ∘ Called Tillaux/Chaput's tubercle; origin of AITFL ∘ Called posterior malleolus; origin of PITFL
Medial malleolus ∘ Anterior colliculus ∘ Posterior colliculus				• Deltoid ligament attaches to medial malleolus ∘ Superficial deltoid attaches to anterior colliculus ∘ Deep deltoid attaches to posterior colliculus
CALCANEUS				
Body ∘ Tuberosity · Medial process · Lateral process ∘ Peroneal tubercle	**Primary** Body **Secondary** Tuberosity	6mo (fetal) 9yr	13-15yr 13-15yr	• Largest tarsal bone • Provides support for lateral column of foot • Bohler's angle (normal 25-40°) • Gissane's critical angle (normal 95-105°) • Peroneal tubercle separates peroneal tendons
Sustentaculum tali				• Prominent medially, supports the medial facet • Fulcrum for FHL tendon (on inferior surface)
Multiple facets ∘ Posterior: largest ∘ Medial: on sust. tali ∘ Anterior				• Posterior facet most often involved in fractures

• Borders of ankle mortise: superior: tibia (plafond), medial: medial malleolus (tibia), lateral: lateral malleolus (fibula)

Lateral view

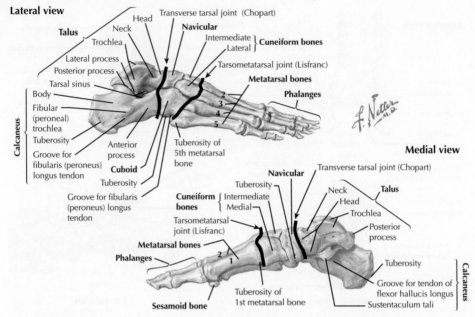

Medial view

CHARACTERISTICS	OSSIFY	FUSE	COMMENTS
TALUS			
Head	Primary		• Talar head is supported by the spring ligament
			• Convex head forms tight articulation w/navicular
Neck			• Neck is site of entry for most of the blood supply
Body/trochlea (dome)	Body	7mo (fetal)	13-15yr • Body is mostly covered with articular cartilage
			• AVN is a concern owing to retrograde blood supply
Posterior process			• Body weight is transmitted from tibia to dome
Medial tubercle			• FHL tendon runs between med. & lat.tubercles
Lateral tubercle			• Os trigonum may be an unfused lateral tubercle
Lateral process			• Lateral process often fractured by snowboarders
NAVICULAR			
• Curved/ "boat" shape	Primary	4yr	13-15yr • Forms "acetabulum pedis" for talar head (along
• Multiple facets			with strong plantar ligaments)
○ Proximal: concave for talus			• Is the "keystone" of the transverse arch of foot
○ Distal: facet for each cunei-			• Posterior tibialis tendon inserts on tuberosity
form & cuboid			• Susceptible to stress fracture
• Tuberosity: medial/plantar			• Kohler's disease: osteonecrosis of navicular
CUBOID			
• Tuberosity; inferiorly	Primary	Birth	13-15yr • Most lateral tarsal bone
• 4 facets: calcaneus, lat.			• Peroneus longus tendon passes through groove
cuneiform, 4th & 5th MTs			on inferior surface
• Cuboid groove; inferiorly			
CUNEIFORMS			
• Three bones	Primary		• 2nd MT "keys" into recess of short intermediate
○ Medial: largest		3yr	bone; can lead to fracture of MT base
○ Intermediate: shortest		4yr	13-15yr • TA, PL, PT tendons partially insert on medial cu-
○ Lateral		1yr	neiform
• Trapezoidal			• Trapezoidal shape strengthens transverse arch

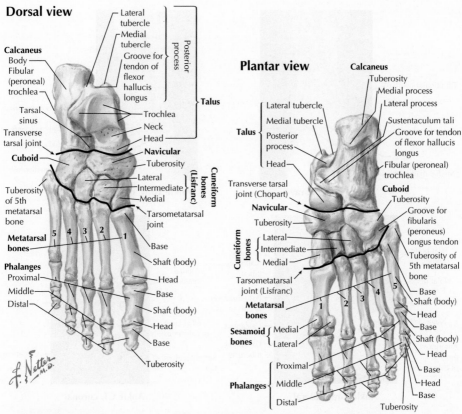

Dorsal view

Calcaneus
Body
Fibular (peroneal) trochlea
Tarsal sinus
Transverse tarsal joint
Cuboid
Tuberosity of 5th metatarsal bone
Metatarsal bones 5 4 3 2 1
Phalanges
Proximal
Middle
Distal

Lateral tubercle
Medial tubercle
Groove for tendon of flexor hallucis longus
}Posterior process
}Talus
Trochlea
Neck
Head
Navicular
Tuberosity
Lateral
Intermediate
Medial
}Cuneiform bones (Lisfranc)
Tarsometatarsal joint
Base
Shaft (body)
Head
Base
Shaft (body)
Head
Base
Tuberosity

f. Netter M.D.

Plantar view

Talus {
Lateral tubercle
Medial tubercle
Posterior process
Head

Transverse tarsal joint (Chopart)
Navicular
Tuberosity
Cuneiform bones {
Lateral
Intermediate
Medial
Tarsometatarsal joint (Lisfranc)
Metatarsal bones 1 2 3 4 5
Sesamoid bones { Medial / Lateral
Phalanges {
Proximal
Middle
Distal

Calcaneus
Tuberosity
Medial process
Lateral process
Sustentaculum tali
Groove for tendon of flexor hallucis longus
Fibular (peroneal) trochlea
Cuboid
Tuberosity
Groove for fibularis (peroneus) longus tendon
Tuberosity of 5th metatarsal bone
Base
Shaft (body)
Head
Base
Shaft (body)
Head
Base
Head
Base
Tuberosity

CHARACTERISTICS	OSSIFY		FUSE	COMMENTS
METATARSALS				
• Long bone characteristics • Base of 2nd MT keys into tarsal recess • 1st MT head has crista that separates two sesamoids	**Primary** Shaft **Secondary** Epiphysis	9wk (fetal) 5-8yr	Birth 14-18y	• Numbered medial to lateral, I to V • Only one physis per bone (in neck) except in 1st metatarsal (in base) • Peroneus brevis inserts on base of 5th MT (avulsion fracture can occur)
PHALANGES				
• Toes 2-5 have three phalanges • Great toe has only two phalanges	**Primary** Body **Secondary** Epiphysis	10wk (fetal) 2-3yr	14-18yr 14-18yr	• 14 total phalanges in each foot • Only one physis per bone (in the base) • Sesamoid bones with other toes can occur as a normal variant (usually b/w MT head)
• Ossification of each tarsal bone occurs from a single center (except calcaneus) • Tarsal tunnel: a fibroosseous tunnel formed by the posterior medial malleolus, medial walls of calcaneus and talus, and flexor retinaculum. Contents: tendons (TP, FDL, FHL), posterior tibial artery, tibial nerve (can be compressed in tunnel)				
OSSICLES				

Sesamoids
  Medial (tibial)
  Lateral (fibular)
Accessory navicular
Os trigonum
				• Separated by cristae plantarly (1st MT head)
				• Part of flexor mechanism (in FDB tendons)
				• Can be fractured or dislocated
				• Can cause medial foot prominence/pain
				• Can cause heel pain (e.g., ballet dancers)

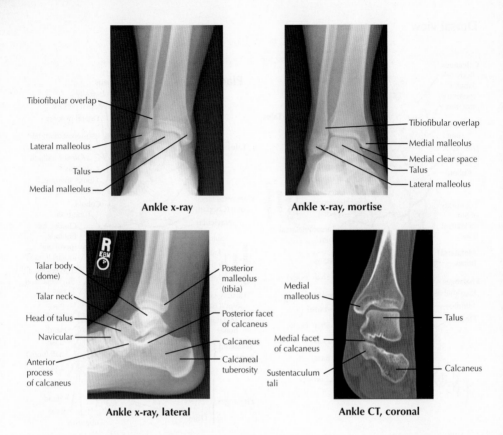

Ankle x-ray

- Tibiofibular overlap
- Lateral malleolus
- Talus
- Medial malleolus

Ankle x-ray, mortise

- Tibiofibular overlap
- Medial malleolus
- Medial clear space
- Talus
- Lateral malleolus

Ankle x-ray, lateral

- Talar body (dome)
- Talar neck
- Head of talus
- Navicular
- Anterior process of calcaneus
- Posterior malleolus (tibia)
- Posterior facet of calcaneus
- Calcaneus
- Calcaneal tuberosity

Ankle CT, coronal

- Medial malleolus
- Medial facet of calcaneus
- Sustentaculum tali
- Talus
- Calcaneus

RADIOGRAPH	TECHNIQUE	FINDINGS	CLINICAL APPLICATION
ANKLE			
Anteroposterior (AP)	Beam aimed between malleoli	Ankle (distal tibia, fibula, and talus)	Fractures, malalignment, arthritis
Lateral	Beam aimed laterally at malleolus	Tibia (anterior lip & posterior malleolus), talar dome, calcaneus, subtalar joint	Fractures: tibia, talus, calcaneus; Bohler's angle (nl: 25-40°)
Mortise view	AP with 15° of internal rotation	Best view of ankle mortise, plafond	Fractures; widening = ligament injury
Stress view	Mortise with external stress	ER: syndesmosis widening (nl <6mm) Medial clear space widening (nl<4mm) Inversion/tilt: joint space widening Anterior/drawer: ant. talus subluxation	ER: syndesmosis injury, deltoid ligament injury Inv: lateral ligament (CFL) injury Ant: lateral ligament (ATFL) injury
OTHER STUDIES			
CT	Axial, coronal, sagittal	Articular congruity, fracture fragments	Intraarticular or comminuted fxs
MRI	Sequence protocols vary	Ligaments, tendons, and cartilage	OCD lesions, ligament or tendon tears
Bone scan		All bones evaluated	Stress fractures, infection

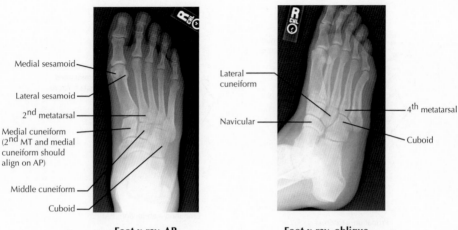

Foot x-ray, AP

Medial sesamoid
Lateral sesamoid
2nd metatarsal
Medial cuneiform (2nd MT and medial cuneiform should align on AP)
Middle cuneiform
Cuboid

Foot x-ray, oblique

Lateral cuneiform
Navicular
4th metatarsal
Cuboid

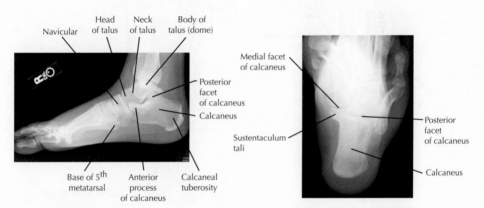

Foot x-ray, lateral

Navicular
Head of talus
Neck of talus
Body of talus (dome)
Posterior facet of calcaneus
Calcaneus
Base of 5th metatarsal
Anterior process of calcaneus
Calcaneal tuberosity

Foot x-ray, calcaneus

Medial facet of calcaneus
Posterior facet of calcaneus
Sustentaculum tali
Calcaneus

RADIOGRAPH	TECHNIQUE	FINDINGS	CLINICAL APPLICATION
FOOT			
Anteroposterior (AP)	Beam perpendicular to midfoot; WB used to evaluate deformity	Tarsals, metatarsals, and phalanges; 2nd MT should align w/medial cuneiform	Fractures/dislocations mid & forefoot; used to measure hallux valgus angles
Lateral	Beam aimed laterally at tarsals	Hind, mid, and forefoot	Fractures and dislocations
Oblique	AP with 45° of internal rotation	Mid & forefoot, TMT jt.	4th MT aligns with cuboid
Harris	DF foot, beam 45° to heel	Calcaneal tuberosity, post. facet	Calcaneus fractures
Canale	15° foot eversion, tilt beam 15°	Talar neck	Talar neck fractures
Broden	IR leg 40°, tilt beam 10, 20, 30, 40°	Posterior subtalar facet	Fx of posterior facet or sustentaculum
Stress views	AP with abd/add or inv/eversion	Bony and joint alignment	Lisfranc fracture/dislocations
Axial/sesamoid view	DF hallux, beam along foot axis	Shows sesamoid bones/ articulation	Sesamoid fracture or dislocation

Lauge-Hansen Classification of Ankle Fractures

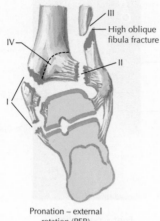

III — High oblique fibula fracture

IV

II

I

Pronation – external rotation (PER)

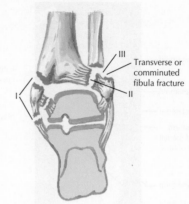

III — Transverse or comminuted fibula fracture

II

I

Pronation – abduction (PA)

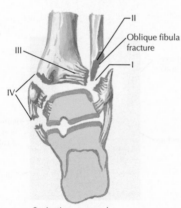

II

Oblique fibula fracture

III

I

IV

Supination – external rotation (SER)

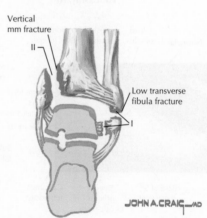

Vertical mm fracture

II

Low transverse fibula fracture

I

Supination – adduction (SA)

JOHN A. CRAIG—AD

DESCRIPTION	EVALUATION	CLASSIFICATION	TREATMENT
ANKLE FRACTURE			

• Very common in all ages
• One or both malleoli involved
• 1 malleolus fx: usually stable
• Bimalleolar fx OR lateral malleolus fx with medial ligament rupture: unstable
• Congruent mortise required
• Fibular length & rotation must be correct
	Hx: Trauma, pain, swelling, +/– inability to bear weight
	PE: Effusion, soft tissue swelling. One or both malleoli TTP +/– proximal fibula tenderness
	XR: Ankle trauma series
	Stress XR: If stability of fx is in question (esp. Weber B/SER II)
		Weber/AO: location of fibula fx
		  A: distal to plafond
		  B: at the plafond
		  C: above the plafond
		Lauge-Hansen: based on foot position & mechanism
		  SA: supination/adduction I-II
		  SER: supination/ER I-IV
		  PER: pronation/ER I-IV
		  PA: pronation/abduction I-III
			• Dislocation: reduce joint immediately
			• Stable/nondisplaced/avulsion: short leg cast for 4-6wk
			• Unstable/displaced: ORIF. Restore congruent mortise & fibular length. Add syndesmosis fixation for unstable syndesmosis.

COMPLICATIONS: Posttraumatic osteoarthritis/pain, limited range of motion, nonunion/malunion, instability, RSD			
See Chapter 9, Knee/Leg for pilon fracture and Maisonneuve fracture			

Intraarticular Fracture of Calcaneus

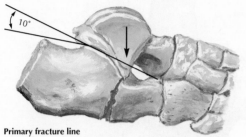

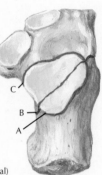

Primary fracture line
Talus driven down into calcaneus, usually by fall and landing on heel. Böhler angle narrowed

Primary fracture line runs across posterior facet, forming antero-medial and posterolateral fragments

Saunders classified this fratcture A-C (lateral to medial)

Essex-Lopresti

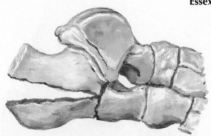

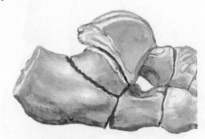

Secondary fracture line
Often extends through tuberosity of calcaneus to produce **tongue-type fracture**

If secondary fracture line extends to dorsal aspect of calcaneus, **joint depression-type** fracture results

DESCRIPTION	EVALUATION	CLASSIFICATION	TREATMENT
CALCANEUS FRACTURE			

• Most common tarsal fracture
• Mechanism: high energy/axial load (e.g., MVA, high fall)
• Most fractures intraarticular
• Intraarticular fractures affect subtalar joint (esp. posterior facet)
• Skin at risk from extensive edema
• Rule out spine injury in a fall
• Associated with poor outcomes and long-term disability
	Hx: Trauma, pain, swelling, inability to bear weight
	PE: Marked edema & arch swelling, +/− fx blisters. Widened heel. Check nerve function and pulses.
	XR: AP, lateral (Böhler's angle nl 25-40°), Harris view
	CT: To better define fx lines, displacement, comminution
		Extraarticular
		• Body, tuberosity, anterior or medial process, sustentaculum tali
		Intraarticular
		• *Essex-Lopresti*
		  ∘ Joint depression
		  ∘ Tongue type
		• *Sanders:* per coronal CT
		  ∘ I-IV: how many fragments/fracture lines?
		  ∘ A-C: lateral to medial
			Extraarticular
			• Nondisplaced: cast 10-12wk
			• Displaced: perc. pinning
			Intraarticular
			• Nondisplaced: cast 12 wk
			• Displaced: ORIF
			• Comminuted, low demand/elderly, smokers: closed reduction, cast
			• Comminuted, laborer: primary subtalar fusion

COMPLICATIONS: Skin/wound slough (delay surgery until edema has resolved), malunion (varus), subtalar OA, pain			

Fracture of Talar Neck

Usual cause is impact
on anterior margin
of tibia due to
forceful dorsiflexion

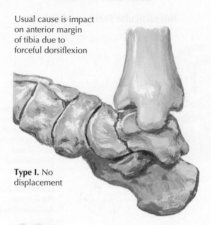

Type I. No
displacement

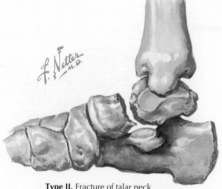

Type II. Fracture of talar neck
with subluxation or dislocation
of subtalar joints

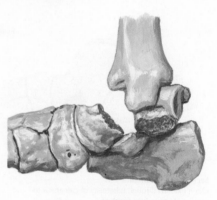

Type III. Fracture of talar neck
with dislocation of subtalar and
tibiotalar joints

DESCRIPTION	EVALUATION	CLASSIFICATION	TREATMENT
TALUS FRACTURE			

• Mechanism: high energy (e.g., MVA, fall from height)
• Neck fractures #1
• Talus has tenuous blood supply
• Neck fx can result in AVN
• Displaced neck fractures are a surgical emergency
• AVN decreased with ORIF
• Hawkins sign = no AVN
• Lateral process fx: snowboarders
	Hx: Trauma, pain, swelling, inability to bear weight
	PE: Edema, tenderness, +/− deformity. Check pulses.
	XR: AP, lateral, Canale (neck) & Broden (post. facet) views
	Hawkins sign: resorption of subchondral bone (lucency on XR) indicates fracture healing
	CT: To better define fx lines
		Body (dome)
		  Osteochondral fx/ injury
		Head
		Process: lateral, posterior
		Neck: Hawkins (predicts risk of AVN)
		  I: Nondisplaced (<10%)
		  II: Subtalar dx (40%)
		  III: II + tibiotalar dx (90%)
		  IV: III + talonavicular dx (100%)
			Body/head/process fractures
			• Nondisplaced: cast
			• Displaced: ORIF
			Osteochondral fx/injury
			• Large bony piece: repair
			• Small/mostly cartilaginous: arthroscopic debride/drilling
			Neck fractures
			• Type I: percutaneous pin
			• Types II-IV: ORIF

COMPLICATIONS: Ankle or subtalar osteoarthritis/pain, malunion (varus #1), osteonecrosis, arthrofibrosis/stiffness			

Lisfranc fracture/dislocation

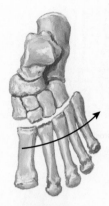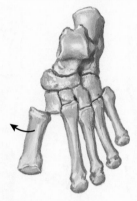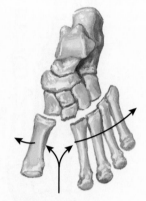

Homolateral dislocation. All five metatarsals displaced in same direction. Fracture of base of 2nd metatarsal

Isolated dislocation. One or two metatarsals displaced; others in normal position

Divergent dislocation. 1st metatarsal displaced medially, others superolaterally

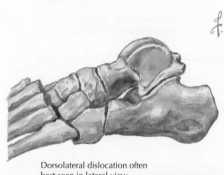

Dorsolateral dislocation often best seen in lateral view

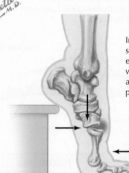

Injury may occur from seemingly trivial event, eg, misstep into a hole with axial compression and abduction force on plantarflexion foot.

DESCRIPTION	EVALUATION	CLASSIFICATION	TREATMENT
TARSOMETATARSAL (LISFRANC) FRACTURE/DISLOCATIONS			
• Mechanism: torque of fixed foot or axial load to vertical foot • Recessed 2nd MT base gives stability to joint • Can have fx or purely ligamentous injury • "Fleck" sign is avulsion of Lisfranc ligament from 2nd MT base • Easily missed injury • Assoc. w/other injuries including tarsal fractures	**Hx:** Trauma to planted foot, pain, swelling **PE:** Edema & ecchymosis. Careful vascular exam. **XR:** AP, lateral, oblique; >2mm b/w 2nd MT base and cuneiform is pathologic. WB/stress views if needed; consider comparison view **CT:** Usually not needed	**By direction** • Isolated: a single metatarsal is affected (usu. 1st or 2nd) • Homolateral: all metatarsals dislocate in same direction • Divergent: metatarsals dislocate in different directions *Many different combinations are possible.*	**Nondisplaced (no widening)** • NWB cast: 8wk • >2mm needs surgical fixation **Minimally displaced** • Closed reduction and percutaneous pinning **Displaced** • ORIF (screws and K-wires) • External fixation if needed preliminarily
COMPLICATIONS: Posttraumatic arthritis/pain, altered gait/limp, compartment syndrome (1st intermetatarsal br. of DPA)			

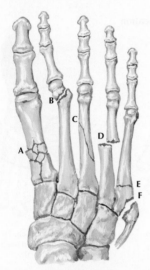

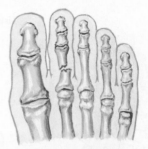

Fracture of proximal phalanx

Types of fractures of metatarsal: A. Comminuted fracture. B. Displaced neck fracture. C. Oblique fracture. D. Displaced transverse fracture. E. Fracture of base of 5th metatarsal. F. Avulsion of tuberosity of 5th metatarsal

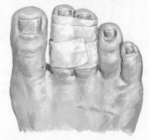

Fracture of phalanx splinted by taping to adjacent toe (buddy taping)

Proximal fifth metatarsal fracture

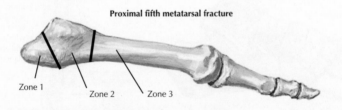

Zone 1   Zone 2   Zone 3

DESCRIPTION	EVALUATION	CLASSIFICATION	TREATMENT
METATARSAL FRACTURES			

• Common injuries: most benign
• Prox. 5th MT is watershed area. Nutrient artery injury can result in nonunion
• Prox. 5th MT avulsion fx by lateral plantar aponeurosis or peroneus brevis tendon
• Stress fractures in runners
	Hx: Trauma, pain, swelling
	PE: Edema & ecchymosis, TTP
	XR: AP, lateral, oblique
	BS: To evaluate for stress fx
		Location:
		Head, neck, shaft, base
		5th MT base fracture:
		Zone 1: avulsion fx
		Zone 2: metadiaphyseal jxn
		Zone 3: proximal diaphysis
			• Nondisplaced: hard shoe/cast
			• Displaced/angulated: PCP or ORIF
			• 5th MT base:
			  ○ Zone 1: hard shoe
			  ○ Zone 2: SLNWC 6-8wk
			  ○ Zone 3: SLNWC 8wk/ORIF; zones 2&3: ORIF in elite athletes

COMPLICATIONS: Nonunion (esp. proximal 5th metatarsal), malunion, posttraumatic osteoarthritis/pain			
PHALANGEAL FRACTURES			
• Common injuries: most benign • Usually from "stubbing" toe or dropping object on toe • Rarely need surgical treatment	**Hx:** Trauma, pain, swelling **PE:** Edema & ecchymosis, TTP **XR:** AP, lateral, oblique	Location Head Shaft Base	• Non/minimally displaced: buddy tape & hard shoe • Displaced/unstable: PCP • Intraarticular hallux fx: ORIF

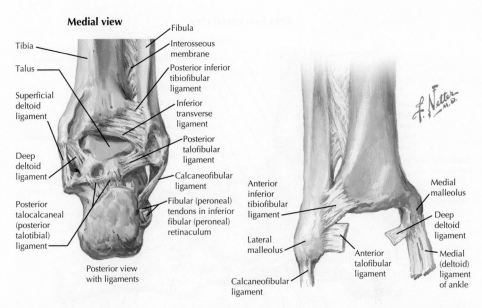

Medial view

Tibia
Talus
Superficial deltoid ligament
Deep deltoid ligament
Posterior talocalcaneal (posterior talotibial) ligament

Fibula
Interosseous membrane
Posterior inferior tibiofibular ligament
Inferior transverse ligament
Posterior talofibular ligament
Calcaneofibular ligament
Fibular (peroneal) tendons in inferior fibular (peroneal) retinaculum

Posterior view with ligaments

Anterior inferior tibiofibular ligament
Lateral malleolus
Calcaneofibular ligament

Anterior talofibular ligament

Medial malleolus
Deep deltoid ligament
Medial (deltoid) ligament of ankle

LIGAMENTS	ATTACHMENTS	COMMENTS
DISTAL TIBIOFIBULAR		
Syndesmosis	Primary support of ankle	Injured in Weber C fx & "high" ankle sprains
○ Anterior inferior tibiofibular (AITFL)	Anterior tibia (ant. tubercle) to distal fibula	Strong, oblique ligament. Avulsion yields "Tillaux" fracture/fragment
○ Posterior inferior tibiofibular (PITFL)	Posterior tibia to distal fibula	Weaker; originates on posterior malleolus
○ Inferior transverse ligament (ITL)	Inferior & deep to PITFL	Gives posterior support to ankle mortise
○ Interosseous ligament (IOL)	Lateral tibia to medial fibula	Strong distal thickening of interosseous memb.
If the syndesmosis is torn, the ankle mortise is disrupted. The fibula (& firmly attached talus) will displace laterally.		
ANKLE		
The ankle is ginglymus, or hinge joint. It primarily provides plantarflexion & dorsiflexion motion. ROM: DF 20°, PF 50°		
Capsule	Tibia and fibula to talus	Gives varying amount of support to the ankle
Lateral	Lateral malleolus to:	ATFL & PTFL are capsular thickenings
○ **Anterior talofibular** (ATFL)	Neck of talus	Resists anterior translation. #1 injured ligament in ankle sprains.
○ **Calcaneofibular** (CFL)	Calcaneus (peroneal tub.)	Deep to peroneal tendons. Resists inversion. #2 in ankle sprains.
○ Posterior talofibular (PTFL)	Talus (posterior process)	Strong. Rarely torn. Attaches to lateral tubercle of posterior process.
Medial: deltoid ligament (4 parts)		Origin on medial malleolus (MM)
Superficial deltoid	Anterior colliculus of MM to:	Resists eversion of the ankle
○ Anterior tibiotalar	Anteromedial talus	Weak ligament. Can cause impingement
○ Tibionavicular	Navicular tuberosity	Restraint to medial migration of talar head
○ Tibiocalcaneal	Sustentaculum tali	Strongest portion of the superficial deltoid, resists valgus
Deep deltoid	Posterior colliculus of MM to:	Resists external rotation and lateral migration
○ Posterior tibiotalar	Medial talus & medial tubercle	Nearly horizontal; strongest portion of deltoid

Right foot: lateral view

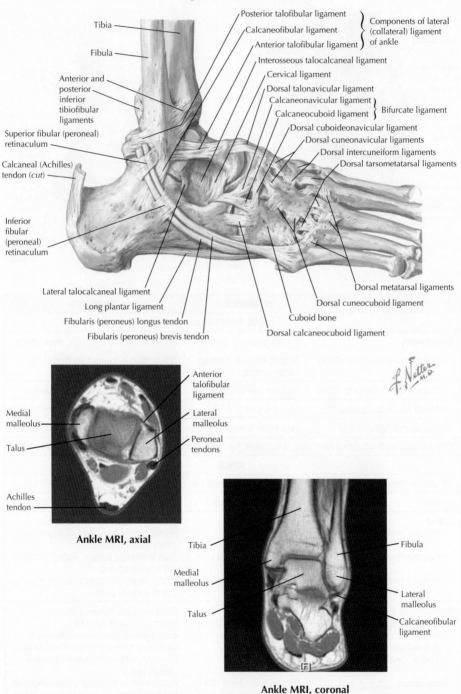

Posterior talofibular ligament
Calcaneofibular ligament } Components of lateral (collateral) ligament
Anterior talofibular ligament } of ankle
Interosseous talocalcaneal ligament
Cervical ligament
Dorsal talonavicular ligament
Calcaneonavicular ligament }
Calcaneocuboid ligament } Bifurcate ligament
Dorsal cuboideonavicular ligament
Dorsal cuneonavicular ligaments
Dorsal intercuneiform ligaments
Dorsal tarsometatarsal ligaments

Tibia
Fibula
Anterior and posterior inferior tibiofibular ligaments
Superior fibular (peroneal) retinaculum
Calcaneal (Achilles) tendon (cut)
Inferior fibular (peroneal) retinaculum

Lateral talocalcaneal ligament
Long plantar ligament
Fibularis (peroneus) longus tendon
Fibularis (peroneus) brevis tendon

Dorsal metatarsal ligaments
Dorsal cuneocuboid ligament
Cuboid bone
Dorsal calcaneocuboid ligament

Anterior talofibular ligament
Medial malleolus
Talus
Achilles tendon

Lateral malleolus
Peroneal tendons

Ankle MRI, axial

Tibia
Medial malleolus
Talus

Fibula
Lateral malleolus
Calcaneofibular ligament

Ankle MRI, coronal

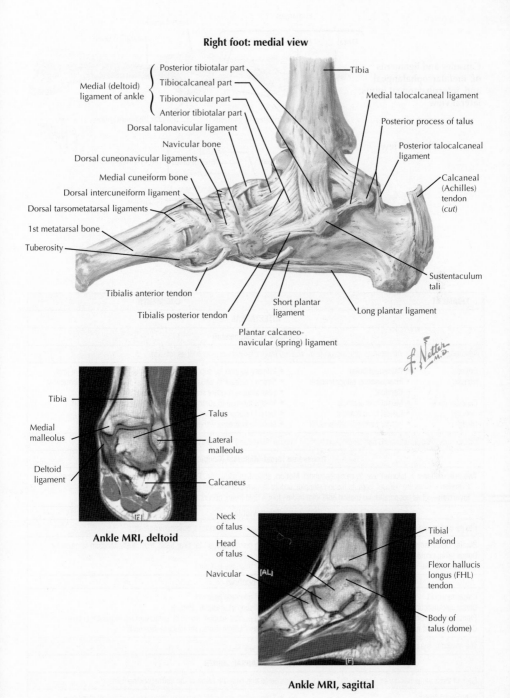

Right foot: medial view

Medial (deltoid) ligament of ankle
- Posterior tibiotalar part
- Tibiocalcaneal part
- Tibionavicular part
- Anterior tibiotalar part

Dorsal talonavicular ligament
Navicular bone
Dorsal cuneonavicular ligaments
Medial cuneiform bone
Dorsal intercuneiform ligament
Dorsal tarsometatarsal ligaments
1st metatarsal bone
Tuberosity
Tibialis anterior tendon
Tibialis posterior tendon
Plantar calcaneo-navicular (spring) ligament
Short plantar ligament
Long plantar ligament

Tibia
Medial talocalcaneal ligament
Posterior process of talus
Posterior talocalcaneal ligament
Calcaneal (Achilles) tendon (cut)
Sustentaculum tali

Tibia
Medial malleolus
Deltoid ligament
Talus
Lateral malleolus
Calcaneus

Ankle MRI, deltoid

Neck of talus
Head of talus
Navicular
Tibial plafond
Flexor hallucis longus (FHL) tendon
Body of talus (dome)

Ankle MRI, sagittal

Phalanges

Joint capsule

Distal   Middle   Proximal

Metatarsal bone

Capsules and ligaments of metatarsophalangeal and interphalangeal joints: lateral view

Collateral ligaments

Plantar ligament (plate)

f. Netter.
M.D.

Plantar view

Tarsometatarsal joint

Medial
Intermediate } Cuneiform bones
Lateral

Metatarsal bones

Navicular

1

2

Intermetatarsal lig.

Lisfranc lig.

LIGAMENT	COMMENTS
INTERTARSAL	
Subtalar (Talocalcaneal)	
Articulation of 3 facets. Allows inversion/version (e.g., walking on uneven surfaces) as well as rotation.	
Extrinsic — **• Calcaneofibular**	• Primary support for subtalar joint. Also a main support for ankle joint.
Intrinsic — **• Interosseous talocalcaneal**	• Strong stabilizer in sinus tarsi. Injury can be cause of chronic instability.
• Cervical	• Less stout secondary stabilizer. Also in sinus tarsi.
Capsular thick- — • Medial talocalcaneal	• Medial tubercle to sustentaculum tali. Provides minimal support.
enings — • Lateral talocalcaneal	• Deep to calcaneofibular. Provides minimal support.
Other — • Inferior peroneal retinaculum	• Multiple insertions within sinus tarsi.
Dislocations: Closed reductions can be blocked by: EDB (medial dislocation) or PT tendon (lateral dislocation)	
Transverse Tarsal/Midtarsal (Chopart's)	
Two articulations: 1. talonavicular, 2. calcaneocuboid. **Motion:** abduction/adduction. **Function** depends on foot/subtalar position: **Eversion**—joints are parallel, permits motion (supple), occurs in early stance/"heel strike". **Inversion**—joints not parallel, no motion (stiff joint makes foot a rigid lever), occurs in late stance/"toe off."	
Talonavicular	
Highly congruent "ball & socket" type joint. Convex talar head in concave navicular ("acetabulum pedis")	
Plantar calcaneonavicular (Spring)	• Strong plantar support for talar head, from sustentaculum to navicular
Dorsal talonavicular	• Dorsal support
Calcaneonavicular	• Half of bifurcate ligament
Calcaneocuboid	
Calcaneocuboid	• Half of bifurcate ligament
Dorsal calcaneocuboid	• Dorsal support, minimal strength
Plantar calcaneocuboid (short plantar)	• Strong plantar support, from sustentaculum tali to plantar cuboid
Calcaneocuboid metatarsal (long plantar)	• Crosses multiple joints with multiple insertions
The tendon of the peroneus longus also crosses this joint and adds support.	
OTHER INTERTARSAL JOINTS	
Each of these joints has dorsal, plantar, and interosseous ligaments that bear the name of the corresponding joint.	
Cuboideonavicular	• These joints are small, have very little motion or clinical significance.
Cuneonavicular	• The plantar ligaments are the strongest.
Intercuneiform	
Cuneocuboid	

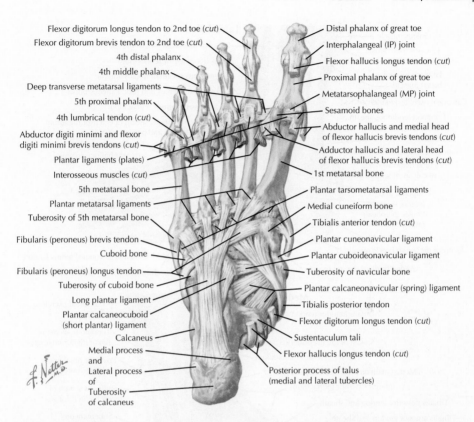

Flexor digitorum longus tendon to 2nd toe (*cut*)
Flexor digitorum brevis tendon to 2nd toe (*cut*)
4th distal phalanx
4th middle phalanx
Deep transverse metatarsal ligaments
5th proximal phalanx
4th lumbrical tendon (*cut*)
Abductor digiti minimi and flexor digiti minimi brevis tendons (*cut*)
Plantar ligaments (plates)
Interosseous muscles (*cut*)
5th metatarsal bone
Plantar metatarsal ligaments
Tuberosity of 5th metatarsal bone
Fibularis (peroneus) brevis tendon
Cuboid bone
Fibularis (peroneus) longus tendon
Tuberosity of cuboid bone
Long plantar ligament
Plantar calcaneocuboid (short plantar) ligament
Calcaneus
Medial process and Lateral process of Tuberosity of calcaneus

Distal phalanx of great toe
Interphalangeal (IP) joint
Flexor hallucis longus tendon (*cut*)
Proximal phalanx of great toe
Metatarsophalangeal (MP) joint
Sesamoid bones
Abductor hallucis and medial head of flexor hallucis brevis tendons (*cut*)
Adductor hallucis and lateral head of flexor hallucis brevis tendons (*cut*)
1st metatarsal bone
Plantar tarsometatarsal ligaments
Medial cuneiform bone
Tibialis anterior tendon (*cut*)
Plantar cuneonavicular ligament
Plantar cuboideonavicular ligament
Tuberosity of navicular bone
Plantar calcaneonavicular (spring) ligament
Tibialis posterior tendon
Flexor digitorum longus tendon (*cut*)
Sustentaculum tali
Flexor hallucis longus tendon (*cut*)
Posterior process of talus (medial and lateral tubercles)

LIGAMENTS	COMMENTS
OTHER JOINTS	
Tarsometatarsal (Lisfranc)	
Gliding joints. Make up the transverse arch of foot. 2nd MT base is the "keystone"	
Intermetatarsal Lisfranc: medial cuneiform to 2nd MT base Dorsal, plantar, interosseous tarsometatarsal	• B/w 2nd & 5th metatarsal bases. No ligament b/w 1st & 2nd MT • Primary stabilizer of articulation. Avulsion of ligament = "fleck" sign • Plantar ligaments are the strongest.
Metatarsophalangeal	
Condyloid joint	
Collateral Plantar plate Deep transverse metatarsal Intersesamoidal Abd. & add. hallucis tendons	• Strong medial and lateral support; limits varus and valgus • Primary support. Loose origin on MT neck to strong insertion on P1 • Injured (avulsion from MT) in hyperextension injury/turf toe • Sesamoids adherent to plantar plate (within FHB tendon) • B/w metatarsal heads. Can compress nerve = Morton's neuroma • The 1st/2nd ligament also attaches to and stabilizes lateral sesamoid • Runs between the two sesamoid bones, stabilizing them • Tendinous insertions on P1 add medial and lateral joint stability
Interphalangeal	
Hinge (ginglymus) joint	
Capsule Collateral and plantar plate	• Gives primary support • Additional support medial, lateral, and plantar

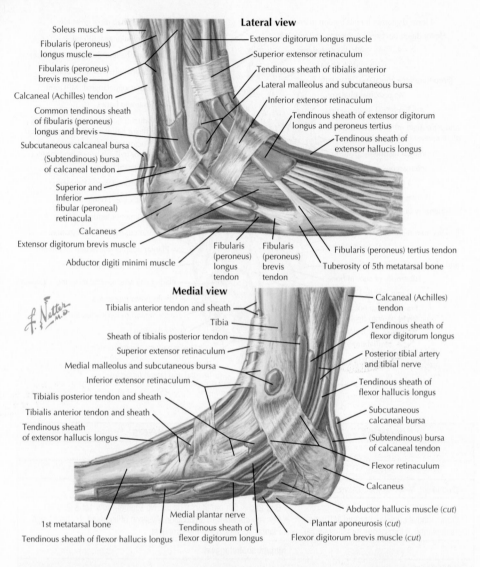

Lateral view

Soleus muscle
Fibularis (peroneus) longus muscle
Fibularis (peroneus) brevis muscle
Calcaneal (Achilles) tendon
Common tendinous sheath of fibularis (peroneus) longus and brevis
Subcutaneous calcaneal bursa
(Subtendinous) bursa of calcaneal tendon
Superior and Inferior fibular (peroneal) retinacula
Calcaneus
Extensor digitorum brevis muscle
Abductor digiti minimi muscle

Extensor digitorum longus muscle
Superior extensor retinaculum
Tendinous sheath of tibialis anterior
Lateral malleolus and subcutaneous bursa
Inferior extensor retinaculum
Tendinous sheath of extensor digitorum longus and peroneus tertius
Tendinous sheath of extensor hallucis longus

Fibularis (peroneus) longus tendon
Fibularis (peroneus) brevis tendon
Fibularis (peroneus) tertius tendon
Tuberosity of 5th metatarsal bone

Medial view

Tibialis anterior tendon and sheath
Tibia
Sheath of tibialis posterior tendon
Superior extensor retinaculum
Medial malleolus and subcutaneous bursa
Inferior extensor retinaculum
Tibialis posterior tendon and sheath
Tibialis anterior tendon and sheath
Tendinous sheath of extensor hallucis longus

Calcaneal (Achilles) tendon
Tendinous sheath of flexor digitorum longus
Posterior tibial artery and tibial nerve
Tendinous sheath of flexor hallucis longus
Subcutaneous calcaneal bursa
(Subtendinous) bursa of calcaneal tendon
Flexor retinaculum
Calcaneus
Abductor hallucis muscle (*cut*)
Plantar aponeurosis (*cut*)
Flexor digitorum brevis muscle (*cut*)

1st metatarsal bone
Tendinous sheath of flexor hallucis longus
Medial plantar nerve
Tendinous sheath of flexor digitorum longus

STRUCTURE	FUNCTION	COMMENT
Superior extensor retinaculum	Covers tendons, nerves, vessels of anterior compartment at ankle	Distal fibula to medial tibia
Inferior extensor retinaculum	Surrounds & covers tendons, etc. of anterior compartment in foot	"Y" shaped; calcaneus to medial malleolus and navicular
Flexor retinaculum	Covers tendons of posterior compartment	Medial malleolus to calcaneus; roof of tarsal tunnel
Superior & inferior peroneal retinaculum	Covers tendons & sheaths of lateral compartment at hind foot	Superior: lateral malleolus to calcaneus Inferior: inf. extensor retinaculum to calcaneus
Plantar aponeurosis (plantar fascia)	Supports longitudinal arch	Inflamed: plantar fasciitis; can develop nodules

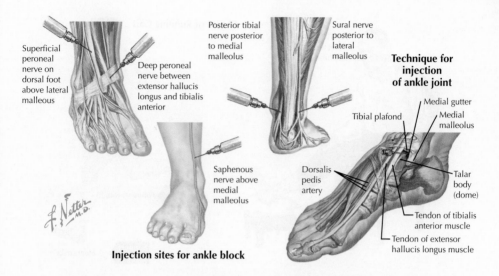

Technique for injection of ankle joint

Injection sites for ankle block

STEPS
ANKLE ARTHROCENTESIS
1. Ask patient about allergies
2. Plantarflex foot, palpate medial malleolus and sulcus between it and the tibialis anterior tendon.
3. Prep skin over ankle joint (iodine/antiseptic soap).
4. Anesthetize skin locally (quarter size spot).
5. Insert 20-gauge needle perpendicularly into the sulcus/ankle joint (medial to the tendon, inferior to distal tibia articular surface, lateral to medial malleolus). Gentle ankle distraction may assist in entering the joint. Aspirate fluid. If suspicious for infection, send fluid for gram stain and culture. Alternatively, may inject into the joint. The fluid should flow easily if needle is in joint.
6. Dress aspiration/injection site.
ANKLE BLOCK
Five separate nerves are blocked. Based on the necessary anesthesia, a complete or partial block can be performed.
1. Ask patient about allergies.
2. Prep skin (iodine/antiseptic soap) circumferentially around the ankle immediately above and below the malleoli.
3. Prepare syringe with 22- to 25-gauge needle with local anesthetic.
4. **Superficial peroneal nerve:** raise a wheal at least 3-4cm across anterolateral ankle from LM to midline.
5. **Deep peroneal nerve:** palpate TA and EHL tendons. Insert needle between tendons to bone, then withdraw slightly. Aspirate to ensure the needle is not in anterior tibial artery. Inject 2-3ml of local anesthetic.
6. **Saphenous nerve:** raise a wheal at least 2-3cm across the anteromedial ankle anterior to medial mall.
7. **Tibial nerve:** palpate posterior tibial artery pulse, FHL (if possible), and Achilles tendon behind the MM. Insert needle posterior to artery, anterior to FHL/Achilles tendon down to bone, then withdraw slightly. Aspirate to ensure the needle is not in the posterior tibial artery. Pull back from bone slightly and inject 2-3ml.
8. **Sural nerve:** raise a subcutaneous wheal at least 2-3cm across the posterolateral ankle b/w LM and Achilles tendon.
9. Dress each injection site.
DIGITAL BLOCK
1. Ask patient about allergies.
2. Prep skin (iodine/soap) over the proximal dorsal toe and adjacent web space(s).
3. Prepare syringe with local without epinephrine and 25-gauge needle.
4. Insert needle along medial and lateral borders of the proximal phalanx to plantar surface. Aspirate to confirm needle is not in a vessel. Slowly inject as you withdraw the needle dorsally. 2-3ml of local should be adequate on either side. Raising a wheal dorsally across the proximal toe may improve the block.
5. Take care not to inject too much fluid into this closed space.
6. Dress the injection sites.

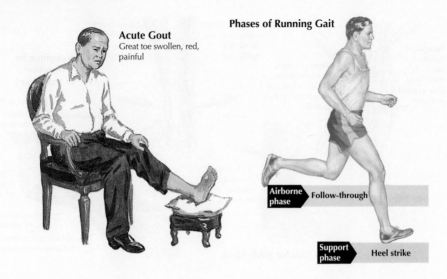

Acute Gout
Great toe swollen, red, painful

Phases of Running Gait

Airborne phase   Follow-through

Support phase   Heel strike

QUESTION	ANSWER	CLINICAL APPLICATION
1. Age	Young	Sprain, fractures
	Middle aged–elderly	Overuse injuries, arthritis, gout, hallux valgus, hammertoes
2. Pain		
a. Onset	Acute (less common)	Fracture, sprain, dislocation
	Chronic	Most foot/ankle disorders are chronic, runners
	After ankle sprain	Talar OCD, subluxating peroneal tendons or tendon tear, lateral process (talus) fracture, SPN injury
b. Location	Ankle	Fracture, osteoarthritis, instability, posterior tibial tendinitis
	Hind foot	Fracture, retrocalcaneal bursitis, Achilles tendinitis, arthritis
	Plantar foot	Plantar fasciitis, nerve compression, ulcer, metatarsalgia
	Midfoot	Osteoarthritis of the tarsus, fracture (Lisfranc), PTTD
	Forefoot	Fractures, metatarsalgia, Morton's neuroma, hammertoes
	1st MTPJ	Hallux vagus, hallux rigidus, sesamoiditis, fx, turf toe, gout
	Bilateral	Consider systemic illness, RA, CMT
c. Occurrence	Morning pain	Plantar fasciitis (improves with stretching)
	With activity	Overuse type injuries: stress fx, tendinitis, bursitis
3. Stiffness	Without locking	Ankle sprain, RA, osteoarthritis
	With locking	Loose body
4. Swelling	Yes	Fracture sprain, arthritis, gout
5. Trauma	Can bear weight	Sprain, contusion, minor fracture
	Cannot bear weight	Fracture: ankle, tarsal, metatarsal
	Fall	Calcaneus fracture, pilon fracture
6. Activity/occupation	Sports, repetitive motion	Achilles tendinitis, overuse injuries (e.g., stress fx)
	Standing all day	Overuse injuries: tendinitis, bursitis
7. Shoe type	Tight/narrow toe box	Hallux valgus (bunion most common in women)
8. Neurologic symptoms	Pain, numbness, tingling	Tarsal tunnel syndrome, diabetic neuropathy, other nerve compression
9. History of systemic disease	Manifestations in foot	Diabetes mellitus, gout, peripheral vascular disease, RA, Reiter's syndrome.

Anterior View

Bunion/Hallux Valgus

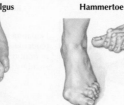

Hammertoe

Plantar View

Callus

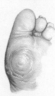

Medial View

Pes Planus

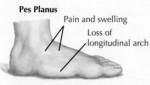

Pain and swelling

Loss of longitudinal arch

Medial view of pronated foot reveals flattened longitudinal arch

Cavovarus Foot

Plantar View

Ulcer

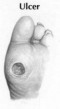

f. Netter M.D.

JOHN A.CRAIG—AD

D. Mascaro

Posterior View

"Too many toes" sign

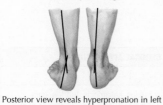

Cavovarus Foot

Pump bump

Tender, slightly red nodule just lateral to calcaneal attachment of Achilles (calcaneal) tendon

Posterior view reveals hyperpronation in left foot. In normal foot, midlines of calcaneus and leg are aligned or deviate less than 2°

Posterior view clearly shows varus deformity of affected right foot.

EXAM	TECHNIQUE	CLINICAL APPLICATION/DDX
INSPECTION		
Foot (weight-bearing)	Anterior view	Hallux valgus (bunion), hammertoes, other deformities (clubfeet, MT adductus)
	Posterior view	Slight valgus is normal; "pump-bump" seen with Achilles tendinitis Increased valgus: posterior tibialis dysfunction, tarsal coalition, planovalgus Varus alignment: neurologic disease (e.g., Charcot-Marie-Tooth)
	Medial view	Pes planus (flat foot): posterior tibialis dysfunction, tarsal coalition, pediatric pes planovalgus Pes cavus (high arch): neurologic disease (e.g., Charcot-Marie-Tooth)
Foot (non-WB)	Plantar view	Ulcers (esp. in diabetics), callus, transfer lesions (callus under 2nd MT head)
Swelling	Ankle Foot: Dorsal Medial Diffuse	Sprain, fracture Fracture, contusion Posterior tibialis dysfunction Consider cardiovascular etiology
Skin	Color Hair	Pallor may indicate vascular disease; congestion may indicate venous insufficiency Decreased hair may indicate peripheral vascular disease
Shoes	Narrow toe box Abnormal wear	Associated with hallux valgus (esp. in women) May indicate malalignment (e.g., pes planus or cavus) or dysfunction (e.g., foot drop)

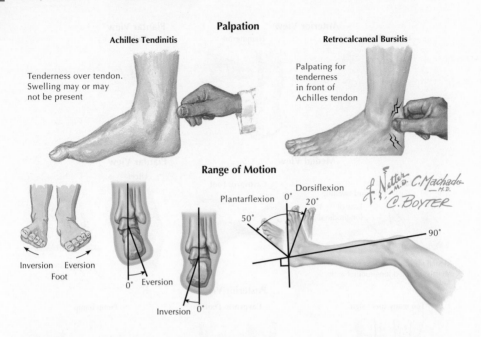

Palpation

Achilles Tendinitis

Tenderness over tendon. Swelling may or may not be present

Retrocalcaneal Bursitis

Palpating for tenderness in front of Achilles tendon

Range of Motion

Inversion Eversion
Foot

0° Eversion

Inversion 0°

Plantarflexion 0°

Dorsiflexion

20°

50°

90°

EXAM	TECHNIQUE	CLINICAL APPLICATION
PALPATION		
Bony structures	1st MP joint/MT& head	Bunion, pain: hallux rigidus, sesamoids, turf toe, gout
	Lesser MPT joint/MT	Pain: metatarsalgia, Freiberg's infraction, fx, tailor's bunion (5th MT head)
	Tarsal bones/midfoot	Tenderness suggests fracture, osteoarthritis, dislocation
	Calcaneus/heel	Pain: fracture; posterior: bursitis (pump bump); plantar: spur, plantar fasciitis; medial: nerve entrapment
	Malleoli	Pain indicates fracture, syndesmosis injury in leg
Soft tissue	Skin	Cool: peripheral vascular disease
		Swelling: trauma/infection vs venous insufficiency
	Between metatarsal heads	Pain: neuroma
	Medial ankle ligaments	Pain suggests ankle sprain (deltoid ligament)
	Tendons (at med. malleolus)	Pain indicates tendinitis, rupture
	Lateral ankle ligaments	Pain suggests ankle sprain (ATFL, CFL, PTFL [rare])
	Peroneal tendons (LM)	Pain indicates tendinitis, tear, dislocation/subluxation
	Achilles tendon	Pain: tendinitis; defect suggests Achilles rupture
RANGE OF MOTION		
Ankle: dorsiflex/plantarflex	Stabilize subtalar joint	Normal: flex 50°/extend 25°
Subtalar: inversion/ eversion	Stabilize tibia	Normal: invert 5-10°/evert 5°
Transverse/midtarsal: adduction/abduction	Stabilize heel/hind foot, give abd./add. stress	Normal: adduct 20°/abduct 10°
Great toe: MTP: flex/extend IP: flex/extend	Stabilize foot, flex/extend Stabilize foot, flex/extend	Normal: flex 75°/extend 75°; decreased in hallux rigidus Normal: flex 90°/extend 0°
Combine motions; Pronation: dorsiflexion, eversion, abduction; Supination: plantarflexion, inversion, adduction		

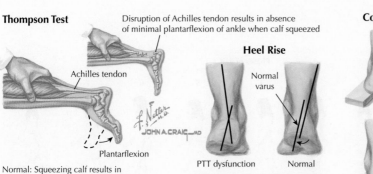

Thompson Test

Disruption of Achilles tendon results in absence of minimal plantarflexion of ankle when calf squeezed

Coleman Block Test

Achilles tendon

Heel Rise

Normal varus

Plantarflexion

Flexible cavovarus

Normal: Squeezing calf results in gastrocnemius and soleus contraction causing plantarflexion of ankle joint if Achilles tendon is intact

PTT dysfunction   Normal

On toe standing, normal PTT function pulls heel into varus. PTT dysfunction allows heel to remain in valgus poisition

Fixed cavovarus

EXAM	TECHNIQUE	CLINICAL APPLICATION
NEUROVASCULAR		
Sensory		
Saphenous (L4)	Medial foot (med. cutaneous)	Deficit indicates corresponding nerve or root lesion
Tibial (L4-S1)	Plantar foot (med. & lat./plantar)	Deficit indicates corresponding nerve or root lesion
Superficial peroneal	Dorsal foot	Deficit indicates corresponding nerve or root lesion
Deep peroneal (L5)	1st dorsal web space	Deficit indicates corresponding nerve or root lesion
Sural (S1)	Lateral foot	Deficit indicates corresponding nerve or root lesion
Motor		
Deep peroneal (L4)	Foot inversion/dorsiflexion	Weakness = tibialis anterior or corresponding nerve or root lesion
Deep peroneal (L5)	Great toe dorsiflex	Weakness = extensor hallucis longus or nerve or root lesion
Tibial (S1)	Foot plantarflexion	Weakness = gastrocnemius or nerve or root lesion
Superficial peroneal	Foot eversion	Weakness = peroneus muscles or nerve or root lesion
Reflex		
S1	Achilles reflex	Hypoactive/absence indicates S1 radiculopathy
Upper motor neuron	Babinski reflex	Upgoing toes indicates an upper motor neuron disorder
Pulses	Dorsalis pedis (on dorsum)	Decreased pulses = trauma/vascular compromise, peripheral vascu-
	Post. tibial (post. med. mall.)	lar disease
SPECIAL TESTS		
Thompson	Prone: squeeze calf	Absent foot plantarflexion indicates Achilles tendon rupture.
Anterior drawer	Stabilize tibia, PF foot, anterior force on heel	Tests lateral ligaments (esp. ATFL). Increased laxity indicates ligament injury.
Talar tilt	Stabilize tibia, DF foot, invert foot	Tests lateral ligaments (esp. CFL). Increased laxity indicates ligament injury.
Ext. rotation stress	Stabilize tibia, ER foot	Tests deep deltoid & syndesmotic ligs. Laxity indicates ligament injury
Eversion stress	Stabilize tibia, evert foot	Tests superficial deltoid ligament. Incr. laxity indicates ligament injury
Squeeze	Compress distal tibia/fibula	Pain may suggest a syndesmosis injury (sprain or complete rupture).
Heel rise	Standing, rise onto toes	Heel should go into varus. No varus in PTTD and fixed deformities. Inability to do single heel rise indicates PTTD.
Coleman block	Lateral foot and heel on block; 1st ray hangs free	Flexible hind foot varus: ankle will go into valgus or neutral when on block. Fixed hind foot varus: ankle will stay in varus on the block.
Tinel's sign	Tap nerve posterior to MM	Paresthesias/tingling indicate tibial nerve entrapment (in tarsal tunnel).
Compression	Squeeze foot at MT heads	Pain (or numbness/tingling): interdigital neuroma (Morton's neuroma)

Phases of gait

| 1 | 2 | 3 | 4 | 5 | 6 | 7 | 8 |

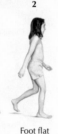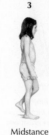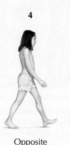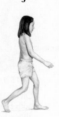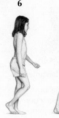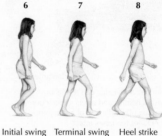

Heel strike · Foot flat · Midstance · Opposite heel strike · Preswing · Initial swing · Terminal swing · Heel strike

C.Machado
— M.D.

GAIT CYCLE
General
Complex interaction of multiple muscles and joints within both lower extremities to produce propulsion of the body
Definitions
Gait: the manner in which a person walks Step: from heel strike of one foot to heel strike of the opposite foot Stride: from heel strike of one foot to the subsequent heel strike of the same foot
Phases
Stance (62%): Part of gait when foot is in contact with ground. Can be subdivided into 3 (or 5) subcategories • Initial phase—double stance (12%): both feet in stance, opposite foot in toe off • Intermediate phase—single stance (38%): opposite foot in swing phase • Terminal phase—double stance (12%): both feet in stance, opposite foot in heel strike **Swing** (38%): Part of gait with foot in air, advancing forward
Sequence
1. Heel strike: Ankle is plantar flexed against the eccentrically contracting TA. The subtalar joint begins everting, allowing IR of tibia. 2. Foot flat: The gastrocnemius fires eccentrically to limit DF of ankle. The foot pronates and subtalar joint everts, resulting in a parallel and supple transverse tarsal joint, which allows the foot to accept the weight and accommodates for uneven surfaces. 3. Midstance: Body weight is over stance leg. The ankle is neutral. The foot begins to transition to a rigid position to allow for push off. 4. Heel off: The posterior tibialis (PT) initiates subtalar inversion (making the transverse tarsal joint unparallel and rigid). The foot supinates, the tibia externally rotates, and the gastrocnemius concentrically contracts producing plantarflexion of the ankle/heel off. 5. Toe off: The passive dorsiflexion of the toes initiates the windlass mechanism, which tightens the plantar fascia, deepening the arch and further inverting the subtalar joint, locking the transverse tarsal joint making the foot a rigid lever upon which to push off. 6. Preswing: the knee flexes to begin to give clearance for the swinging foot. 7. Midswing: knee and hip flexion as well as concentric anterior compartment (TA) contraction provide foot clearance 8. Terminal swing: The transition to heel strike begins

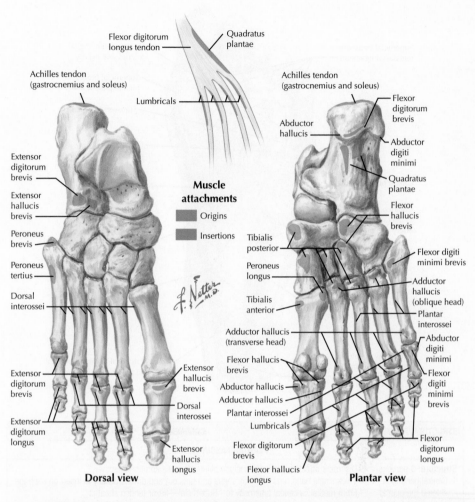

Muscle attachments

| | Origins |
| | Insertions |

Dorsal view

Flexor digitorum longus tendon
Quadratus plantae
Achilles tendon (gastrocnemius and soleus)
Lumbricals
Extensor digitorum brevis
Extensor hallucis brevis
Peroneus brevis
Peroneus tertius
Dorsal interossei
Extensor digitorum brevis
Extensor digitorum longus
Extensor hallucis brevis
Dorsal interossei
Extensor hallucis longus

Plantar view

Achilles tendon (gastrocnemius and soleus)
Flexor digitorum brevis
Abductor hallucis
Abductor digiti minimi
Quadratus plantae
Flexor hallucis brevis
Tibialis posterior
Peroneus longus
Tibialis anterior
Flexor digiti minimi brevis
Adductor hallucis (oblique head)
Plantar interossei
Abductor digiti minimi
Flexor digiti minimi brevis
Adductor hallucis (transverse head)
Flexor hallucis brevis
Abductor hallucis
Adductor hallucis
Plantar interossei
Lumbricals
Flexor digitorum brevis
Flexor hallucis longus
Flexor digitorum longus

CALCANEUS	METATARSAL	PHALANGES—DORSAL	PHALANGES—PLANTAR	FDL TENDON
Dorsal	**Dorsal**	Extensor hallucis brevis	Adductor hallucis (transverse head)	Lumbrical
Extensor hallucis brevis	Peroneus brevis	Extensor hallucis longus	Abductor hallucis	Quadratus plantae
Extensor digitorum brevis	Peroneus tertius	Extensor digitorum brevis	Flexor hallucis brevis	
	Dorsal interosseous		Adductor hallucis	
Plantar		Extensor digitorum longus	Flexor hallucis longus	
Flexor digitorum brevis	**Plantar**	Dorsal interosseous	Flexor digitorum brevis	
Abductor hallucis	Tibialis anterior		Flexor digitorum longus	
Abductor digiti minimi	Peroneus longus		Flexor digiti minimi brevis	
	Adductor hallucis (oblique head)		Abductor digiti minimi	
Posterior	Flexor digiti minimi brevis		Lumbricals	
Gastrocnemius/soleus (Achilles tendon)	Plantar interosseous		Plantar interosseous	
	Adductor hallucis (transverse head)			

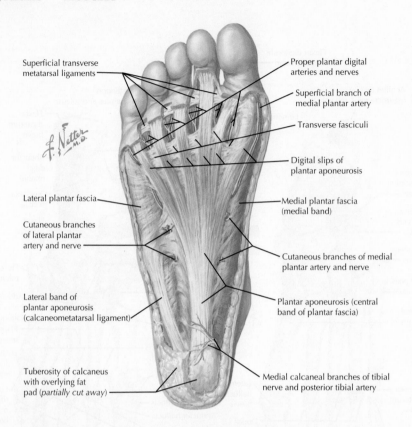

Superficial transverse
metatarsal ligaments

Proper plantar digital
arteries and nerves

Superficial branch of
medial plantar artery

Transverse fasciculi

Digital slips of
plantar aponeurosis

Lateral plantar fascia

Cutaneous branches
of lateral plantar
artery and nerve

Medial plantar fascia
(medial band)

Cutaneous branches of medial
plantar artery and nerve

Lateral band of
plantar aponeurosis
(calcaneometatarsal ligament)

Plantar aponeurosis (central
band of plantar fascia)

Tuberosity of calcaneus
with overlying fat
pad (*partially cut away*)

Medial calcaneal branches of tibial
nerve and posterior tibial artery

STRUCTURE/FUNCTION	COMMENT
PLANTAR FASCIA	
Structure: 3 portions 1. Central band (considered the plantar aponeurosis) 2. Medial band 3. Lateral band	Disorders affecting the fascia include plantar fasciitis and fibromatosis Thick single band runs from calcaneus and fans out and divides distally to insert on each toe From medial calcaneal tuberosity to: Superficial—flexor tendon sheaths Deep—deep transverse metatarsal ligaments Supports the abductor hallucis muscle Supports the abductor digiti minimi muscle Inserts on the base of 5th metatarsal. Can be cause of avulsion fracture
Function 1. Stabilizes longitudinal arch 2. Protects underlying structures 3. Stabilizes foot in gait via the windlass mechanism	
LAYER	**STRUCTURES**
LAYERS OF THE FOOT	
Plantar fascia	3 bands—see above
1: 3 muscles	Abductor hallucis, flexor digitorum brevis, abductor digiti minimi
2: 2 muscles	Quadratus plantae, lumbricals (2 tendons: FHL and FDL)
3: 3 muscles	Flexor hallucis brevis, adductor hallucis, flexor digiti minimi brevis
4: 2 muscles	Plantar interossei, dorsal interossei (2 tendons: PL and PT)

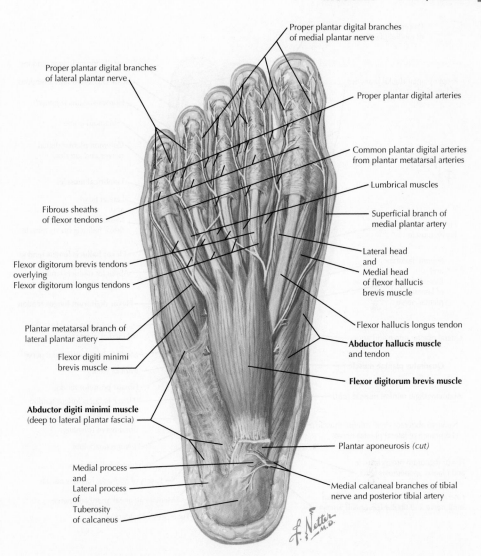

Proper plantar digital branches
of medial plantar nerve

Proper plantar digital branches
of lateral plantar nerve

Proper plantar digital arteries

Common plantar digital arteries
from plantar metatarsal arteries

Lumbrical muscles

Fibrous sheaths
of flexor tendons

Superficial branch of
medial plantar artery

Lateral head
and
Medial head
of flexor hallucis
brevis muscle

Flexor digitorum brevis tendons
overlying
Flexor digitorum longus tendons

Plantar metatarsal branch of
lateral plantar artery

Flexor hallucis longus tendon

Abductor hallucis muscle
and tendon

Flexor digiti minimi
brevis muscle

Flexor digitorum brevis muscle

Abductor digiti minimi muscle
(deep to lateral plantar fascia)

Plantar aponeurosis *(cut)*

Medial process
and
Lateral process
of
Tuberosity
of calcaneus

Medial calcaneal branches of tibial
nerve and posterior tibial artery

MUSCLE	ORIGIN	INSERTION	NERVE	ACTION	COMMENT
FIRST LAYER					
Abductor hallucis	Calcaneal tuberosity, medial process	Through med. sesamoid to proximal phalanx of great toe	Medial plantar	Abducts great toe	Fascia can entrap nerve to ADM
Flexor digitorum brevis (FDB)	Calcaneal tuberosity, medial process	Sides of middle phalanges: lateral 4 toes	Medial plantar	Flexes lateral 4 toes	Supports longitudinal arch
Abductor digiti minimi (ADM)	Calcaneal tuberosity, medial & lateral processes	Lateral base of proximal phalanx: 5th toe	Lateral plantar (1st branch)	Abducts small toe	Nerve can be entrapped by abd. h. fascia

Proper plantar digital branches of medial plantar nerve

Proper plantar digital branches of lateral plantar nerve

Flexor digiti minimi brevis muscle

Superficial branch and Deep branch of lateral plantar nerve

Lateral plantar nerve and artery

Quadratus plantae muscle

Abductor digiti minimi muscle (cut)

Nerve to abductor digiti minimi muscle (1st branch of lateral plantar nerve)

Flexor digitorum brevis muscle and plantar aponeurosis (cut)

Lateral calcaneal nerve and artery (from sural nerve and fibular [peroneal] artery)

Flexor digitorum longus tendons

Flexor digitorum brevis tendons

Fibrous sheaths (opened)

Sesamoid bones

Common plantar digital nerves and arteries

Lumbrical muscles

Lateral head and Medial head of flexor hallucis brevis muscle

Flexor hallucis longus tendon

Abductor hallucis tendon and muscle (cut)

Flexor digitorum longus tendon

Superficial and deep branches of medial plantar artery

Medial plantar artery and nerve

Knot of Henry

Tibialis posterior tendon

Flexor hallucis longus tendon

Posterior tibial artery and tibial nerve (dividing)

Flexor retinaculum

Abductor hallucis muscle (cut)

Fascia of abductor hallucis muscle

Medial calcaneal artery and nerve

Tuberosity of calcaneus

MUSCLE	ORIGIN	INSERTION	NERVE	ACTION	COMMENT
SECOND LAYER					
Quadratus plantae	Medial and lateral plantar calcaneus	Lateral FDL tendon	Lateral plantar	Assists FDL with toe flexion	Two heads/bellies join on FDL tendon
Lumbricals	Separate FDL tendons	Proximal phalanges, extensor expansion	1: medial plantar 2-4: lateral plantar	Flex MTP joint, extend IP joint	1st lumbrical attaches to only 1 FDL tendon

- Medial and lateral plantar nerves are terminal branches of the tibial nerve; they run in the 2nd layer.
- Tendons of FHL and FDL also pass through in the second layer.
- FHL tendon courses between tubercles of posterior process of talus, under sustentaculum tali, then deep to FDL at knot of Henry (crossing of FHL & FDL).

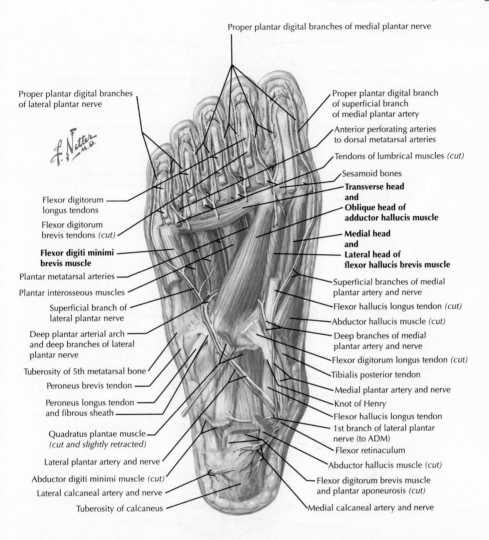

Proper plantar digital branches of medial plantar nerve

Proper plantar digital branches of lateral plantar nerve

Flexor digitorum longus tendons

Flexor digitorum brevis tendons *(cut)*

Flexor digiti minimi brevis muscle

Plantar metatarsal arteries

Plantar interosseous muscles

Superficial branch of lateral plantar nerve

Deep plantar arterial arch and deep branches of lateral plantar nerve

Tuberosity of 5th metatarsal bone

Peroneus brevis tendon

Peroneus longus tendon and fibrous sheath

Quadratus plantae muscle *(cut and slightly retracted)*

Lateral plantar artery and nerve

Abductor digiti minimi muscle *(cut)*

Lateral calcaneal artery and nerve

Tuberosity of calcaneus

Proper plantar digital branch of superficial branch of medial plantar artery

Anterior perforating arteries to dorsal metatarsal arteries

Tendons of lumbrical muscles *(cut)*

Sesamoid bones

Transverse head and Oblique head of adductor hallucis muscle

Medial head and Lateral head of flexor hallucis brevis muscle

Superficial branches of medial plantar artery and nerve

Flexor hallucis longus tendon *(cut)*

Abductor hallucis muscle *(cut)*

Deep branches of medial plantar artery and nerve

Flexor digitorum longus tendon *(cut)*

Tibialis posterior tendon

Medial plantar artery and nerve

Knot of Henry

Flexor hallucis longus tendon

1st branch of lateral plantar nerve (to ADM)

Flexor retinaculum

Abductor hallucis muscle *(cut)*

Flexor digitorum brevis muscle and plantar aponeurosis *(cut)*

Medial calcaneal artery and nerve

MUSCLE	ORIGIN	INSERTION	NERVE	ACTION	COMMENT
THIRD LAYER					
Flexor hallucis brevis (FHB)	Cuboid, lateral cuneiform	Through sesamoids to proximal phalanx of great toe	Medial plantar	Assists great toe flexion at MTPJ	Sesamoid bones are within the tendons
Adductor hallucis	Oblique: base 2-4 MT Transverse: lateral 4 MTP	Through lateral sesamoid to lateral proximal phalanx of great toe	Lateral plantar	Adducts great toe	2 heads have different orientations; contributes to hallux valgus deformity
Flexor digiti minimi brevis (FDMB)	Base of 5th metatarsal	Base of proximal phalanx of small toe	Lateral plantar	Flex small toe	Small, relatively insignificant muscle

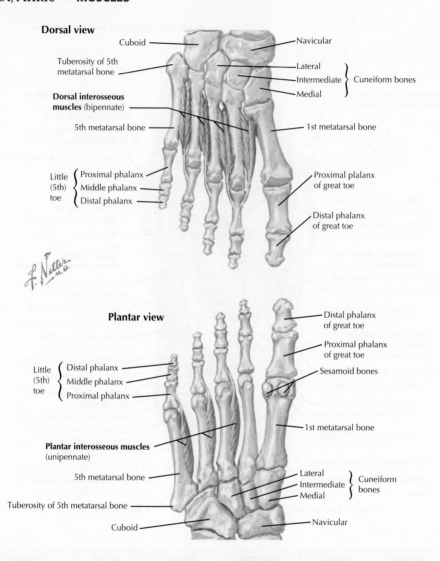

Dorsal view

Cuboid
Navicular
Tuberosity of 5th metatarsal bone
Lateral
Intermediate } Cuneiform bones
Medial
Dorsal interosseous muscles (bipennate)
5th metatarsal bone
1st metatarsal bone
Little (5th) toe { Proximal phalanx / Middle phalanx / Distal phalanx
Proximal plalanx of great toe
Distal phalanx of great toe

Plantar view

Distal phalanx of great toe
Proximal phalanx of great toe
Little (5th) toe { Distal phalanx / Middle phalanx / Proximal phalanx
Sesamoid bones
1st metatarsal bone
Plantar interosseous muscles (unipennate)
5th metatarsal bone
Lateral
Intermediate } Cuneiform bones
Medial
Tuberosity of 5th metatarsal bone
Cuboid
Navicular

MUSCLE	ORIGIN	INSERTION	NERVE	ACTION	COMMENT
FOURTH LAYER					
Plantar interossei (3)	Medial 3rd, 4th, 5th MTs	Medial proximal phalanges: toes 3-5	Lateral plantar	Adduct toes, flex MTPJ; extend LPJ	Attachment to MT is medial for all 3
Dorsal interossei (4)	Adjacent MT shafts	Medial proximal phalanx (2nd toe) Lateral proximal phalanx (toes 2-4)	Lateral plantar	Abduct toes	Larger than the plantar interossei (bipennate)

Peroneus longus and tibialis posterior tendons pass through the fourth layer.
PAD = Plantar ADduct, DAB = Dorsal ABduct (the 2nd digit is reference point for abduction/adduction in the foot).

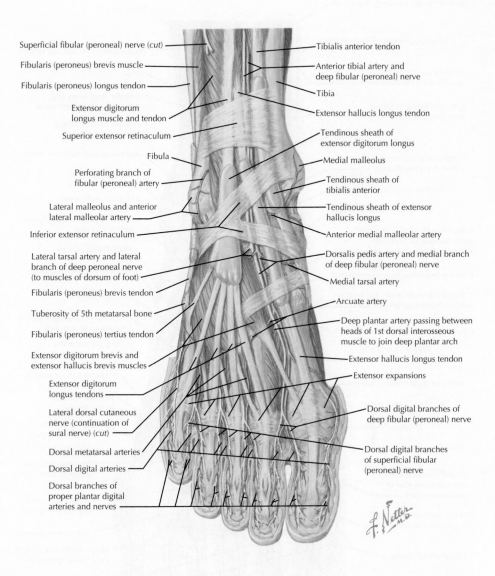

Superficial fibular (peroneal) nerve (*cut*)

Fibularis (peroneus) brevis muscle

Fibularis (peroneus) longus tendon

Extensor digitorum longus muscle and tendon

Superior extensor retinaculum

Fibula

Perforating branch of fibular (peroneal) artery

Lateral malleolus and anterior lateral malleolar artery

Inferior extensor retinaculum

Lateral tarsal artery and lateral branch of deep peroneal nerve (to muscles of dorsum of foot)

Fibularis (peroneus) brevis tendon

Tuberosity of 5th metatarsal bone

Fibularis (peroneus) tertius tendon

Extensor digitorum brevis and extensor hallucis brevis muscles

Extensor digitorum longus tendons

Lateral dorsal cutaneous nerve (continuation of sural nerve) (*cut*)

Dorsal metatarsal arteries

Dorsal digital arteries

Dorsal branches of proper plantar digital arteries and nerves

Tibialis anterior tendon

Anterior tibial artery and deep fibular (peroneal) nerve

Tibia

Extensor hallucis longus tendon

Tendinous sheath of extensor digitorum longus

Medial malleolus

Tendinous sheath of tibialis anterior

Tendinous sheath of extensor hallucis longus

Anterior medial malleolar artery

Dorsalis pedis artery and medial branch of deep fibular (peroneal) nerve

Medial tarsal artery

Arcuate artery

Deep plantar artery passing between heads of 1st dorsal interosseous muscle to join deep plantar arch

Extensor hallucis longus tendon

Extensor expansions

Dorsal digital branches of deep fibular (peroneal) nerve

Dorsal digital branches of superficial fibular (peroneal) nerve

MUSCLE	ORIGIN	INSERTION	NERVE	ACTION	COMMENT
DORSUM					
Extensor hallucis brevis (EHB)	Dorsolateral calcaneus	Base of proximal phalanx of great toe	Deep peroneal	Extends great toe at MCPJ	Assists EHL with its action
Extensor digito-rum brevis (EDB)	Dorsolateral calcaneus	Base of proximal phalanx: toes 2-4	Deep peroneal	Extends lesser toes at MCPJ	No tendon to small toe

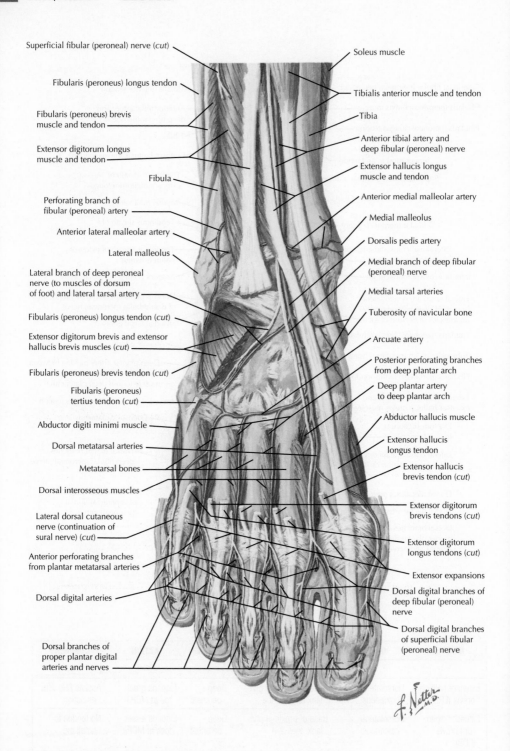

Superficial fibular (peroneal) nerve (*cut*)

Fibularis (peroneus) longus tendon

Fibularis (peroneus) brevis muscle and tendon

Extensor digitorum longus muscle and tendon

Fibula

Perforating branch of fibular (peroneal) artery

Anterior lateral malleolar artery

Lateral malleolus

Lateral branch of deep peroneal nerve (to muscles of dorsum of foot) and lateral tarsal artery

Fibularis (peroneus) longus tendon (*cut*)

Extensor digitorum brevis and extensor hallucis brevis muscles (*cut*)

Fibularis (peroneus) brevis tendon (*cut*)

Fibularis (peroneus) tertius tendon (*cut*)

Abductor digiti minimi muscle

Dorsal metatarsal arteries

Metatarsal bones

Dorsal interosseous muscles

Lateral dorsal cutaneous nerve (continuation of sural nerve) (*cut*)

Anterior perforating branches from plantar metatarsal arteries

Dorsal digital arteries

Dorsal branches of proper plantar digital arteries and nerves

Soleus muscle

Tibialis anterior muscle and tendon

Tibia

Anterior tibial artery and deep fibular (peroneal) nerve

Extensor hallucis longus muscle and tendon

Anterior medial malleolar artery

Medial malleolus

Dorsalis pedis artery

Medial branch of deep fibular (peroneal) nerve

Medial tarsal arteries

Tuberosity of navicular bone

Arcuate artery

Posterior perforating branches from deep plantar arch

Deep plantar artery to deep plantar arch

Abductor hallucis muscle

Extensor hallucis longus tendon

Extensor hallucis brevis tendon (*cut*)

Extensor digitorum brevis tendons (*cut*)

Extensor digitorum longus tendons (*cut*)

Extensor expansions

Dorsal digital branches of deep fibular (peroneal) nerve

Dorsal digital branches of superficial fibular (peroneal) nerve

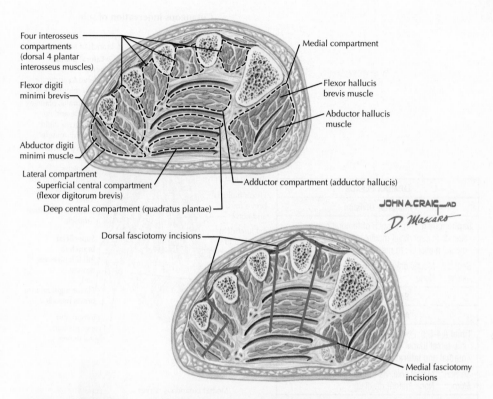

Four interosseus compartments (dorsal 4 plantar interosseus muscles)

Flexor digiti minimi brevis

Abductor digiti minimi muscle

Lateral compartment

Superficial central compartment (flexor digitorum brevis)

Deep central compartment (quadratus plantae)

Medial compartment

Flexor hallucis brevis muscle

Abductor hallucis muscle

Adductor compartment (adductor hallucis)

Dorsal fasciotomy incisions

Medial fasciotomy incisions

JOHN A.CRAIG—AD
D. Mascaro

COMPARTMENT	CONTENTS
COMPARTMENTS (9)	
Medial	Abductor hallucis, flexor hallucis brevis, FHL tendon
Lateral	Abductor digiti minimi, flexor digiti minimi
Superficial central	Flexor digitorum brevis, lumbricals (4), FDL tendons
Deep central (calcaneal)	Quadratus plantae, posterior tibial neurovascular bundle
Adductor	Adductor hallucis
Interosseous (1-2)	Dorsal interosseous muscle
Interosseous (2-3)	Dorsal and plantar interosseous muscles
Interosseous (3-4)	Dorsal and plantar interosseous muscles
Interosseous (4-5)	Dorsal and plantar interosseous muscles
Deep central (calcaneal) compartment communicates with the deep posterior compartment of the leg.	
FASCIOTOMIES	
Incisions	3 incisions (2 dorsal and 1 medial) can release all compartments.
Dorsal (1)	Over 2nd metatarsal, dissect on both sides: release medial 2 interosseous, adductor, deep central
Dorsal (2)	Over 4th metatarsal, dissect on both sides: release lateral 2 interosseous, lateral, and both central
Medial	Along medial border of hind foot & midfoot: release medial, superficial, and deep central compartments

Cutaneous innervation of sole

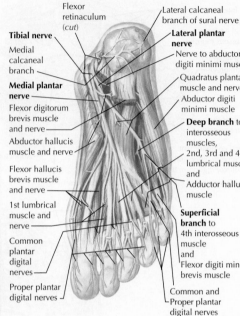

Flexor retinaculum (*cut*)

Tibial nerve

Medial calcaneal branch

Medial plantar nerve

Flexor digitorum brevis muscle and nerve

Abductor hallucis muscle and nerve

Flexor hallucis brevis muscle and nerve

1st lumbrical muscle and nerve

Common plantar digital nerves

Proper plantar digital nerves

Lateral calcaneal branch of sural nerve

Lateral plantar nerve

Nerve to abductor digiti minimi muscle

Quadratus plantae muscle and nerve

Abductor digiti minimi muscle

Deep branch to interosseous muscles, 2nd, 3rd and 4th lumbrical muscles and Adductor hallucis muscle

Superficial branch to 4th interosseous muscle and Flexor digiti minimi brevis muscle

Common and Proper plantar digital nerves

LUMBAR PLEXUS
Posterior Division
Saphenous (L2-4): Branch of femoral nerve, descends in superficial medial leg then anterior to medial malleolus to medial arch of foot.
Sensory: Medial ankle and foot (arch)   *Motor:* None

SACRAL PLEXUS
Anterior Division
Tibial (L4-S3): Posterior to medial malleolus, into tarsal tunnel, divides on plantar surface into **medial** and **lateral plantar nerves.**
Sensory: Medial heel, via **medial calcaneal nerve**   *Motor:* None (before dividing)
Medial plantar: Runs medially in foot within the 2nd plantar layer. Compression can cause medial foot/arch pain (esp. in runners).
Sensory: Medial plantar foot and toes   *Motor:* • First plantar layer   ∘ Abductor hallucis   ∘ Flexor digitorum brevis (FDB)   • Second plantar layer   ∘ Lumbricals (medial 2)   • Third plantar layer   ∘ Flexor hallucis brevis (FHB)
Lateral plantar: Gives branch to ADM (can be entrapped by abductor hallucis fascia), then runs laterally within the 2nd plantar layer.
Sensory: Lateral plantar foot and toes   *Motor:* • First plantar layer   ∘ Abductor digiti minimi (ADM): via **1st branch** (Baxter's n.)   • Second plantar layer   ∘ Quadratus plantae   ∘ Lumbricals (lateral 2)   • Third plantar layer   ∘ Adductor hallucis   ∘ Flexor digiti minimi brevis   • Fourth plantar layer   ∘ Dorsal interosseous   ∘ Plantar interosseous

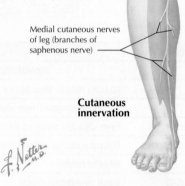

Medial cutaneous nerves of leg (branches of saphenous nerve)

Cutaneous innervation

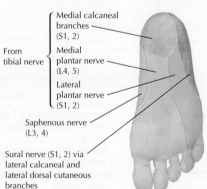

Medial calcaneal branches (S1, 2)

From tibial nerve { Medial plantar nerve (L4, 5)

Lateral plantar nerve (S1, 2)

Saphenous nerve (L3, 4)

Sural nerve (S1, 2) via lateral calcaneal and lateral dorsal cutaneous branches

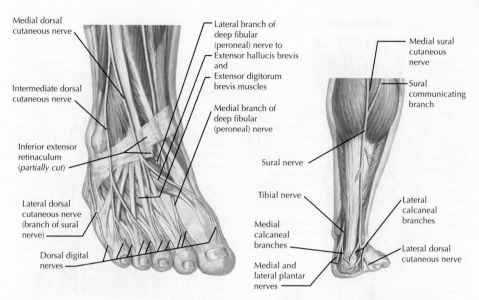

Medial dorsal cutaneous nerve

Intermediate dorsal cutaneous nerve

Inferior extensor retinaculum (*partially cut*)

Lateral dorsal cutaneous nerve (branch of sural nerve)

Dorsal digital nerves

Lateral branch of deep fibular (peroneal) nerve to Extensor hallucis brevis and Extensor digitorum brevis muscles

Medial branch of deep fibular (peroneal) nerve

Sural nerve

Tibial nerve

Medial calcaneal branches

Medial and lateral plantar nerves

Medial sural cutaneous nerve

Sural communicating branch

Lateral calcaneal branches

Lateral dorsal cutaneous nerve

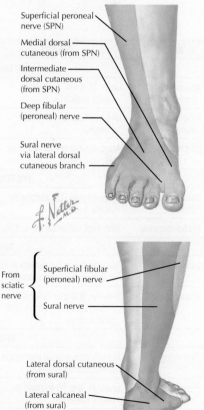

Superficial peroneal nerve (SPN)

Medial dorsal cutaneous (from SPN)

Intermediate dorsal cutaneous (from SPN)

Deep fibular (peroneal) nerve

Sural nerve via lateral dorsal cutaneous branch

From sciatic nerve

Superficial fibular (peroneal) nerve

Sural nerve

Lateral dorsal cutaneous (from sural)

Lateral calcaneal (from sural)

SACRAL PLEXUS
Posterior Division
Deep peroneal: Runs in anterior compartment of leg with anterior tibial artery, under inferior extensor retinaculum (can entrap nerve), then divides into motor (lateral) and sensory (medial) branches. *Sensory:* 1st/2nd toe interdigital space via **medial** branch *Motor:* Via **lateral** branch ○ Extensor hallucis brevis (EHB) ○ Extensor digitorum brevis (EDB)
Superficial peroneal: Runs in lateral compartment of leg, crosses anteriorly 12cm above LM to dorsal foot, then divides into 2 nerves. Can be injured during ORIF of ankle or by anterolateral arthroscopy portal. *Sensory:* Dorsal foot: **intermediate dorsal cutaneous n.** Medial hallux: via **medial dorsal cutaneous** nerve *Motor:* None (in foot and ankle)
Other
Sural: Formed from medial sural cutaneous (tibial nerve) and lateral sural cutaneous (peroneal nerve), runs subcutaneously in posterolateral leg. Gives a branch to the heel, then terminates in lateral foot and toes. *Sensory:* Lateral heel: via **lateral calcaneal nerve** Lateral foot: via **lateral dorsal cutaneous** nerve *Motor:* None
Dorsal foot sensory innervation: 3 cutaneous nerves (2 from superficial peroneal nerve, 1 from sural nerve)

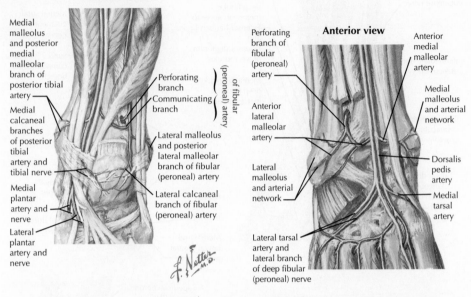

Posterior view

Medial malleolus and posterior medial malleolar branch of posterior tibial artery

Medial calcaneal branches of posterior tibial artery and tibial nerve

Medial plantar artery and nerve

Lateral plantar artery and nerve

Perforating branch
Communicating branch

of fibular (peroneal) artery

Lateral malleolus and posterior lateral malleolar branch of fibular (peroneal) artery

Lateral calcaneal branch of fibular (peroneal) artery

Anterior view

Perforating branch of fibular (peroneal) artery

Anterior lateral malleolar artery

Lateral malleolus and arterial network

Lateral tarsal artery and lateral branch of deep fibular (peroneal) nerve

Anterior medial malleolar artery

Medial malleolus and arterial network

Dorsalis pedis artery

Medial tarsal artery

ARTERY	COURSE	BRANCHES	COMMENT/SUPPLY
ANTERIOR TIBIAL ARTERY			
Anterior medial malleolar	Under TA & EHL tendons to medial malleolus	None	Supplies medial malleolus
Anterior lateral malleolar	Under EDL tendon to lateral malleolus	None	Supplies lateral malleolus
Dorsalis pedis	Along dorsum of foot with deep peroneal nerve	Continuation of anterior tibial artery in foot	Supplies dorsum of foot via multiple branches (see foot table)
POSTERIOR TIBIAL ARTERY			
Posterior medial malleolar	Under PT and FDL tendons to medial malleolus	None	Supplies medial malleolus
Medial calcaneal	With med. calcaneal nerve (tibial)	None	Supplies heel/calcaneus
Terminal Branches			
Lateral plantar	Between quadratus plantae & FDB in 2nd layer w/lateral plantar n.	Deep plantar arch	Larger of the terminal branches Terminates as deep plantar arch
Medial plantar	Between abductor hallucis and FDB in 2nd layer with medial plantar nerve	Superficial branch 1 proper plantar digital Deep branch	Runs in medial foot Supplies medial plantar hallux Supplies central plantar midfoot
PERONEAL ARTERY			
Perforating artery	Pierces interosseous membrane going to anterior ankle	Branches or contributes to tarsal sinus artery	Joins with ant. lat. malleolus a. Direct supply to posterior talus
Posterior lateral malleolar	Under PL and PB tendons to lateral malleolus	None	Supplies lateral malleolus
Lateral calcaneal	With lat. calcaneal nerve (sural)	None	Supplies heel/calcaneus
Ant. & post. medial malleolar arteries & ant. & post. lateral malleolar arteries form an anastomosis at each malleolus.			

Blood Supply of Talus

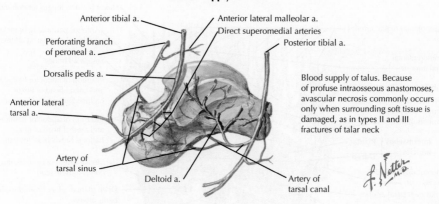

Anterior tibial a.

Perforating branch of peroneal a.

Dorsalis pedis a.

Anterior lateral tarsal a.

Artery of tarsal sinus

Deltoid a.

Anterior lateral malleolar a.

Direct superomedial arteries

Posterior tibial a.

Blood supply of talus. Because of profuse intraosseous anastomoses, avascular necrosis commonly occurs only when surrounding soft tissue is damaged, as in types II and III fractures of talar neck

Artery of tarsal canal

Dorsal view

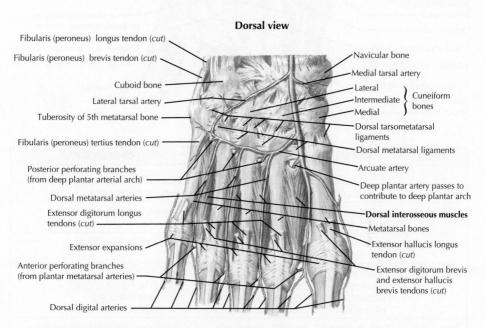

Fibularis (peroneus) longus tendon (*cut*)

Fibularis (peroneus) brevis tendon (*cut*)

Cuboid bone

Lateral tarsal artery

Tuberosity of 5th metatarsal bone

Fibularis (peroneus) tertius tendon (*cut*)

Posterior perforating branches (from deep plantar arterial arch)

Dorsal metatarsal arteries

Extensor digitorum longus tendons (*cut*)

Extensor expansions

Anterior perforating branches (from plantar metatarsal arteries)

Dorsal digital arteries

Navicular bone

Medial tarsal artery

Lateral
Intermediate } Cuneiform bones
Medial

Dorsal tarsometatarsal ligaments

Dorsal metatarsal ligaments

Arcuate artery

Deep plantar artery passes to contribute to deep plantar arch

Dorsal interosseous muscles

Metatarsal bones

Extensor hallucis longus tendon (*cut*)

Extensor digitorum brevis and extensor hallucis brevis tendons (*cut*)

ARTERY	STEM ARTERY	BONE SUPPLIED
BLOOD SUPPLY OF TALUS		
1. Artery of tarsal canal	Posterior tibial (PT)	Body (dome): primary supply of body
2. Deltoid artery	Artery of tarsal canal (or PT)	Medial body; artery pierces deltoid ligament
3. Direct superomedial arteries	Dorsalis pedis	Head and neck
4. Artery of tarsal sinus	Dorsalis pedis and/or Peroneal (perforating br.)	Neck and lateral body, also contributes to head
5. Direct posterior arteries	Peroneal (perforating br.)	Posterior process/body

- Arteries of tarsal canal and tarsal sinus form a primary anastomosis inferior to talar neck that supplies the neck.
- Intraosseous anastomoses allow talus to withstand a less severe vascular injury. Significant vascular injury (e.g., Hawkins type II or III talar neck fracture) often results in AVN.

Plantar view

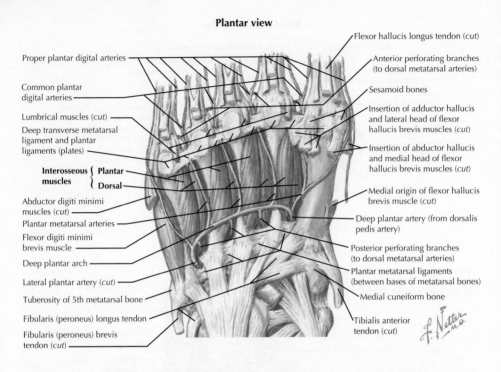

Flexor hallucis longus tendon (*cut*)

Proper plantar digital arteries

Anterior perforating branches
(to dorsal metatarsal arteries)

Common plantar
digital arteries

Sesamoid bones

Lumbrical muscles (*cut*)

Insertion of adductor hallucis
and lateral head of flexor
hallucis brevis muscles (*cut*)

Deep transverse metatarsal
ligament and plantar
ligaments (plates)

Insertion of abductor hallucis
and medial head of flexor
hallucis brevis muscles (*cut*)

Interosseous { **Plantar**
muscles { **Dorsal**

Medial origin of flexor hallucis
brevis muscle (*cut*)

Abductor digiti minimi
muscles (*cut*)

Deep plantar artery (from dorsalis
pedis artery)

Plantar metatarsal arteries

Flexor digiti minimi
brevis muscle

Posterior perforating branches
(to dorsal metatarsal arteries)

Deep plantar arch

Plantar metatarsal ligaments
(between bases of metatarsal bones)

Lateral plantar artery (*cut*)

Medial cuneiform bone

Tuberosity of 5th metatarsal bone

Fibularis (peroneus) longus tendon

Tibialis anterior
tendon (*cut*)

Fibularis (peroneus) brevis
tendon (*cut*)

ARTERY	COURSE	BRANCHES	COMMENT/SUPPLY
DORSALIS PEDIS ARTERY			
Direct talar brs.	Directly into talus	None	Supplies head and neck
Medial tarsal	Across tarsals, under EHL tendon	None	Supplies dorsum & medial tarsus
Lateral tarsal	With lateral br., deep peroneal n.	None	Supplies EDB, lateral tarsus
Arcuate	Transversely across metatarsal bases, under EDL tendons	3 dorsal MT arteries (2, 3, 4) 6 dorsal digital arteries 3 posterior perforating arteries 1 dorsal digital artery	Bifurcate at level of MT base Med. & lat. aspects of toes From deep plantar arch Far lateral vessel to small toe
Deep plantar	Descends between 1st & 2nd MTs	Terminates as deep arch	Forms deep plantar arch with terminal branch of lateral plantar artery
1st dorsal metatarsal		Terminal branch of DP 3 dorsal digital arteries	Medial dorsal hallux & 1st web space
Deep plantar arch	On plantar interosseous muscles in the 4th plantar layer	3 posterior perforating arteries 4 plantar MT arteries 1 common/proper plantar dig. 4 anterior perforating 4 common plantar digital 8 proper plantar digital 1 common/proper plantar	Anastomose with arcuate/dorsal MT Along plantar metatarsal Joins w/terminal br. of med. plantar artery To dorsal metatarsal arteries Continuation after perforators branch Medial, lateral aspects of toes Lateral aspect of small toe

• 10 dorsal digital arteries (8 from the 4 dorsal MT art. plus 2 that branch proximally) do not reach to distal tip of toe.
• 10 proper plantar digital arteries (8 from plantar MT arteries plus 2 that branch proximally) supply the distal tip of toe.
• Each toe has 2 dorsal digital arteries and 2 proper plantar digital arteries.

Achilles Tendinitis

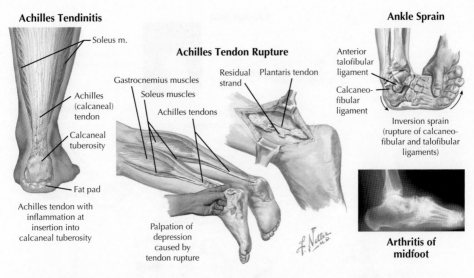

Achilles Tendon Rupture

Ankle Sprain

Soleus m.

Achilles (calcaneal) tendon

Calcaneal tuberosity

Fat pad

Achilles tendon with inflammation at insertion into calcaneal tuberosity

Residual strand Plantaris tendon

Gastrocnemius muscles

Soleus muscles

Achilles tendons

Palpation of depression caused by tendon rupture

Anterior talofibular ligament

Calcaneo-fibular ligament

Inversion sprain (rupture of calcaneo-fibular and talofibular ligaments)

Arthritis of midfoot

DESCRIPTION	Hx & PE	WORKUP/FINDINGS	TREATMENT
ACHILLES TENDINITIS			
• Occurs at or above insertion of Achilles tendon • Microtrauma to insertion	**Hx/PE:** Heel pain, worse with push off; tender to palpation	**XR:** Standing lateral: +/− spur at Achilles insertion **MR:** Fusiform tendon	1. Rest, NSAIDs, heel lift 2. Excise—tendinosus 3. Reconstruct w/FHL tendon
ACHILLES TENDON RUPTURE			
• "Weekend warriors"—middle-aged men/athletics • Occurs with eccentric load	**Hx:** "Pop" sensation **PE:** Defect, + Thompson test	**XR:** Standing AP/lateral; usually normal	1. Casting (in equinus) vs 2. Surgical repair (decrease re-rupture)
ANKLE INSTABILITY			
• Multiple/recurrent sprains • Associated with varus heel • Can be from subtalar joint	**Hx:** Pain and instability **PE:** ATFL/CFL TTP, check for varus heel; + ant. drawer/talar tilt	**XR:** AP/lateral/oblique **Stress:** Drawer and tilt show subluxation	1. Rest, brace PT: strengthen peroneals 2. Surgical reconstruction (Brostrom) if condition persists
ANKLE SPRAIN			
• #1 musculoskeletal injury • Lateral 90%—ATFL only • 60% with CFL, ("high ankle sprain") w/syndesmosis 5% • Inversion #1 mechanism	**Hx:** "Pop," pain, swelling, +/− ability to bear weight **PE:** Edema, ecchymosis, ATFL (CFL) TTP, +/− ant. drawer, talar tilt tests	**XR:** AP, lateral, mortise: Rule out fracture (only if cannot WB, or bony point tenderness)	1. RICE, NSAIDs 2. Immobilize grade III 3. PT & ROM exercises 4. Surgery: severe injury or persistent instability
ARTHRITIS (OA/DJD)			
• Can occur in any joint (ankle, subtalar, midtarsal, midfoot) • Associated with prior trauma, overuse, AVN, inflammatory arthropathy, obesity	**Hx:** Older; pain, +/− previous trauma **PE:** Pain at affected joint, +/− decreased range of motion	**XR:** Weight-bearing images Ankle: AP/lateral/mortise Foot: AP/lateral/oblique Look for classic OA findings	1. NSAIDs, modify activities 2. Orthotics: cup, AFO or double upright Midfoot: steel shank/rocker 3. Fusion or arthroplasty

Charcot Foot

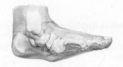
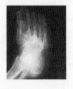

Anteroposterior radiograph
of Charcot ankle joint

C.Machado
_M.D.

Diabetic Foot
Autonomic and Sensory Neuropathy

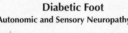
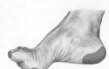

Ulcer   Treatment

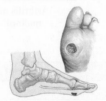
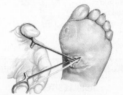
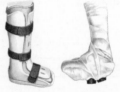
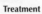

DESCRIPTION	Hx & PE	WORKUP/FINDINGS	TREATMENT
CHARCOT NEUROARTHROPATHY			
• End stage of diabetic foot • Decreased sensation—patient cannot detect fracture or dislocation • Multiple injuries, unhealed or malunited leads to joint destruction and deformity	**Hx:** Diabetes. DO NOT complain of pain because they are insensate **PE:** Red, warm, swollen joint, +/− deformity and/or ulcers (may look like infection)	**XR:** AP(WB)/lateral/oblique Findings: osteopenia, fracture, callus, bony prominences, joint destruction **Indium scan:** r/o osteomyelitis	1. Immobilize, skin checks 2. Brace if possible 3. Treat ulcers as needed 4. Bony prominence excision 5. TAL if indicated 6. Selected fusions
CORN			

• Two types
  ○ Hard: hyperkeratosis—pressure on bones (5th toe #1)
  ○ Soft: interdigit maceration
	Hx/PE: Tight shoes, pain at lesion site	**XR:** AP/lateral: look for bone spurs/bony prominence	1. Wide toe box shoe
			2. Debride callus
			3. Pads relieve pressure
			4. Excise bony prominence

DIABETIC FOOT			
• Ulcers from pressure & neuropathy (sensory & autonomic); patient doesn't feel pain of lesion • Previous ulcer #1 risk for ulcer • 15% of DM pts. have ulcers • 2° infection can occur • Vascular insufficiency leads to decreased healing potential	**Hx:** NO pain, +/−wound drainage **PE:** Skin changes (e.g., hair loss), diminished/absent pulses, decreased sensation (monofilament tests protective sensation: 5.07 or better); ulcer; erythema, swelling, drainage may be present in infection.	**XR:** Look for osteomyelitis **MR/indium scan:** evaluate for osteomyelitis **Labs:** CBC/CRP (infection) *Ulcer Healing Indicators:* Lymphocytes: >1500 Albumin: >3.5 **ABI:** >0.45 (non-Ca⁺⁺ vessels) Toe pressures: >30 mmHg	1. Prevention: skin care, DM shoes 2. Debride ulcer/callus, total contact casting (TCC) 3. Infection: Superficial: debride, antibiotics; Deep: surgical debridement, IV antibiotics Amputation for severe or persistent cases

Gout

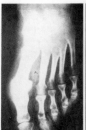
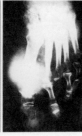
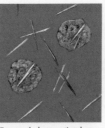

Free and phagocytized monosodium urate crystals in aspirated joint fluid seen on compensated polarized light microscopy

Hallux rigidus

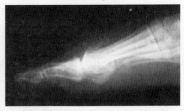

Lateral radiograph showing narrowing of the joint and marked dorsal osteophyte formation

Hallux valgus

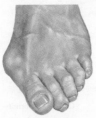

Advanced bunion. Wide (splayed) forefoot with inflamed prominence over 1st metatarsal head. Great toe deviated laterally (hallux valgus), overlaps 2nd toe, and is internally rotated. Other toes also deviated laterally in conformity with great toe. Laterally displaced extensor hallucis longus tendon is apparent

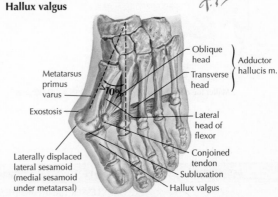

Metatarsus primus varus

Exostosis

Laterally displaced lateral sesamoid (medial sesamoid under metatarsal)

Oblique head
Transverse head
} Adductor hallucis m.

Lateral head of flexor

Conjoined tendon

Subluxation

Hallux valgus

DESCRIPTION	Hx & PE	WORKUP/FINDINGS	TREATMENT
GOUT (PODAGRA)			
• Purine metabolism defect • Monosodium urate, urate crystal deposition create synovitis • 1st MTPJ #1 site	**Hx:** Men; acute & exquisite pain **PE:** Red, swollen toe	**XP:** Erosion on both sides of joint **Labs:** 1. Elevated uric acid; 2. negatively birefringent crystals (in aspirate)	1. NSAIDs/colchicine 2. Rest 3. Allopurinol (prevention) 4. If DJD, fusion
HALLUX RIGIDUS			
• DJD of MTP of great toe • Dorsal metatarsal head osteophyte • Often posttraumatic	**Hx:** Middle age; painful, stiff toe (hallux) **PE:** MTP tender to palpation, decreased ROM	**XR:** standing AP/lateral; dorsal osteophyte or OA findings at 1st MTP	1. NSAID, full length rigid orthosis 2. Cheilectomy 3. Fusion (adv. DJD)
HALLUX VALGUS			
• Deformity: lateral deviation & pronation of hallux, varus 1st MT • Adductor hallucis over pulls hallux • Capsule: medial loose lateral tight • Women (10:1), narrow toe shoes	**Hx:** Pain (worse with shoe wear) **PE:** Valgus deformity/bunion; medial 1st MT head/MTPJ TTP, +/– MTPJ decr. ROM, check for 1st ray hypermobility	**XR:** AP(WB)/lateral/oblique Measure angles: 1. Hallux valgus (nl <15°) 2. Intermetatarsal (nl <9°) 3. Interphalangeal (nl <10°) 4. **DMMA** (nl <15°)	1. Modify shoes: wide toe box 2. Operative: Mild: Chevron or DSTP Severe: Proximal osteotomy/DSTP DJD: 1st MTPJ fusion COMP: recurrence #1

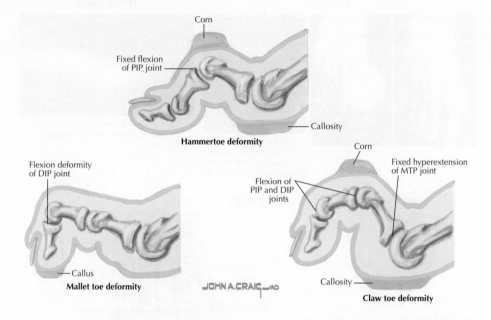

Corn

Fixed flexion
of PIP joint

Callosity

Hammertoe deformity

Flexion deformity
of DIP joint

Corn

Fixed hyperextension
of MTP joint

Flexion of
PIP and DIP
joints

Callus

Mallet toe deformity

JOHN A.CRAIG—AD

Callosity

Claw toe deformity

DESCRIPTION	Hx & PE	WORKUP/FINDINGS	TREATMENT
LESSER TOE DEFORMITIES			
Claw Toes			
• 1° deformity: MTPJ hyperextension (extrinsics overpower weak intrinsic muscles) • 2° deformity: PIP & DIP flexion • Associated with neurologic disease	**Hx:** Toe or plantar foot pain; neuro disease (e.g., DM, CMT) **PE:** Toe deformities, callus on dorsal PIPJ, & plantar MT heads; assess flexibility of deformity	**XR:** AP/lateral/oblique foot; subluxating P1 on MT head **MR:** Spine: r/o neurologic lesion **EMG:** r/o neurologic disease	1. Pads for callus, MT pads or inserts, extra-depth shoes 2. Flexible: FDL to P1 transfer; Fixed: FDL tx, EDB release, lengthen EDL, PIPJ resection
Hammertoes			
• PIPJ flexed w/dorsal callus • MTPJ & DIPJ extended • Assoc. w/tight shoes and long 2nd or 3rd rays (>4mm)	**Hx:** Toe/plantar foot pain **PE:** Toe deformity, callus on dorsal PIPJ, plantar MT head; assess flexibility of deformity	**XR:** WB AP/lateral: Look for joint subluxation Evaluate for long metatarsal	1. Pads, hammertoe braces 2. Flexible: FDL transfer; Fixed: PIPJ resection +/− tx.; extensor release if MTPJ fixed
Mallet Toes			
• Flexion of DIPJ • Assoc. w/long ray in tight shoes & arthritis of DIPJ	**Hx:** Toe pain **PE:** Flexed DIP, dorsal callus over DIPJ	**XR:** AP/lateral/oblique DIPJ deformity	1. Pads, extra-depth shoes 2. FDL tendon release 3. Partial amputation
METATARSALGIA			
• Metatarsal head pain • Etiology: flexor tendinitis, ligament rupture, callus (#1)	**Hx/PE:** Pain under MT head (2nd MT most common)	**XR:** Standing AP/lateral: look for short MT	1. Metatarsal pads 2. Modify shoes 3. Treat underlying cause

Plantar fasciitis

Haglund's disease

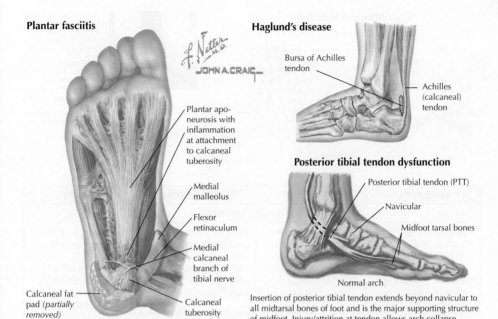

Bursa of Achilles tendon

Achilles (calcaneal) tendon

Plantar apo-neurosis with inflammation at attachment to calcaneal tuberosity

Posterior tibial tendon dysfunction

Posterior tibial tendon (PTT)

Navicular

Midfoot tarsal bones

Medial malleolus

Flexor retinaculum

Medial calcaneal branch of tibial nerve

Calcaneal fat pad *(partially removed)*

Calcaneal tuberosity

Normal arch

Insertion of posterior tibial tendon extends beyond navicular to all midtarsal bones of foot and is the major supporting structure of midfoot. Injury/attrition at tendon allows arch collapse.

DESCRIPTION	Hx & PE	WORKUP/FINDINGS	TREATMENT
MORTON'S NEUROMA (INTERDIGITAL)			
• Fibrosis of irritated nerve • Usually between 2nd and 3rd metatarsals • 5:1 female (shoes)	**Hx:** Pain w/shoes & walking, relief w/rest/no shoes **PE:** MT, web space, TTP, +/− numbness, + compression test	**XR:** Standing AP/lateral: MT heads may be close together	1. Wide toe shoes, steroid injections, MT pads/bars 2. Nerve excision & deep transverse MT lig. release
PLANTAR FASCIITIS			
• Inflammation/degeneration of fascia; female 2:1 • Associated with obesity	**Hx:** AM pain, improves w/ ambulation or stretching **PE:** Medial plantar calcaneus TTP	**XR:** Standing lateral: +/− calcaneal bone spur	1. Stretching, NSAIDs 2. Heel cup 3. Splint (night), casting 4. Partial fascia release
POSTERIOR TIBIALIS TENDON DYSFUNCTION (ACQUIRED FLATFOOT)			

• Failure of post. tib. tendon—foot deformity/loss of arch
• Chronic (attrition) or acute (rupture [hx of trauma])
• Assoc. w/obesity and DM
• 3 stages:
  ○ I: tenosynovitis, no deformity (no pes planus)
  ○ II: pes planus, flexible hind foot; no single heel raise
  ○ III: rigid hind foot +/−DJD
	Hx: Med. foot pain, "weakness"; deformity; lat. foot pain in late stages; hx of trauma in some cases
	PE: + pes planus, valgus heel, PT tendon TTP (b/w MM and navicular-hypovascular area), pain with or unable to do single heel raise, + "too many toes sign"
		XR:
		Foot: AP (WB), lat. oblique; AP: subluxation of talar head;
		Lat: collapse of long. arch
		Ankle: AP & mortise (WB); look for valgus talar tilt (incompetent deltoid lig.) seen in late stages
			Stage:
			I: cast/boot 2-4mo, NSAIDs, custom-molded orthosis
			II: UCBL/AFO orthosis OR tendon transfer (use FDL) & medial slide calcaneal osteotomy
			III: Triple arthrodesis +/− TAL (tendoachilles lengthening)

RETROCALCANEAL BURSITIS (HAGLUND'S DISEASE)			
• Bursitis at insertion of Achilles tendon on calcaneus	**Hx:** Pain on posterior heel **PE:** Red, TTP, "pump bump"	**XR:** Standing lateral: spur at Achilles insertion	1. NSAID, heel lift, casting 2. Excise bone/bursa (rare)

Rheumatoid Arthritis

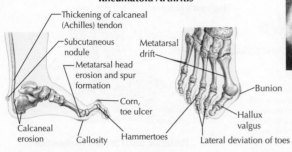

- Thickening of calcaneal (Achilles) tendon
- Subcutaneous nodule
- Metatarsal head erosion and spur formation
- Metatarsal drift
- Corn, toe ulcer
- Calcaneal erosion
- Callosity
- Hammertoes
- Bunion
- Hallux valgus
- Lateral deviation of toes

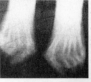

Radiograph reveals severe deformities of forefoot. Hallux valgus, dislocations of metatarsophalangeal joint with lateral deviation of toes. Note also displacement of sesamoids, which results in increased pressure on head of 1st metatarsal

Runner's Foot

2nd metatarsal stress fracture

DESCRIPTION	Hx & PE	WORKUP/FINDINGS	TREATMENT
RHEUMATOID ARTHRITIS			
• Synovitis is 1° problem • Forefoot: 1st MTPJ has HV, lesser claw toe deformities • Hind foot: PT insufficiency and subtalar instability = valgus heel	**Hx:** Pain, swelling, deformity **PE:** Hallux valgus, claw toes with plantar callus; hind foot in valgus	**XR:** AP(WB)/lateral/oblique: evaluate for joint destruction, osteopenia, joint subluxation, hallux valgus (measure angle) **Labs:** Positive RF, ANA	1. Medical mgmt. of RA 2. Wide toe shoes and orthosis 3. Forefoot: 1st MTPJ fusion, 2-5 lesser toe MT head resection 4. Hind foot: triple arthrodesis
RUNNER'S FOOT			
Multiple etiologies • Medial plantar nerve entrapment • Baxter's nerve (1st br LPN) • Stress fracture	**Hx:** Avid runner, pain **PE:** MPN: medial arch pain; Baxter's n.; plantar/lat. pain Bone TTP (MT, nav., etc)	**XR:** AP/lateral/oblique; usually normal **Bone scan:** evaluate for stress fracture	**Based on etiology:** MPN: release at knot of Henry Baxter's: release abductor hallucis fascia Stress fx: immobilize, rest
SERONEGATIVE SPONDYLOARTHROPATHY (REITER'S, AS, PSORIASIS)			
• Inflammatory arthritides: with symptoms in multiple joints • Types: psoriatic arthritis, Reiter's syndrome, ankylosing spondylitis	**Hx:** Foot pain, any joint **PE:** Evaluate whole foot Psoriatic: sausage digit Reiter/ankyl. spondylitis: Achilles/heel pain, bursitis, plantar fasciitis	**XR:** AP/lateral/oblique Psoriatic: pencil/cup deformity; DIPJ joint erosion; Reiter/AS: +/− enthesiophytes **Labs:** Neg. RF, + HLA-B27	1. Medical management 2. Conservative care of arthritis, tendinitis, bursitis, fascitis 3. Surgical intervention is infrequent
TAILOR'S BUNION (BUNIONETTE)			
• Prominent 5th metatarsal head laterally • Bony exostosis/bursitis	**Hx/PE:** Difficulty fitting shoes, painful lateral 5th metatarsal prominence	**XR:** Standing **AP:** 5th toe medially deviated, MT laterally deviated	1. Pads, wide toe box 2. Mild: chevron osteotomy 3. Severe: MT shelf osteotomy
TARSAL TUNNEL			
• Tibial nerve entrapped by flexor retinaculum or space-occupying lesion (e.g., cyst) in tunnel • Clinical diagnosis	**Hx:** Pain, numbness/ tingling **PE:** Pain at tarsal tunnel, +/− sensory changes and Tinel's test	**XR:** AP/lateral; usu. normal **MR:** Mass or lesion in tunnel **EMG:** Confirm clinical diagnosis	1. NSAIDs, steroid inj. 2. Release retinaculum, abductor hallucis fascia, remove any mass (release plantar nerves)
TURF TOE			
• Plantar plate injury (rupture) from MT neck • Hyperextension of 1st MTPJ	**Hx:** Hyperextension, toe (MTP) pain **PE:** Plantar pain, pain with extension (DF), decr. ROM	**XR:** AP/lateral/oblique; usually normal **Bone scan:** r/o stress fx	1. Immobilize, rest, NSAIDs 2. Brace/orthosis to block dorsiflexion during activities

Clubfoot

Plantar flexion (equinus) at ankle joint

Deformity of talus

Tightness of tibionavicular ligament and extensor digitorum longus, tibialis anterior, and extensor hallucis longus tendons

Extreme varus position of forefoot bones
Inversion of calcaneus

Pathologic changes in congenital clubfoot

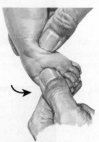

Manipulation of foot in step-by-step correction of varus deformity. (Excessive force must be avoided.)

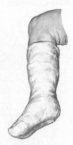

After each stage of manipulation, plaster cast applied to maintain correction

Pes Cavus

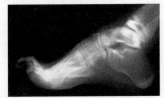

Radiograph shows high arch.

Metatarsus Adductus

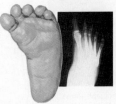

View of sole and radiograph show medial deviation of forefoot

DESCRIPTION	Hx & PE	TREATMENT
CLUBFOOT (TALIPES EQUINOVARUS)		

• Idiopathic, congenital
• Boys 2:1, 50% bilateral, 1:1000
• Multifactorial etiology: genetic, environmental
• Assoc. w/other conditions
• 4 different deformities: **CAVE**
• Also seen in neuromuscular disease
	Hx: Born with deformity
	PE: 4 deformities (mnemonic **CAVE**)
	  Cavus midfoot, forefoot **A**dductus,
	  subtalar **V**arus, hindfoot **E**quinus
	XR: AP/lateral: "parallelism" of talus
	  & calcaneus
	  Lateral: T-C angle: nl >35°
	  AP: T-C angle: nl 20-40°, <20°
	  in clubfoot
		• Ponseti: serial casting + bars
		  ○ **C**avus: dorsiflex 1st ray
		  ○ **A**dductus/**V**arus: talar head is the fulcrum for correction
		  ○ **E**quinus: dorsiflex ankle, TAL
		• Release if persistent >6-9 m.o.
		• Neuromuscular: release 6-12mo

PES CAVUS (HIGH ARCH FOOT)		
• High arch due to muscle imbalance in immature foot (TA and peroneus longus); TA weak, PL & PT strong • Ankle flexed: causes pain • Must rule out neuromuscular disease (e.g., Charcot-Marie-Tooth) • May have claw toes	**Hx:** 8-10yr, ankle pain **PE:** Toe walking, tight heel cord, decreased ankle dorsiflexion **XR:** AP/lateral foot and ankle **EMG/NCS:** Test for weakness **MR:** Spine: r/o neuromuscular disease	• Braces/inserts/AFO as needed (used w/mixed results) • Various osteotomies • Tendon transfer and balance
METATARSUS ADDUCTUS		
• Forefoot adduction (varus) • #1 pediatric foot disorder • Assoc. w/intrauterine position or other "packaging" disorders	**Hx:** Parent notices deformity **PE:** "Kidney bean" deformity, negative thigh/foot angle, + intoeing gait	• Most spontaneously resolve with normal development • Serial casing • Abductor hallucis release • Rarely, midfoot osteotomies

Tarsal Coalition

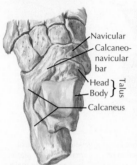

- Navicular
- Calcaneo-navicular bar
- Head } Talus
- Body }
- Calcaneus

Calcaneonavicular coalition

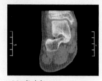

Solid, bony calcaneonavicular coalition evident on oblique radiograph

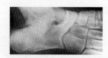

Medial facet talocalcaneal coalition

Pes Planovalgus

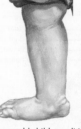

Lateral radiograph of same child's foot

2 year old child, condition more apparent when patient stands.

f. Netter M.D.

Vertical Talus

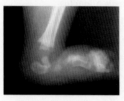

Lateral radiograph shows vertical position of talus, plantar flexion of hindfoot, and dorsiflexion of forefoot

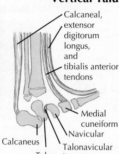

- Calcaneal, extensor digitorum longus, and tibialis anterior tendons
- Medial cuneiform
- Navicular
- Talonavicular ligament
- Talus
- Calcaneus

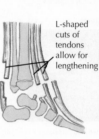

L-shaped cuts of tendons allow for lengthening

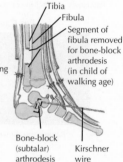

- Tibia
- Fibula
- Segment of fibula removed for bone-block arthrodesis (in child of walking age)
- Bone-block (subtalar) arthrodesis
- Kirschner wire

DESCRIPTION	EVALUATION	TREATMENT
FLEXIBLE FLATFOOT		
Pes Planovalgus (Pes Planus)		
• Normal variant • Almost always bilateral • Foot flat only with weight-bearing; forms an arch when non-weight-bearing	**Hx:** Usually asymptomatic, +/− pain w/activity **PE:** Pes planus when WB. NonWB arch reconstitutes; heel goes into varus on heel rise **XR:** Decreased arch, otherwise normal	1. Observation, parental reassurance, no special shoes 2. Arch supports may help if sx mild 3. Calc. osteotomy for persistent pain
RIGID FLATFOOT		
Tarsal Coalition		

• Congenital fusion of 2 tarsal bones
• Calcaneonavicular #1 (younger children)
• Talocalcaneal (subtalar) #2 (older)
• Coalitions can be fibrous, bony, or cartilaginous
	Hx: Older child/adolescent with insidious onset of pain, worse w/activity
	PE: Rigid flat foot, peroneal spasm
	XR: Anteater sign (calcaneonavicular)
	CT: Best study to identify and measure coalition
		1. Cast, orthosis, NSAIDs
		2. Persistent or recurrent pain
		  C-N: coalition resection
		  T-C: <50% involved: resection
		  >50% involved: subtalar fusion

Congenital Vertical Talus		
• Talus plantarflexed. Irreducible dorsolateral talonavicular dislocation • Also seen in neuromuscular disorders	**Hx/PE:** Convex/rockerbottom sole, rigid flatfoot (always flat), +/− calcaneovalgus appearance **XR:** PF lateral: talar axis line below cuneiform MT joint	1. Initial casting (in PF) for stretching 2. Complete release at 6-18mo 3. Talectomy in resistant cases

Anterolateral approach to ankle joint

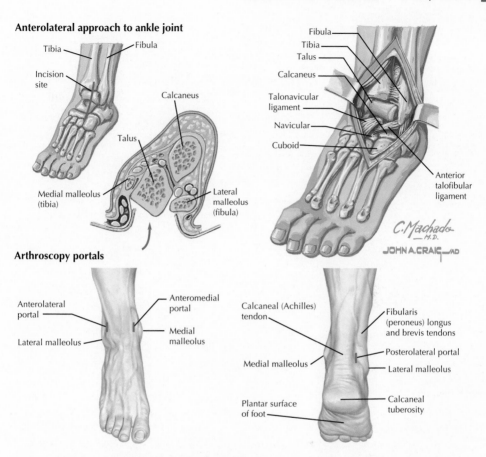

Arthroscopy portals

C. Machado
_M.D._

JOHN A. CRAIG_MD

USES	INTERNERVOUS PLANE	DANGERS	COMMENT
ANKLE: ANTEROLATERAL APPROACH			
• Fusions/triple arthrodesis • Fractures (e.g., pilon, talus) • Intertarsal joint access	• Peroneals (superficial peroneal) • EDL (deep peroneal)	• Deep peroneal nerve • Anterior tibial artery	• Can access hind foot • Preserving fat pad (sinus tarsus) helps wound healing
ARTHROSCOPY PORTALS			
Uses: synovectomy, loose body removal, osteochondral lesions, impingement, chondroplasty, some arthrodeses			
Anteromedial	Medial to tibialis anterior (TA) tendon at or just proximal to joint	Saphenous nerve & vein	Least risky portal, should be established first
Anterolateral	Lateral to peroneus tertius tendon at or just proximal to joint	Superficial peroneal nerve	Can establish with needle under direct visualization
Posterolateral	Lateral edge of Achilles tendon 1cm proximal to fibula tip	Sural nerve, lesser saphenous vein	Can establish with needle under direct visualization
Anterocentral, posterocentral, posteromedial portals have been described but are not recommended due to NV risks.			
FASCIOTOMIES			
See page 369			

Abbreviations

A

a.	artery
abd	abduct
abx	antibiotics
AC	acromioclavicular, anterior column
ACJ	acromioclavicular joint
ACL	anterior cruciate ligament
ADI	atlantodens interval
ADM	abductor digiti minimi
AGRAM	arthrogram
AIIS	anterior inferior iliac spine
AIN	anterior interosseous nerve
aka	also known as
ALL	anterior longitudinal ligament
AMBRI	Atraumatic, Multidirectional, Bilateral instability, Rehabilitation, Inferior capsular shift
ANA	antinuclear antibody
ant.	anterior
AP	anteroposterior
APB	abductor pollicis brevis
APC	anterior-posterior compression
APL	abductor pollicis longus
art.	artery
AS	ankylosing spondylitis
ASIS	anterior superior iliac spine
assoc.	associated
ATFL	anterior talofibular ligament
ATP	adenosine triphosphate
AVN	avascular necrosis
AW	anterior wall

B

BG	bone graft
br.	branch
BR	brachioradialis
BTB	bone-tendon-bone
b/w	between

C

CA	cancer
Ca++	ionic calcium
CBC	complete blood cell count
CC	coracoclavicular
CHL	coracohumeral
CL	capitate-lunate joint
CMC	carpometacarpal
CMCJ	carpometacarpal joint

CNS	central nervous system
c/o	complains of
CPK	creatine phosphokinase
CPPD	calcium pyrophosphate dihydrate crystals
CRP	C-reactive protein
CR-PCP	closed reduction, percutaneous pinning
C-spine	cervical spine
CT	carpal tunnel, computed tomography
CTL	capitotriquetral ligament
CTS	carpal tunnel syndrome
cut.	cutaneous

D

°	degree
DAB	dorsal abduct
DDD	degenerative disc disease
decr.	decreased
DF	dorsiflex, dorsiflexion
DIC	dorsal intercarpal ligament
DIO	dorsal interossei
DIPJ	distal interphalangeal joint
DISI	dorsal intercalated segment instability
DJD	degenerative joint disease
DR	distal radius
DRC	dorsal radiocarpal ligament
DRG	dorsal root ganglion
DRUJ	distal radioulnar joint
DVT	deep vein thrombosis
dx	dislocation, diagnosis

E

ECRB	extensor carpi radialis brevis
ECRL	extensor carpi radialis longus
ECU	extensor carpi ulnaris
EDC	extensor digitorum communis
EDL	extensor digitorum longus
EDM	extensor digiti minimi
EHL	extensor hallucis longus
EIA	external iliac artery
EIP	extensor indicis proprius
EMG	electromyogram, electromyography
EPB	extensor pollicis brevis
EPL	extensor pollicis longus

Abbreviations *cont.*

ER	external rotation		IV	intravenous
esp.	especially		IVIG	intravenous immunoglobulin
ESR	erythrocyte sedimentation rate			
EUA	exam under anesthesia		**J**	
ext.	extension, extensor		jt	joint

F

FCR	flexor carpi radialis		**L**	
FCU	flexor carpi ulnaris		LAC	long arm cast
FDB	flexor digitorum brevis		lat.	lateral
FDL	flexor digitorum longus		LB	loose bodies
FDMB	flexor digiti minimi brevis		LBP	low back pain
FDP	flexor digitorum profundus		LC	lateral compression
FDS	flexor digitorum superficialis		LCL	lateral collateral ligament
FHB	flexor hallucis brevis		LE	lower extremity
FHL	flexor hallucis longus		LFCN	lateral femoral cutaneous
fix.	fixation			nerve
flex.	flexion, flexor		LH	long head
FPB	flexor pollicis brevis		lig.	ligament
FPL	flexor pollicis longus		LRL	long radiolunate
fx, fxs	fracture, fractures		lsr	lesser
fxn	function		LT	lunotriquetral

G

			M	
GAG	glycosaminoglycans		MC	metacarpal
GH	glenohumeral		MCL	medial collateral ligament
GI	gastrointestinal		MCP	metacarpophalangeal
gtr	greater		MCPJ	metacarpophalangeal joint
GU	genitourinary		MDI	multidirectional instability
			mech.	mechanism/mechanism
H				of injury
HNP	herniated nucleus pulposus		med.	medial
HO	heterotopic ossification		MEN	multiple endocrine neoplasia
HTO	high tibial osteotomy		MF	middle finger
hx	history		MPFL	medial patellofemoral ligament
			MRI	magnetic resonance imaging
I			MT	metatarsal
			MTPJ	metatarsophalangeal joint
I&D	incision and drainage,		MUA	manipulation under anesthesia
	irrigation and debridement		MVA	motor vehicle accident
IF	index finger			
IJ	internal jugular		**N**	
IM	intramedullary		n.	nerve
incr.	increased		NCS	nerve conduction study
inf.	inferior		nl	normal (within normal limits)
inj.	injury		NSAID	nonsteroidal anti-inflammatory
IP	interphalangeal			drug
IR	internal rotation		NV	neurovascular
ITB	iliotibial band		NWB	non-weight-bearing

O

OA	osteoarthritis
OP	opponens pollicis muscle
ORIF	open reduction, internal fixation

P

PAD	palmar adduct
PC	posterior column
PCL	posterior cruciate ligament
PCP	percutaneous pinning
PE	physical examination
pect.	pectoral
peds	pediatrics/pediatric patients
PF	plantarflex, plantarflexion
PFCN	posterior femoral cutaneous nerve
PFS	patellofemoral syndrome
PG	proteoglycan
PIN	posterior interosseous nerve
PIPJ	proximal interphalangeal joint
PL	palmaris longus
PLC	posterolateral corner complex
PLL	posterior longitudinal ligament
PLRI	posterolateral rotary instability
PMHx	past medical history
PMRI	posteromedial rotary instability
PO	per oral, postoperatively
poll.	pollicus
post.	posterior
PQ	pronator quadratus
prox.	proximal
PRUJ	proximal radioulnar joint
PSIS	posterosuperior iliac spine
PT	posterior tibialis, pronator teres
PTH	parathyroid hormone
pts.	patients
PTTD	posterior tibialis tendon dysfunction
PVNS	pigmented villonodular synovitis
PW	posterior wall

Q

Q	quadriceps

R

RA	rheumatoid arthritis
RAD	radiation absorbed dose
RC	rotator cuff
RCL	radioscaphocapitate ligament
RF	rheumatoid factor, ring finger
RH	radial head
RICE	rest, ice, compression, and elevation
r/o	rule out
ROM	range of motion

RSC	radioscaphocapitate
RSD	reflex sympathetic dystrophy
RSL	radioscapholunate ligament
RTL	radiolunotriquetral ligament

S

SAC	short arm cast
SC	scaphocapitate, sternoclavicular
SCM	sternocleidomastoid
SF	small finger
SFA	superficial femoral artery
SGN	superior gluteal nerve
SH	short head
SI	sacroiliac
SIJ	sacroiliac joint
SL	scapholunate
SLAC	scapholunate advanced collapse
SLAP	superior labrum anterior/posterior
SLNWC	short leg non weightbearing cast
SPN	superficial peroneal nerve
sRL	short radiolunate
SS	supraspinatus
STT	scaphotrapeziotrapezoid
sup.	superior
sx	symptom
synd.	syndrome

T

TA	tibialis anterior
TAL	transverse acetabular ligament, transverse atlantal ligament
TC	triquetrocapitate
TCL	transverse carpal ligament
Td	tetanus and diphtheria toxoid
TFC	triangular fibrocartilage
TFCC	triangular fibrocartilage complex
TFL	tensor fascia lata
TH	triquetrohamate
THA	total hip arthroplasty
THC	triquetrohamocapitate
TIG	tetanus immunoglobulin
TKA	total knee arthroplasty
TLSO	thoracolumbosacral orthosis
TP	tibialis posterior
TTP	tenderness to palpation
TUBS	Traumatic, Unilateral instability, Bankart lesion, Surgery
tx	treatment

Abbreviations *cont.*

U

UE	upper extremity
UL	ulnolunate
UMN	upper motor neuron
usu.	usually
UT	ulnotriquetral

V

VIO	volar interosseus
VISI	volar intercalated segment instability
VMO	vastus medialis obliquus

W

w/	with
WB	weight bearing
WBAT	weight bear as tolerated
WBC	white blood cell count

X-Z

XR	x-ray
XRT	radiation therapy
y.o.	year old

Index

A

Abduction, 91
Abductor digiti minimi, 207, 363, 368
Abductor hallucis, 363, 368
Abductor magnus/longus/brevis, 265
Abductor pollicis longus, 167
Accessory lateral collateral ligament, 119
Acetabular ligament, 258
Acetabulum, 222, 224, 230–231
Acetylcholine (ACh), 23
Acetylcholinesterase, 23
Achilles tendon, 26
   rupture of, 375
   tendonitis of, 358, 375
   topographic anatomy of, 338
Acromioclavicular joint
   arthrosis of, 102
   injection of, 88
   ligaments of, 87
   radiography of, 78
   separation of, 81, 89
   topographic anatomy of, 76
Acromion, 76
Actin, 24
Active compression (O'Brien's) test, 93
Adductor brevis/longus/magnus, 237, 267
Adductor compartment, 207, 209
Adductor hallucis, 308
Adductor pollicis, 308
Adhesive capsulitis, 102
Adson's test, 93
Alignment radiography, of leg, 291
Allen test, 160, 204
Allis maneuver, 254
Allis' sign, 264
Anatomic snuffbox, 140, 184
Anconeus, 166
Animal bites, 200, 215
Ankle. *See also* Foot/ankle.
   arteries of, 372–373
   arthrocentesis of, 355
   arthroscopy portals of, 383
   block of, 355
   fractures of, 344
   history-taking, 356
   injections in, 355
   instability of, 375
   ligaments of, 349–351
   physical examination, 357–359
   radiography of, 342, 350, 351
   range of motion of, 358

Ankle *(Continued)*
   sprain of, 375
   surgical approaches to, 383
   topographic anatomy of, 338
Ankle clonus, 51
Ankylosing spondylitis, 380
Annular ligament, 119
Annulus fibrosis, 46
Ansa cervicalis, 64
Anterior cruciate ligament, 297, 307,
   311, 326
Anterior drawer test, 311, 359
Anterior interosseous syndrome, 175
Anterior spinal artery syndrome, 42
Anteroposterior view
   ankle, 342
   cervical spine, 37
   elbow, 113
   femur, 253
   foot, 343
   hand, 186
   hip, 253
   leg/knee, 290–291
   lumbar spine, 38
   pelvis, 225, 253
   shoulder, 79
   wrist, 143
Aorta, 244
Aortic arch, 65
Apley's compression, 311
Appositional ossification, 6
Apprehension (Fairbank) test, 93, 311
Arcade of Struthers, 121
Arcuate artery, 374
Arcuate ligament, 299
Arcuate line, 223
Arm
   arteries of, 133
   compartments of, 130
   disorders of, 134–136
   fasciotomies of, 130
   history-taking, 123
   joints of, 119–120
   minor procedures in, 122
   muscles of, 127–130
   nerves of, 130–132
   origins and insertions of, 127
   osteology of, 111–112
   other structures of, 121
   pediatric disorders of, 136
   physical examination of, 124–126

Arm *(Continued)*
  radiography of, 113
  range of motion of, 125
  surgical approaches to, 137–138
  topographic anatomy of, 110
  trauma of, 114–118
Arthritis. *See* Osteoarthritis; Rheumatoid
    arthritis.
Arthrocentesis
  ankle, 355
  elbow, 122
  knee, 306
Arthroplasty
  elbow, 134
  total hip, 277–278
  total knee, 330–331
Arthroscopy
  ankle, 383
  elbow, 138
  hip, 284
  knee/patellar, 324, 336
  shoulder, 87, 106–107
  wrist, 182
Articular cartilage, 16–19
Articularis genu, 266
Atlantoaxial joint, 39, 43
Atlas (C1 vertebra), 31, 32, 39, 43
ATP, in muscle contraction, 25
Avascular necrosis (osteonecrosis),
    of hip, 276
Avascular tendon, 26
Axial/sesamoid view, of foot, 343
Axial/sunrise view, of leg/knee, 290
Axilla, 97
Axillary artery, 100, 101, 133
Axillary lateral view, of shoulder, 79
Axillary nerve, 92, 99, 100, 126
Axis (C2 vertebra), 31, 32, 43
Axon, 21
Axonotmesis, 22

B
Babinski reflex, 51
Back, muscles of, 56–58
Bankart lesion, 104
Barlow's (dislocation) test, 264
Belly press, 93
Bennett fracture, 187
Biceps aponeurosis, 121
Biceps brachii
  cross section, 130
  origins and insertions of, 94, 127
  physical examination of, 93
  topographic anatomy of, 110
Biceps brachii tendon
  origins and insertions of, 128
  rupture of, 90, 102, 135
  tendonitis of, 102

Biceps femoris, 265, 268, 299
Bites, human/animal, 200, 215
Blount's disease (infantile tibia vara), 332
Body, of vertebra, 31
Bone. *See also specific bones.*
  in calcium metabolism, 8
  cell types of, 5
  composition of, 4
  formation of, 6
  forms of, 2
  fractures of, 12. *See also* Fractures.
  functions of, 2
  healing of, 14–15
  homeostasis of, 10
  microscopic types of, 2
  in phosphate metabolism, 8
  regulation of, 5
  structural types of, 3
Bone mass, regulation of, 5
Bone scan
  ankle, 342
  forearm, 143
  hand, 186
  leg/knee, 291
  shoulder, 79
  spine, 38
  thigh/hip, 253
Bouchard's nodes, 201
Boutonniere deformity, 201, 213
Bowstring test, 52
Boxer fracture, 200
Brachial artery, 133
Brachial nerve, 130
Brachial plexus, 100
  anterior view, 170
  lateral cord, 99, 132, 170, 172
  medial cord, 99, 132, 170, 172, 210
  posterior cord, 99, 131, 171
  posterior view, 171
  roots of, 98
  topographic anatomy of, 30
  upper trunk of, 98
Brachialis, 128, 130
Brachiocephalic trunk, 65
Brachioradialis, 166
Broden view, of foot, 343
Brown-Sequard syndrome, 42
Brudzinski test, 52
Bryan/Morrey approach, to elbow, 138
Bulge sign, 309
Bunion (hallux valgus), 357, 377
Bunionette, 380
Bunnell-Littler test, 205
Bursitis
  ischial, 235
  knee, 308
  prepatellar, 308, 325
  retrocalcaneal, 358, 379

Internal iliac artery, 244
Internal rotation, 91, 92
Interosseous ligament, 349
Interosseous muscles, dorsal/plantar, 208,
    366, 368, 373, 374
Interosseous nerve, anterior, 170
Interphalangeal joints
    finger, 338
    flexion/extension of, 195
    ligaments of, 194, 353
    osteoarthritis of, 201
    proximal, 194, 338
    radiography of, 186
    thumb, 338
Interspinales, 58
Intertarsal joint, 352
Intertransversarii, 58
Intertransverse ligament, 44
Intertrochanteric fracture, 256
Intervertebral articulation, 44
Intervertebral disc, 44, 46
Intramembranous ossification, 2, 6
Intraspinous ligament, 44
Ischial bursitis, 235, 246
Ischial spine, 223
Ischial tuberosity, 220, 223, 250
Ischiofemoral ligament, 258
Isokinetic contraction, 25
Isometric contraction, 25
Isotonic contraction, 25

J
J sign, 311
Jefferson fracture, of atlas, 39
Jerk test, 93
Jersey finger, 189
Joint line tenderness, 311
Junctura tendinae, 196

K
Kanavel, cardinal signs of, 202
Kernig test, 52
Kienböck's disease, 178
Knee
    anterior, 16
    arthroscopy portals for, 336
    aspiration/arthrocentesis of, 306
    dislocation of, 292
    disorders of, 324–328
    injection of, 306
    kinematics of, 296
    ligaments of, 297–301, 304, 326–327
    meniscus of, 302–303
    range of motion of, 310
    structure of, 296
    surgical approaches to, 335
    total arthroplasty of, 330–331
    trauma of, 307

Kocher approach, to elbow, 137
Kocher-Langenbeck approach, to pelvis, 248

L
L1 vertebrae, 31
L2 vertebra, 35
L3 vertebrae, 31, 35
L4 vertebrae, 31, 35
Labrum, 258
Lachman test, 311
Lamellar bones, 2
Laminectomy, 68
Lateral bands, of hand, 196
Lateral (radial) collateral ligament, 119
Lateral (ulnar) collateral ligament, 119
Lateral collateral ligaments, knee, 299, 327
Lateral epicondyle, 110
Lateral epicondylitis (tennis elbow), 122, 124,
    126, 134
Lateral patellar compression syndrome, 324
Lateral slip, of hand, 196
Lateral view
    ankle, 342
    cervical spine, 37
    elbow, 113
    femur, 253
    foot, 343
    hand, 186
    leg/knee, 290–291
    lumbar spine, 38
    thigh/hip, 253
    wrist, 143
Latissimus dorsi, 56, 95
Lauge-Hansen classification, of ankle
    fractures, 344
Leash of Henry, 121
Leg length, 263
Legg-Calve-Perthes disease, 280
Leg/knee. See also Knee.
    alignment of, 289
    arteries of, 322
    compartments of, 315
    disorders of, 323–329
    fasciotomies of, 315
    history-taking, 307
    joints of, 305. See also Knee.
    minor procedures in, 306
    muscles of
        anterior compartment, 316
        deep posterior compartment, 319
        lateral compartment, 317
        origins and insertions of, 314
        superficial posterior compartment,
            318
    nerves of, 320–321
    osteology of, 287–289
    pediatric disorders of, 332–334
    physical examination of, 308–310

P

Paget's disease, 11
Palmar arch, deep/superficial, 212
Palmar crease, proximal/distal, 184
Palmar digital arteries, 212
Palmar digital nerves, 212
Palmar interosseous compartment, 209
Palmar radioulnar joint, 153
Palmaris brevis, 207
Palmaris longus, 163
Palmaris longus tendon, 140, 184
Palpation
    elbow, 124
    fingers, 202
    foot/ankle, 358
    forearm, 158
    leg/knee, 309
    pelvis, 235
    shoulder, 90
    spine, 49
    thigh/hip, 261
Panner's disease (osteochondrosis of
        capitellum), 135, 136
Parathyroid hormone, 8, 9
Parona space, 197, 214
Paronychia, 198, 214
Patella
    displacement of, 311
    fractures of, 292
    osteology of, 287
    structure and function of, 304
    subluxation and dislocation of, 304, 325
    tendonitis of, 325
    topographic anatomy of, 286
Patella apprehension, 311
Patella compression/grind, 311
Patellar retinaculum, 286, 299, 300, 304
Patellar tendon, 286, 304, 329
Patellofemoral joint
    ligaments of, 299, 300, 304
    special tests for, 311
    stress syndrome of, 324
    structure and function of, 304
Patellomeniscal ligaments, 304
Patellotibial ligaments, 304
Patrick (FABER) test, 236, 263
Pavlik harness, 279
Pectineus, 237, 240, 265, 267
Pectoral nerve, lateral, 92
Pectoralis major
    actions of, 97
    origins and insertions of, 97, 127, 128
    rupture of, 104
    topographic anatomy of, 76
Pectoralis minor, 94, 97
Pelvic inlet view, 225, 226
Pelvic outlet view, 225, 226
Pelvic ring fractures, 228–229

Pelvic rock test, 236
Pelvis
    arteries of, 244–245
    disorders of, 246
    history-taking, 234
    joints of, 232–233
    landmarks of, 223
    ligaments of, 233
    muscles of, 237–240
    nerves of, 241–243
    origins and insertions of, 237
    osteology of, 221–224
    physical examination of, 235
    radiography of, 225–226, 240
    range of motion of, 235
    stability of, 232
    surgical approaches to, 247–248
    topographic anatomy of, 220
    trauma of, 227–231, 234
Perforating artery, 372
Perilunate, 147
Perineurium, 21
Periosteum, 7
Peripheral nerve, 21
Perkin's line, 279
Peroneal artery, 322, 372
Peroneal nerve
    common, 272, 321
    deep/superficial, 321, 371
    physical examination of, 310
Peroneus brevis/longus, 317
Peroneus tertius, 316
Pes anserinus, 286
Pes cavus, 381
Pes planovalgus, 382
Pes planus, 357, 382
Phalanges
    arteries and nerves of, 198
    cross section, 198
    fractures of, 187–189, 348
    osteology of, 185, 340, 341
    radiography of, 186
    sagittal section, 198
    trauma of, 187–189, 348
Phalen test, 160
Phosphate, 8, 9
Phrenic nerve, 64, 100
Physis, 7
"Piano key" test, 160
Pillar view, of cervical spine, 37
Pilon fracture, 295
Pinch grip, 126
Piriformis
    anatomic relationships of, 243, 245
    origins and insertions of, 237, 239, 265
    physical examination of, 263
Pisiform, 142, 152
Pisohamate ligament, 151, 152

Pisometacarpal ligament, 151, 152
Pivot shift test, 126, 311, 312
Plafond, 339
Plantar artery, 372, 374
Plantar fascia, 362
Plantar fascitis, 379
Plantar foot, 338
Plantar nerve, medial/lateral, 370
Plantaris, 318
Platysma, 53, 54
Plica, synovial, 325
Podagra (gout), 20, 377
Polydactyly, 217
Popliteal artery, 322
Popliteal fossa, 250, 286
Popliteal ligament, oblique, 298
Popliteofibular ligament, 299
Popliteus, 299, 319
Popliteus tendon, 299
POP's IQ mnemonic, 223, 243
Posterior column syndrome, 42
Posterior cruciate ligament
    attachments of, 298
    function of, 298
    injury of, 307
    rupture of, 327
    special tests for, 313
Posterior drawer test, 312, 313
Posterior interosseous syndrome, 176
Posterior lateral drawer test, 313
Posterior longitudinal ligament, 44
Posterior medial drawer test, 313
Posterior oblique ligament, 300
Posterior sag sign, 312, 313
Posterior spinal artery, 66
Posterior tibialis tendon
    dysfunction, 379
Posteromedial compartment, of
    knee, 298
Preaxial polydactyly, 217
Prestyloid recess, 153
Pretracheal fascia, 53
Prevertebral fascia, 53
Primary ossification center, 6
Princeps pollicis artery, 212
Profunda brachii, 133
Profunda femoris (deep femoral
    artery), 273–274
Profundus test, 205
Proliferative zone, of physis, 7
Pronator quadratus, 165
Pronator syndrome, 175
Pronator teres, 163
Proteoglycan, 4, 18
Pseudarthrosis, congenital, 333
Pseudogout, 20
Psoas major/minor, 238, 265
Psoriasis, 380

Pubic crest, 20
Pubic symphysis, 220, 233
Pubofemoral ligament, 258
Pudendal nerve, 236, 242, 243
Pulp, 198
Pump bump, 357

Q
Q angle, 310
Quadrangular space, of shoulder, 96
Quadrate ligament, 119
Quadratus femoris
    anatomic relationships of, 242, 243, 245
    origins and insertions of, 237, 239, 265
Quadratus plantae, 364
Quadriceps, 250, 286, 308
Quadriceps active test, 313
Quadriceps tendon
    attachments of, 304
    rupture of, 309, 329
    topographic anatomy of, 250, 286

R
Radial artery, 133, 168, 173, 212
Radial bursa, 197
Radial club hand (radial hemimelia), 179
Radial nerve
    anatomic relationships of, 99, 121,
        130, 168
    blocks of, 156
    branches of, 210, 211
    compression of, 176
    physical examination of, 126, 204
    posterior view, 131
Radial tunnel syndrome, 176
Radialis indicis artery, 212
Radiocapitellar view, elbow, 113
Radiocarpal joint, 150, 152
Radiocarpal ligament, dorsal, 150, 151
Radiolunate ligaments, short/long, 150
Radioscaphocapitate ligament, 150
Radioulnar joint, distal, 153
Radioulnar ligament, dorsal/palmar,
    151, 153
Radioulnar synostosis, 136
Radius
    anterior view, 141
    distal, fractures of, 146–148, 158
    head
        congenital dislocation of, 136
        fractures of, 117
        subluxation of, 118, 124
        topographic anatomy of, 140
    osteology of, 141
    posterior view, 141
    proximal, 112, 161–162
    shaft, fractures of, 144–145
    topographic anatomy of, 110

Snapping hip (coxa saltans), 275
Soft callus, in fracture healing, 14
Soleus, 26, 318
Speed's test, 93
Spinal accessory nerve, 92, 98
Spinal artery, anterior/posterior, 66
Spinal branch artery, 66
Spinal cord, 42, 50–51, 59
Spinal nerves, 60
Spinal stenosis, 68
Spinalis, 57
Spine
   arteries of, 65–67
   cervical. See Cervical spine.
   disorders of, 68–72
   fascia layers of, 53
   history-taking, 48
   joints of, 43–47
   lumbar. See Lumbar spine.
   muscles of, 54–58
   nerves of, 59–64
   osteology of, 31–36
   pediatric disorders of, 72
   physical examination of, 49–52
   radiography of, 37–38
   range of motion, 49
   regions of, 31
   stability of, 41
   thoracic. See Thoracic spine.
   topographic anatomy of, 30
   trauma of, 39–42
Splenius capitis/cervicis, 57
Spondyloarthropathy, seronegative, 380
Spondylolisthesis, 71
Spondylosis, 70–71
Spongiosa, 7
Sporotrichosis, 214
Sprain, 17
Sprengel's deformity, 105
Spurling maneuver/test, 52, 93
Stance, 360
Stenor lesion, 189
Stenosing tenosynovitis, 202, 215
Sternoclavicular joint, 76, 85
Sternocleidomastoid, 30, 53, 54
Sternohyoid, 54
Stimson maneuver, 83
Stinchfield test, 263
Straight leg 90/90 test, 52, 263
Stress views
   ankle, 342
   foot, 343
   shoulder, 79
Stryker notch radiograph, shoulder, 79
Stylohyoid, 54
Subacromial space, 88
Subclavian artery, 65, 101
Subclavian vein, 65

Subclavius, 97
Subcoracoid dislocation, 82
Subcostal nerve, 241
Sublimus test, 205
Suboccipital triangle, 55
Subscapular nerve, 92, 99
Subscapularis, 96
Subtalar ligament, 352
Subtrochanteric fracture, 257
Sulcus test, 93
Sunrise radiograph, of knee, 290
Superior labral tear, 104
Superior transverse scapular ligament, 87
Supinator, 167
Supraclavicular nerve, 64, 98
Suprapatellar pouch, 304
Suprascapular nerve, 92, 98, 99
Supraspinatus, 93, 96
Supraspinatus outlet view, of shoulder, 79
Sural nerve, 310, 321, 371
Swan-neck deformity, 201, 213
Swimmer's view, of cervical spine, 37
Swing, in gait, 360
Sympathetic trunk, 53
Symphysis pubis, 220, 233
Syndactyly, 216
Syndesmosis, 349
Synovial fluid, 16, 20
Synovial joints, 16, 17
Synovial plica, 325
Synovitis, transient, 280
Synovium, 16, 17

T
T3 vertebrae, 31
T6 vertebra, 34
T7-9 vertebrae, 31, 34
T10 vertebrae, 31
T12 vertebrae, 34
Tailor's bunion, 380
Talar tilt test, 359
Talipes equinovarus (clubfoot), 381
Talocalcaneal ligament, 352
Talofibular ligament, 349
Talonavicular joint, 352
Talus, 340, 346, 373, 382
Tarsal artery, medial/lateral, 374
Tarsal coalition, 382
Tarsal tunnel syndrome, 380
Tarsometatarsal (Lisfranc) joint, 347, 353
Tendon, 26. See also specific tendons.
Tennis elbow (lateral epicondylitis), 122, 124,
      126, 134
Tenosynovitis, 202, 214, 215
Tensor fascia latae, 239, 240
Teres major/minor, 96
Terminal extensor tendon, 196
Terrible triad, 326

Ulna *(Continued)*
  osteology of, 141
  posterior view, 141
  proximal, 112, 161–162
Ulnar artery, 133, 138, 173, 212
Ulnar bursa, 197
Ulnar deviation, 143
Ulnar nerve
  anatomic relationships of, 100, 121, 130, 168, 172
  blocks of, 156
  branches of, 210, 211
  compression of, 123, 176, 201
  submuscular transposition of, 134
  testing of, 126, 204
  zones of, 154
Ulnar styloid, 140
Ulnar tunnel (Guyon's canal), 154
Ulnar tunnel/Guyon's canal syndrome, 176, 177
Ulnocapitate ligament, 150
Ulnolunate ligament, 150, 153
Ulnotriquetral ligament, 153
Uncovertebral joints, 47
Unmyelinated nerve fiber, 21

V
Vaginal examination, after spinal injury, 236
Valgus heel, 338
Valgus stress test, 313
Varus stress test, 313
Vascular leash of Henry, 176
Vastus lateralis/intermedius/medialis, 265, 266
Vertebra, 31, 44
Vertebral artery, 65
Vinculum breve/longa, 26
Vitamin D 1,25 (OH), 8, 9
Volkmann's canals, 3

W
Waddell signs, 52
Wartenbergs's syndrome, 176

Watson test, 160
Watson-Jones approach, to hip, 282
West point radiograph, shoulder, 79
Wilmington portal, 106, 107
Winquist/Hansen classification, of femoral shaft fractures, 256
Wolff's law, 252
Woven bones, 2
Wright's test, 93
Wrist. *See also* Forearm.
  in anatomical position, 149
  anterior view, 142
  arteries of, 173
  arthroscopy portals for, 182
  articular surface, 141
  aspiration/injection of, 156
  dislocation of, 158
  disorders of, 174–178
  distal row, 142
  in extension, 149
  in flexion, 149
  fractures of, 147
  joints of, 150
  ligaments of, 149–151
  minor procedures in, 156
  posterior view, 142
  proximal row, 142
  radiography of, 143, 152
  range of motion of, 149
  special tests, 160
  surgical approaches to, 180–182
Wrist block, 156

X
X-body adduction, 93

Y
Yergason's test, 93
Young and Burgess classification, of pelvic fractures, 228–229

Z
Zanca radiograph, shoulder, 79